Advances in Intelligent and Soft Computing 65

Editor-in-Chief: J. Kacprzyk

Advances in Intelligent and Soft Computing

Further volumes of this series can be found on our homepage: springer.com

Vol. 49. J.M. Corchado, F. de Paz, M.P. Rocha, F. Fernández Riverola (Eds.)
2nd International Workshop on Practical Applications of Computational Biology and Bioinformatics (IWPACBB 2008), 2009
ISBN 978-3-540-85860-7

Vol. 50. J.M. Corchado, S. Rodriguez, J. Llinas, J.M. Molina (Eds.)
International Symposium on Distributed Computing and Artificial Intelligence 2008 (DCAI 2008), 2009
ISBN 978-3-540-85862-1

Vol. 51. J.M. Corchado, D.I. Tapia, J. Bravo (Eds.)
3rd Symposium of Ubiquitous Computing and Ambient Intelligence 2008, 2009
ISBN 978-3-540-85866-9

Vol. 52. E. Avineri, M. Köppen, K. Dahal, Y. Sunitiyoso, R. Roy (Eds.)
Applications of Soft Computing, 2009
ISBN 978-3-540-88078-3

Vol. 53. E. Corchado, R. Zunino, P. Gastaldo, Á. Herrero (Eds.)
Proceedings of the International Workshop on Computational Intelligence in Security for Information Systems CISIS 2008, 2009
ISBN 978-3-540-88180-3

Vol. 54. B.-y. Cao, C.-y. Zhang, T.-f. Li (Eds.)
Fuzzy Information and Engineering, 2009
ISBN 978-3-540-88913-7

Vol. 55. Y. Demazeau, J. Pavón, J.M. Corchado, J. Bajo (Eds.)
7th International Conference on Practical Applications of Agents and Multi-Agent Systems (PAAMS 2009), 2009
ISBN 978-3-642-00486-5

Vol. 56. H. Wang, Y. Shen, T. Huang, Z. Zeng (Eds.)
The Sixth International Symposium on Neural Networks (ISNN 2009), 2009
ISBN 978-3-642-01215-0

Vol. 57. M. Kurzynski, M. Wozniak (Eds.)
Computer Recognition Systems 3, 2009
ISBN 978-3-540-93904-7

Vol. 58. J. Mehnen, A. Tiwari, M. Köppen, A. Saad (Eds.)
Applications of Soft Computing, 2009
ISBN 978-3-540-89618-0

Vol. 59. K.A. Cyran, S. Kozielski, J.F. Peters, U. Stańczyk, A. Wakulicz-Deja (Eds.)
Man-Machine Interactions, 2009
ISBN 978-3-642-00562-6

Vol. 60. Z.S. Hippe, J.L. Kulikowski (Eds.)
Human-Computer Systems Interaction, 2009
ISBN 978-3-642-03201-1

Vol. 61. W. Yu, E.N. Sanchez (Eds.)
Advances in Computational Intelligence, 2009
ISBN 978-3-642-03155-7

Vol. 62. B. Cao, T.-F. Li, C.-Y. Zhang (Eds.)
Fuzzy Information and Engineering Volume 2, 2009
ISBN 978-3-642-03663-7

Vol. 63. Á. Herrero, P. Gastaldo, R. Zunino, E. Corchado (Eds.)
Computational Intelligence in Security for Information Systems, 2009
ISBN 978-3-642-04090-0

Vol. 64. E. Tkacz, A. Kapczynski (Eds.)
Internet–Technical Development and Applications, 2009
ISBN 978-3-642-05018-3

Vol. 65. E. Kącki, M. Rudnicki, J. Stempczyńska (Eds.)
Computers in Medical Activity, 2009
ISBN 978-3-642-04461-8

Edward Kącki, Marek Rudnicki, and
Joanna Stempczyńska (Eds.)

Computers in Medical Activity

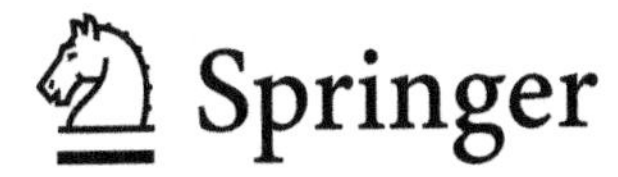

Editors

Prof. Dr. D.Sc. Edward Kącki
Department of Expert Systems and
Artificial Intelligence
College of Computer Science
Rzgowska Str. 17A
93-008 Lódz
Poland
E-mail: ekacki@ics.p.lodz.pl

Associate Prof. Dr. M. Joanna Stempczyńska
Department of Expert Systems and
Artificial Intelligence
College of Computer Science
Rzgowska Str. 17A
93-008 Lódz
Poland
E-mail: Joasia52@poczta.onet.pl

Prof. Dr. D.Sc. Marek Rudnicki
Department of Expert Systems and
Artificial Intelligence
College of Computer Science
Rzgowska Str. 17A
93-008 Lódz
Poland
E-mail: Rudnicki@isc.p.lodz.pl

ISBN 978-3-642-04461-8 e-ISBN 978-3-642-04462-5

DOI 10.1007/978-3-642-04462-5

Advances in Intelligent and Soft Computing ISSN 1867-5662

Library of Congress Control Number: 2009937144

Typeset & Cover Design: Scientific Publishing Services Pvt. Ltd., Chennai, India.

Printed in acid-free paper

5 4 3 2 1 0

springer.com

Preface

First reports in Poland aimed at the computer aided medicine support already appeared at the beginning of sixties of the twentieth century. They were presented on many seminars and scientific conferences: however, they did not find then the practical application. They were difficult in use and that is why they were not accepted by doctors, nurses and hospital administration. Just appearing personal computers, local computer networks and Internet along with multimedia equipment and the virtual reality software allowed to develop a considerable number of computer systems aiding the medical care in the wide range effectively. They were friendly systems and therefore were accepted by workers of hospitals, clinics, medical universities and scientific institutes.

Never ending development of the computer technology, operating systems and the programming languages creates more and more possibilities for new conceptions regarding better utilization of computer systems in the various fields of the medical activity. This concerns both medical education and scientific research and prophylaxis, diagnostics, therapy, convalescence and hospital administration as well.

For many years in all medical universities in Poland students have been learning the practical use of computers within the so-called medical computer science. Computerized clinics and chairs of medical universities provide students with the access to computers and Internet.

It is worthwhile noting that special part in disseminating the newest achievements in the range of the medicine computerization, both among the health service and the patients can be attributed to scientific societies. Three following organizations deserve on the distinction among them: Polish Society of Medical Computer Science put in year 1988, Polish Association of Medical Internet formed in the year 1997 and Polish Society of Biomedical Engineering existing since 1999.

The issues of the wide range medicine computerization taking into account the utilization of the Internet also constitute the cardinal current of interests and related activities of the Polish Society of Medical Computer Science.

Papers selected to the present monograph are only a small piece of subjects being investigated in Poland in the range of medical computer science. Their summaries and preliminary results were presented during the international conference „Computers in Medical Activity" organized by the College of Computer Science in Lodz with the collaboration of the Polish Society of Medical Computer Science in Poland in 2007.

The subject matter of the monograph is mainly steered on employing the computer systems in the diagnostics (chapter 3), then the equipment of the medical activity (chapter 5) and the general problems connected with the organization the medical care (chapter 6).

A single paper (2.1) is concerned with the prophylaxis. The preventive examination method with reference to allergic diseases has been presented. The paper concerns the problem of analyzing the reliability of preventive examination of allergic diseases. In the final part of the paper, the preliminary results of experiments are presented.

There are ten papers presented within the diagnostics chapter (3.1 –3.10). The first one (3.1) proposes type-2 fuzzy decision trees in application to medical diagnosis.

This means that attribute values employed in the tree structures may be characterized by type-2 fuzzy sets. Three medical benchmark data sets, available on the Internet, have been used to illustrate results of diagnosis obtained by this method.

The authors of the second paper (3.2) claim that medical knowledge in the form of causal sequences of diseases can be used in designing ranked models. Considered ranked models are based on linear transformation of multivariate feature vectors on a line that preserves in a best possible way a causal order between diseases. Clinical data sets from particular diseases supplied with a causal order within pairs of these diseases may be used in the definition of the convex and piecewise linear (CPL) criterion function. The linear ranked transformations can be designed through minimization of the CPL criterion functions.

The aim of the work 3.3 is to present the method of a comparative analysis of SPECT images of the left and right cerebral hemispheres in patients with diagnosed epileptic symptoms. Advantage of this technique lies in possibility of brain activity map acquisition at the time of radiotracer injection during seizures though the image registration is done one hour after seizure. The SPECT imaging method makes possible a more accurate spatial localization of seizure source than analysis of EEG signals.

The work 3.4. shows that the rough sets, surrounded by two approximation sets filled with sure and possible members constitute perfect mathematical tools of the classification of some objects. In this work has been adopted the rough technique to verify diagnostic decisions concerning a sample of patients whose symptoms are typical of a considered diagnosis. The objective is to extract the patients who surely suffer from the diagnosis, to indicate the patients who are free from it, and even to make decisions in undefined diagnostic cases.

In the work 3.5 the MoDeRi program for aiding in wireless capsule endoscopy (WCE) video interpretation is presented. It implements the model of deformable rings (MDR), which is a dedicated technique applied to extract certain information from the video. The MDR performs a motion analysis of the video, produces a map of the gastro-intestinal system, estimates a longitudinal velocity of the capsule and detects strong mixing contractions. The extracted data allows for quick identification of gross pathologies and serves as a reference to the video fragments. Preliminary studies have proven usefulness of the MoDeRi program.

The paper 3.6 is focused on segmentation of biomedical images, including textured ones. A segmentation method which is based on network of synchronised oscillators is presented. The proposed method was tested on several biomedical images acquired based on different modalities. Principles of operation of oscillator network are described and discussed. Obtained segmentation results for sample 2D and 3D biomedical images were presented and compared to multilayer perceptron network (MLP) image segmentation technique.

In the work 3.7 a MaZda software package for 2D and 3D image texture analysis with referenc to biomedical objects is presented. The software has been used for research within framework of COST B11 and COST B21 multi-center international projects and it has proven to be an efficient tool for quantitative analysis of magnetic resonance images (MRI) – an aid to more accurate and objective medical diagnosis.

In the paper 3.8 a novel idea and CMOS implementation of power-efficient 1-D and 2-D finite-impulse-response (FIR) filters based on a current-mode Gilbert-vector-multiplier (GVM) for medical diagnostics have been proposed. As an example, a time-domain 1-D 3rd order filter has been presented which dissipates 8-μW of power enabling a 2-MHz sampling frequency (fS). Another example is a 2-D filter with the frame resolution of 6x1 pixels that dissipates 7-μW at the data rate of 1 Mframe/s.

The study presented in the paper 3.9 deals with a method of biomedical images segmentation by discrimination of textures based on their morphological spectra. Their properties making possible to characterize basic morphological structures independently on spatial orientation or shifts of the analyzed specimens are described. Analysis of two types of biomedical images: aorta tissue and pancreas tissue, based on comparison of histograms of selected spectral components values illustrate the presented methods.

Two papers (4.1 and 4.2) are devoted to the prognosis problems. The paper 4.1 presents a determine method of survival time of patients with a bladder cancer and in the work 4.2 prognosis deals with drag side-effects of chemotherapy application. Artificial neural networks have been used in both cases.

In the paper 5.1 a set of software procedures for the Symbian OS mobile smartphone making the device more easily usable for a blind user is described in the paper. The application was written in the Carbide C++ environment, tested both on the S60 series phone emulator and the phone platform itself. The main task was to create a dedicated speech enabled menu, rather than a simple screen reader. Along with ordinary phone functions (calls, SMSs) the programmed phone can be used as a speech recorder, a web browser (RSS feeds are used), and a colour recognizer in images captured by the phone's camera. Added functionality makes the smartphone a very useful personal assistance tool for the blind who tested the developed application.

The paper 5.2 presents an environment for ECG signal visualization, learning of its analysis, diagnostic interpretation and ECG software testing. The functional description of the system is given with focus on analysis module based on energy measure of fuzziness and the interpretation eveluation unit. In the latter, some evaluation criteria have been proposed. We also describe a proposal of testing ECG interpretation algorithm by means of artificial generation of ECG parameters. Some design ideas ensuring flexibility and reusability of our system are also suggested.

In the paper 5.3 the problem of Inverse magnetic modeling in computer tomography is analyzed. The problem of optimizing the magnetic field gradients required for NMR tomography is considered. In particular, a double magnetic quadrupole made of inner and outer parts which is intended for producing a magnetic gradient of given distribution is analyzed. The strict requirements on the magnetic field distribution: non-purity and non-linearity related to the quality of tomographic images are taken into account.

In the paper 5.4 a new idea as well as CMOS implementation of a pulse-shaping filter useful in nuclear medicine to realize a multi-element detection by means of a multichannel readout front-end ASIC have been presented. The filter changes the shape of pulses delivered by a charge amplifier in order to increase the detection speed and robustness. By canceling falling edges of the pulses, a significant increase in the pulse counting rate has been reached (between 3 and 10 MSps in a single channel). The filter takes advantage of a RESET function that is controlled by an asynchronous multiplexer. Including only two resistors, two capacitors and four configuration transistors, it is simpler than other solutions reported to overcome this problem. The proposed shaper together with a peak detector, that receives the shaper signals, dissipates a small amount of power (about 80 μW) for 1V supply voltage. When being inactive, i.e. waiting for the next pulse, the circuit consumes only 200 nW of power.

The survey paper 5.5 deals with a stimulated emission of radiation in media where a population inversion occurs. The change of a particle energy from a higher-energy state to a lower-energy state is a result of an electron moving to a lower orbital. The laser phenomenon is interesting due to the specific light it emits. It is a well focused monochromatic beam, it has a well-defined wavelength and high energy density. Laser light is very useful in many areas (medicine) because it is monochrome, focused and because of its coherence and very high power density.

The paper 6.1 is concerned with computer aiding and virtual integration of the medical activities with regard to the healthcare reform. The authors discuss elaboration of information systems directed on consideration rationalization of medical care, medical personnel works, availability of modern equipment, medical apparatus and data about human wellbeing state. In new solutions we have to do with computer integrated activities organization in the environment of structures of mutual data exchange and the problem domain.

The paper 6.2 is concerned with expert systems in the medical insurance industry, The authors present the expert system for the medical insurance industry which has been developed at the College of Computer Science in cooperation with Technical University of Lodz. The system has been implemented and tested in an insurance company. The system reduces resources, costs and improves reliability of the insurance decision-making process. The time required to insure a customer has been reduced by eight times. The system is an ideal teacher for beginners, and can be used when educating new employees.

In the paper 6.3 a transfer of medical data over P2P network is considered. They are transfer between the nodes representing medical systems. Although only some of the nodes can produce, process or integrate data, all of the nodes are able to propagate them to their neighbors. The cost of building the transmission lines is high, so an optimum network topology is being searched. The random graphs with bounded degree are used for modeling of such networks. The process of transferring data over network is examined by means of the original algorithm RST for searching rooted spanning trees.

The article 7.1 is devoted to the examination of the influence of upper respiratory system disease in humans on the functioning of voice recognition systems. To recognize the speaker by their voice, such systems must be prepared in advance for recognition of the person's voice on the basis of recorded sound samples. Then the recognition system analyzes a new voice sample and verifies whether it has been spoken by the same person. However, often in life there are situations when the human voice is changed. The paper is concerned with a situation when the speaker's voice has been modified between the system's phase of preparation for recognition, and the actual recognition of the speaker. For the research purposes, the focus has been restricted to voice deformation of Polish speaking persons, caused by an acute disease of the upper respiratory system

The article 7.2 presents selected aspects on the research on synthesis of static mages of melanocytic skin lesions. Some algorithms to synthesize static images of melanocytic skin lesions are briefly outlined. The key approach in the elaborated synthesis methodology of images is a semantic conversion of textual description of melanocytic skin lesions - by an inhouse developed system - into hybrid (vector-raster) images. It was found, that the developed methodology can be successfully used in the process of teaching of dermatology students and also in training of preferred medical doctors.

The paper 7.3 presents the study on a possible solution to the questions concerning the classical theory of pressure-volume (PV) hysteresis and determines the role of alveolar recruitment phenomena in it. The primary purpose of the present study is to see, whether this physical process, which can be solved by model analysis, might explain a number of experimental observations on lung and airway dynamics in term of pressure-volume and flow relationships.

In the paper 7.4 authors report on test of three skeletonization algorithms, which could be used as centreline generators for 3D colon images. Two of them belong to the topological thinning group of skeletonization algorithms and the last one to the distance mapping group. After adaptation to centreline generation task the algorithms were tested on a real 3D colon image and obtained results are reported along with the characteristics of each algorithm performance. What is more the authors have made some improvements to the algorithms in order to obtain better results. The improved algorithms were also tested and results are reported. Moreover the paper contains comparison of the new algorithms with their original counterparts. Final discussion and presentation of future works are also included in the paper.

The article 7.5 deals with treelike structures. They are defined as structures which bifurcate but do not form any cycles. Apart from trees examples of such structure are neurons, snow flakes, river deltas, bronchial trees, corals, cardiovascular systems and many more. One of the aims of mathematical modeling of the natural systems is establishment of effective description and generation methods of treelike structures. In the midst of such methods Diffusion Limited Aggregation, L-systems as well as heuristics dedicated to certain issues produce desired results. A great deal of treelike structures reveals self-similarity features that indicates possibility of fractal geometry utilization in order to their description.

The paper 7.6 describes the computer system for the evaluation of test examinations organized by Centre for Examinations in Medicine. The system consists of the optical mark reader (OMR) and originally developed Windows-based application. The application supports up to 600 multiple choice questions with 4 or 5 answers to choose from. There can be two versions of test with the same questions in different orders. After reading the cards, necessary checks are performed (e.g. for multiple or missing answers). The application allows to efficiently input necessary corrections and then to calculate the individual scores. The statistical features of the whole test are also calculated (including KR20, mean difficulty index, mean discrimination index) as well as characteristics of every question, including its difficulty and point biserial correlation coefficients.

Edward Kącki
Marek Rudnicki
Joanna Stempczyńska

Table of Contents

Prophylasis

Diagnosis

Prognosis

Medical Equipment

General Problems and Healthcare Organization

Another Computer Applications

The Estimation of Reliability in the Preventive Examination of Allergic Diseases with Knowledge Discovery Methods

Bartosz Jędrzejec[2], Ewa Czarnobilska[1], Grzegorz Porębski[1], Krystyna Obtułowicz[1], and Edward Nawarecki[3]

[1] Department of Clinical and Environmental Allergology, Jagiellonian University, Medical College
[2] Division of Informatics and Control, Rzeszów University of Technology
[3] Department of Computer Science, AGH University of Science and Technology

Abtract. The paper concerns the problem of analyzing the reliability of preventive examination of allergic diseases. The authors propose an approach based on the employment knowledge discovery methods to examine data obtained from a questionnaire and tests. As a result of the examination, the association rule model is built. The model describes the relations between the survey answers and the medical test results. The evaluation of the relations provides the answers for the quality and the accuracy of the survey. The Predictive Model Markup Language (PMML) and XQuery language are involved to facilitate an environment for the systematic examination of complex mining models. In the final part of the paper, the preliminary results of experiments are presented.

1 Introduction

A frequently used method of undertaking research in medicine is through the surveys. Many conclusions moreover are based on the statistical examination of such data obtained. But preparing a proper, understandable and easily answered questionnaire is not simple and requires a lot of effort. There is also the problem that respondents who usually complete the questionnaire without the help of a medical specialist, in cases of doubt, may answer the questions incorrectly. For this reason, the accuracy of such a survey should be verified and evaluated by confirmation tests. It is not however straightforward to relate the survey answers to the appropriate test results especially when the number of records is significant. The analysis of the relations enables the estimate of a degree of reliability and accuracy in the survey data.

This paper consists of the following sections. In the second section the allergic diseases and the aim of the study are presented, the third and forth describe knowledge discovery methods and the XML standards which are used. The next section explains the model building and analysis process. The preliminary results of the experiments and conclusions are presented in the last part of the paper.

E. Kącki, M. Rudnicki, J. Stempczyńska (Eds.): Computers in Medical Activity, AISC 65, pp. 1–10.
springerlink.com

2 Allergic Diseases

Allergies are common disorders of childhood affecting about 20% of children's population. The last decade has been noticeable for a high and increasing frequency of prevalence of allergic diseases such as bronchial asthma, atopic dermatitis, rhinitis, particularly in Western Europe and North America.

Bronchial asthma is a predominating chronic disease of childhood and its frequency of occurrence has clearly increased in recent years. Despite common knowledge of asthma, the disproportion of the number of children presenting the symptoms of the illness and the number of children with a settled diagnosis is visible [6].

The second allergic disorder which is difficult for epidemiological diagnostician is dermatitis. It is such general symptom and could escape the attention of responders.

Many children who have suffered from the disease in their first years of life will be unwell for the reminder of their lives.

The investigations of the occurrence of atopic dermatitis in children are not easy because it is hard to establish a diagnosis according to common, defined criteria in epidemiological research, so in individual investigations, authors have described their results optionally from skin changes through eczema to atopic dermatitis.

The essential procedures in the prevention of allergic diseases are to minimize exposure to the allergic factors. Preventative activity may be effective when it concerns pupils, particularly from occupational schools where switching on a preventative program and proper allergological supervision will permit to avoid the development of an occupational allergy [9, 11-12].

The aim of the study was to assess the incidence frequency of allergic diseases in a group of children aged 8-10 and youths aged 16-18, based on questionnaires, case historical, physical examination and in the cases of implied allergic disease, an individual pattern of diagnostic tools was established e.g. spirometry, prick and patch skin tests, serum total IgE (t-IgE) and specific IgE (s-IgE) levels for allergens suspected to allergic symptoms, as well as the estimation of reliability of preventive investigations using knowledge discovery methods.

3 Knowledge Discovery

Knowledge discovery in databases (KDD) is a process which is used for finding, previously unknown, information in data. One of the main parts of KDD – data mining (DM) is a rapidly growing research area relating to the use of artificial intelligence and machine learning methods in advanced data analysis. The result of the mining procedure is a kind of knowledge base, called a mining model, containing useful patterns and characteristics derived from the data. Such models are frequently complex and difficult to interpret – therefore considerable efforts are required generally to evaluate mining results. In a typical case, clever visualization techniques are involved to present the generated patterns with the aim of enabling a better insight into mining results. However, when a model becomes complex, it is not always easy to make exhaustive use of a picture and give it a clear description.

3.1 Association Rules

Association rules are an important type of data mining models [2, 5]. In general, an association rule is an expression in the form A ⇒ B, where A and B are subsets of items (usually called itemsets) taken from some universal set of items I, and A ∩ B = ∅. The rules are normally obtained by analyzing a set D (Fig. 1) of task relevant data consisting of a large number of records T often referred to as transactions. Each transaction is composed of items from I. For any transaction T and an itemset A, we say that T contains A, if A ⊆ T.

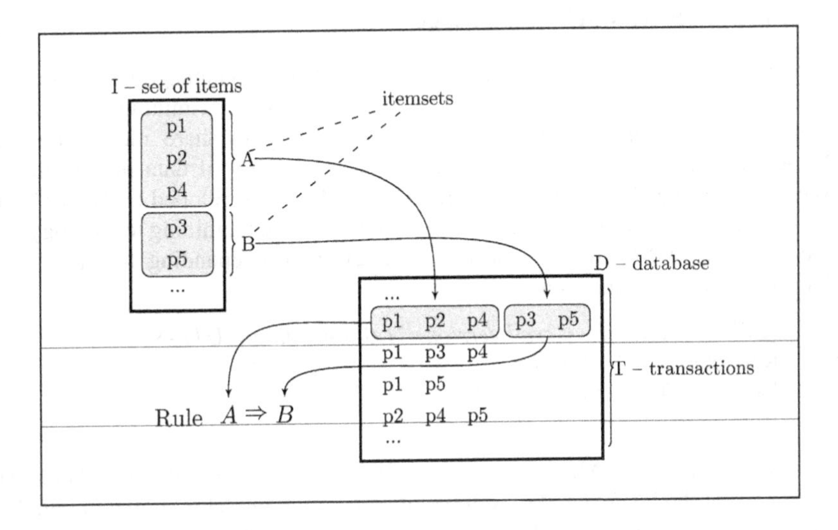

Fig. 1. Association rules

The percentage of transactions in D that contain an itemset A is usually referred to as support of the itemset. An itemset that satisfies minimum support is called frequent itemset. There are two popular interestingness measures for an association rule A ⇒ B i.e.: support and confidence. They are defined as follows:

1. The rule A ⇒ B holds in the transaction set D with support sup, if sup is the percentage of transactions in D that contain both A and B.
2. The rule A ⇒ B has confidence conf in the transaction set D, if conf is the percentage of all transactions containing A, that also contain B.

Minimum support and minimum confidence thresholds are commonly used to control the process of mining association rules. The classic example of association rule mining is market basket analysis, but many other interesting application areas exist, e.g.: business management, click-stream analysis etc.

4 XML Standards in KDD

The eXtensible Markup Language (XML) is a rapidly growing technology, which is widely exploited by applications nowadays. This meta-language, recommended by World Wide Web Consortium (W3C) [4], is used for defining new languages and found application in many areas including: chemistry, multimedia, navigation, music etc. Each of these languages is provided by a document type definition, necessary to build the correct structures. One of the special XML applications, which is utilize in KDD, is Predictive Model Markup Language.

4.1 Predictive Model Markup Language

The Predictive Model Markup Language (PMML) [10] is a language which provides a text-based way for applications to define statistical and data mining models. The essential benefit of such an approach is the possibility to share models between PMML-compliant applications, which denote the portability of data mining models between mining tools from different vendors. PMML was developed by Data Mining Group – an organization which defines new standards for data mining technology.

The structure of PMML file consists of a few parts, depending on the kind of model. The common elements are:

- XML declaration – *<?xml version="1.0" encoding="UTF-8" ?>*
- Root element – *<PMML>*
- Document header – *<HEADER>*
- Data dictionary – *<DataDictionary>*.

The essential part of the PMML document defines one or more of the models allowed in version 2.0 of the language. An example of association model is shown in Fig. 2.

The main element of the PMML-code of the model generated is an *Association-Model*, which attributes describe building parameters of the model such as: minimum support, minimum confidence, number of rules etc. The next elements and their attributes describe model items, itemsets and rules respectively. The rules included in a simple model are:

"final diagnosis doesn't confirm primary" ⇒ "preliminary diagnosis pann"
support = 0.3582 confidence = 0.5200

"preliminary diagnosis pann" ⇒ "final diagnosis doesn't confirm primary"
support = 0.3582 confidence = 0.6617

But such plain and easy understandable models are uncommon. More frequent, association models are complex, consist of hundreds or even thousands of rules, and are difficult to analyse and explain. To get access to and analyse the model in a PMML file we decided to employ XQuery language [7].

4.2 XQuery

A number of techniques and tools have been introduced in the last few years in the area of querying semi-structured data and XML [1]. One of them is XQuery language recently recommended by W3C[3]. The main advantage of this query language is its close similarity to relational databases query language – SQL. A compact and easy to

```
<?xml version="1.0" encoding="UTF-8" ?>
<PMML version="2.0">
    <Header copyright="Copyright (c) 2004 prudsys AG" description="Xelopes mining model">
    <Application version="1.2.3" name="Xelopes" />
    </Header>
    <DataDictionary numberOfFields="2">
        <DataField displayName="transactId" dataType="string" name="transactId" isCyclic="0" optype="categorical" />
        <DataField displayName="itemName" dataType="string" name="itemName" isCyclic="0" optype="categorical"/>
    </DataDictionary>
    <AssociationModel minimumConfidence="0.0" numberOfRules="2"
                minimumSupport="0.3" itemIdName="itemName"
                numberOfTransactions="1445" algorithmName="associationRules"
                numberOfItemsets="4" modelName="Allergic diseases"
                functionName="associationRules" transactIdName="transactId"
                numberOfItems="3">
        <MiningSchema>
            <MiningField missingValueTreatment="asIs" name="transactId" outliers="asIs" usageType="active" />
            <MiningField missingValueTreatment="asIs" name="itemName" outliers="asIs" usageType="active" />
        </MiningSchema>
        <Item value="preliminary diagnosis pann" id="0" />
        <Item value="preliminary diagnosis azs" id="1" />
        <Item value="final diagnosis doesn't confirm primary" id="2" />
        <Itemset numberOfItems="1" support="0.3253" id="1">
            <ItemRef itemRef="0" />
        </Itemset>
        <Itemset numberOfItems="2" support="0.2152" id="2">
            <ItemRef itemRef="0" />
            <ItemRef itemRef="2" />
        </Itemset>
        <Itemset numberOfItems="1" support="0.1869" id="3">
            <ItemRef itemRef="1" />
        </Itemset>
        <Itemset numberOfItems="1" support="0.4138" id="4">
            <ItemRef itemRef="2" />
        </Itemset>
        <AssociationRule confidence="0.5200" support="0.3583" consequent="1" antecedent="4" />
        <AssociationRule confidence="0.6617" support="0.3583" consequent="4" antecedent="1" />
    </AssociationModel>
</PMML>
```

Fig. 2. Association rules model in PMML

understand syntax is also its strong point. Additionally, an important feature is a set of embedded functions, for example set-theoretical operations on query result, and the possibility of writing new ones.

```
for $i in doc("assoc_model_3.xml")//AssociationRule
[@support>=0.3 and consequent=4]
return $i
```

Fig. 3. XQuery example

Fig. 3 shows an example of a query in XQuery language. This query looks up the rule base of the input model and extracts the rules with support greater than or equal to 0.3 and consequent number 4. As the result of the example query, only one rule from the model from Fig. 2 is obtained.

5 Model Building and Analysis

5.1 Model Building

The model building process was divided into a number of steps (Fig. 4).

First of all, the study was performed in the Department of Allergology, University Hospital in Cracow between 2004 – 2006 and was sponsored by the local Healthcare and Promotion Program – "Healthy Cracow". 1918 pupils aged between 8-10 and 16-18 were engaged.

The study was carried out in two stages. In the first stage a questionnaire prepared by Prof K. Obtułowicz, which included questions concerning the occurrence of allergic diseases was used.

On the basis of analysis of the questionnaire filled in by the pupils, their case history and physical examination, 867 children aged 8-10 and 372 aged 16-18 who displayed a positive allergic case history were considered in the second phase of study. In this phase prick tests were performed. The pupils who had an inconsistency of case history with the results of the skin prick tests were examined for confirmation or exclusion of atopic reactions by measuring blood levels of t-IgE and/or s-IgE for allergens suspected to allergic symptoms.

Data obtained from the questionnaire and the tests were inputted into local computer databases by hand and by different people and for their reason special preparations for DM database were needed. The data need to be cleaned, discretized and normalized before transfer to the database for data mining. This part of the model construction procedure is very important because well optimised data increases the chance of correct models.

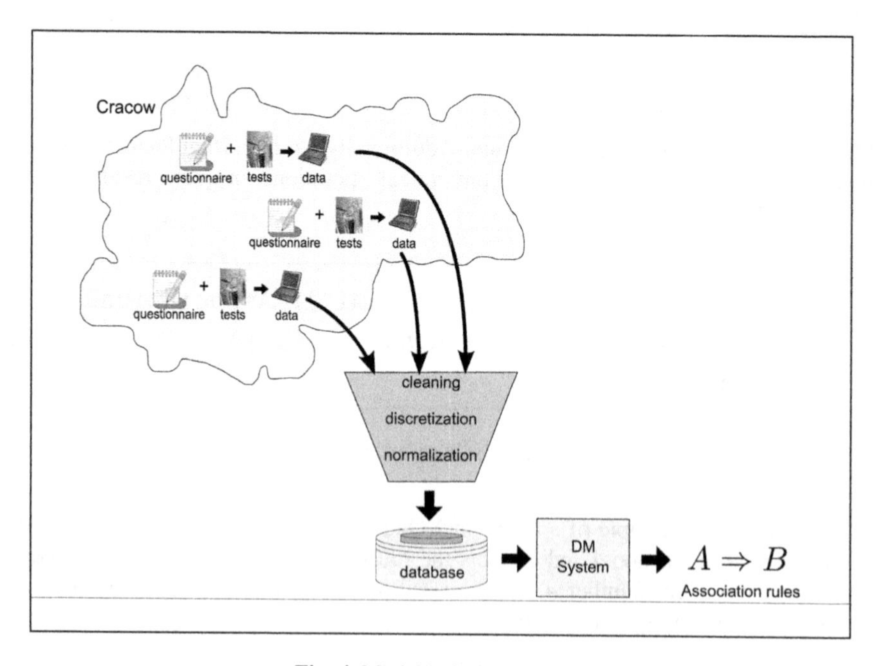

Fig. 4. Model building process

The last step of the process was the association model generating by DM System. In this phase, the attributes for analyse, model threshold parameters, minimum support and confidence, had to be chosen. Too high values for the constraints result in a small, comprehensible, but low-information model. Too low values cause a complex model, with a large number of rules, which is not easy to analyse and understand. However, the advantage of the complex model is that it contains a lot of hidden information. As a store method for the models, the PMML language, described in the previous part of paper, was chosen.

5.2 Model Analysis

The model analysis process, we proposed, is based on the querying data mining model, stored in PMML, by XQuery to extract the interested rules (Fig. 5).

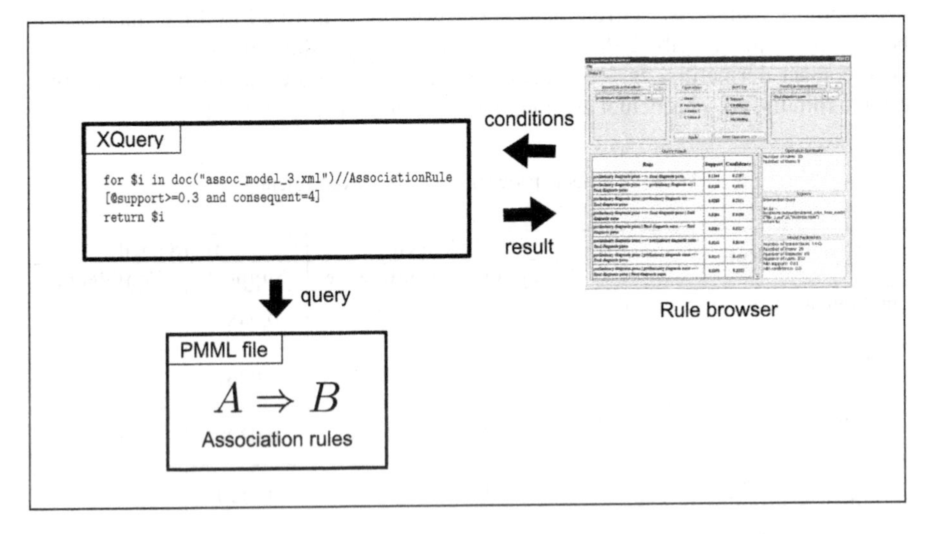

Fig. 5. Model analysis process

To facilitate this procedure, an interactive Association Rule Browser [8] was developed. This program translates the conditions of rules selection into XQuery syntax and executes the query. The query result returns to the browser and is presented as a table of rules. The browser creates a possibility to query the rule base in steps where the subset of rules obtained in the previous step becomes the new rule base for the next query. It is also possible to return to an earlier step and start querying from a prior point of analysis.

6 Experiments and Preliminary Results

The main aim of our experiments focused on estimating the reliability of the survey. To achieve this goal we decided to ascertain what the relations are between the preliminary diagnoses based on the questionnaire and the final diagnoses following the medical tests. In our research, the data for pupils aged 8-10 and 16-18 were analysed separately. The parameters of the models building are presented in Tab. 1.

Table 1. Models parameters

Parameter	Model for pupils aged 8-10	Model for pupils aged 16-18
number of transactions	867	372
number of items	26	18
number of itemsets	88	93
number of rules	352	360
min support	0.01	0.01
min confidence	0.0	0.0

During the model analysis with Rule Browser the search was for the rules in which the preliminary diagnosis in rule antecedent was not confirmed by final diagnosis in the rule consequent. Tab. 2 shows the browsing results (shortcuts: ap – food allergy, wk – contact dermatitis, zs – conjunctivitis, azs – atopic dermatitis, pann – chronic allergic rhinitis, ao – bronchial asthma, oann – acute allergic rhinitis).

Table 2. Models browsing results – experiment 1

Rule	8-10 aged		16-18 aged	
	Support	Confidence	Support	Confidence
preliminary diag. ap ⇒ final diag. not confirm primary	0.0645	0.9333	0.0481	0.5
preliminary diag. wk ⇒ final diag. not confirm primary	0.0195	0.8947	0.0361	0.4090
preliminary diag. zs ⇒ final diag. not confirm primary	0.0253	0.8148	0.0120	0.5
preliminary diag. azs ⇒ final diag. not confirm primary	0.2131	0.6851	0.1124	0.4745
preliminary diag. pann ⇒ final diag. not confirm primary	0.3582	0.6617	0.3574	0.5668
preliminary diag. ao ⇒ final diag. not confirm primary	0.1417	0.6612	0.0361	0.2903
preliminary diag. oann ⇒ final diag. not confirm primary	0.1417	0.6373	0.0923	0.46

Analysing Tab. 2 we can discover that the diagnoses of the 8-10 years old for food allergies provide the worst results because the confidence parameter is the highest. Similar results were obtained for contact dermatitis and conjunctivitis. The reason for these results is probably that parents are overprotective towards their children and all disease symptoms are interpreted as allergic indicators. Better results were achieved among pupils aged 16-18. The reason is probably that the children at this age reveal the youthful spirit of contrariness and try to hide symptoms because they do not want to receive treatment.

In the second experiment for comparison we decided to find out how often the preliminary diagnoses were confirmed by final diagnoses. Tab. 3 presents the results of this experiment. Some rules (e.g. preliminary diagnosis ap ⇒ final diagnosis ap) appeared only in the 16-18 age group. It means that the minimum support threshold was too high to identify any rules or these kinds of relations do not occur in the database.

Table 3. Models browsing results – experiment 2

Rule	**8-10 aged**		**16-18 aged**	
	Support	**Confidence**	**Support**	**Confidence**
preliminary diagnosis ao ⇒ final diagnosis ao	0.0345	0.1612	0.0522	0.4193
preliminary diagnosis ap ⇒ final diagnosis ap	–	–	0.0120	0.125
preliminary diagnosis azs ==> final diagnosis azs	0.0679	0.2185	–	–
preliminary diagnosis oann ⇒ final diagnosis oann	0.0403	0.1813	0.0682	0.34
preliminary diagnosis pann ⇒ final diagnosis pann	0.1244	0.2297	0.2088	0.3312
preliminary diagnosis wk ⇒ final diagnosis wk	–	–	0.0160	0.1818

These preliminary experiments show that the survey is more suitable for older pupils, but still needs to be analysed to achieve better results in the future.

7 Conclusions

In our research we used KDD techniques and methods to analyse the data obtained from the preventive examinations of allergic disease. The PMML standard was presented as a promising method to store data mining models. To process those models XQuery language was proposed. An Association Rule Browser was developed to help query the models and present the results. In future work, it is planned to automate query generation and information retrieval.

It is also proposed to continue the analysis of data and hope that the study will be helpful in the settlement of main risk factors which are responsible for the development of allergic diseases. It is also expected for an answer as to which type of allergy in early childhood (skin or respiratory) would most increase the risk of prevalence of allergic diseases in the future. Preliminary verification of case histories (results of questionnaire) using prick tests and IgE would help to define the influence of laboratory findings on the change or confirmation of preliminary diagnosis or mistakes in the questionnaire.

The answer for the question: do other diseases (and what kind are they) occur in allergic children? will allow an assumption to be made as to which of them can promote allergy.

Detailed analysis of laboratory findings and clinical symptoms of allergic diseases can help to identify if there are any relationships between atopic and contact allergy.

The above analyses would be helpful in:

1. A better understanding of the pathogenesis of allergic diseases,
2. An estimation of the principal risk factors of allergic diseases in childhood,
3. An assessment of additional allergological tests in the diagnosis of allergic diseases,
4. An evaluation of questionnaire credibility.

This work was partly supported by the grant N516 026 31/2545 from the Polish Ministry of Science and Higher Education.

References

[1] Abiteboul, S., Buneman, P., Suciu, D.: Data on the Web. From Relations to Semistructured Data and XML. Morgan Kaufmann, San Francisco (1999)

[2] Agrawal, R., Imieliński, T., Swami, A.: Mining Association Rules between Sets of Items in Large Databases. In: Proc. ACM SIGMOD International Conference on Management of Data, Washington, USA, pp. 207–216 (1993)

[3] Boag, S., Chamberlin, D., Fernandez, M.F., Florescu, D., Robie, J., Simeon, J.: XQuery 1.0: An XML Query Language (2007), `http://www.w3.org/TR/xquery/`

[4] Bray, T., Paoli, J., Sperberg-McQueen, C.E., Maler, E., Yergeau, F.: Extensible Markup Language (XML) 1.0 Third Edition. W3C Recommendation (2004), `http://www.w3.org/TR/2004/REC-xml-20040204/`

[5] Han, J., Kamber, M.: Data Mining. Concepts and Techniques. Morgan Kaufmann, San Francisco (2001)

[6] Lis, G., Bręborowicz, A., Świątły, A., et al.: Występowanie chorób alergicznych u dzieci szkolnych w Krakowie i Poznaniu (na podstawie badań ankietowych ISAAC). Pneumonol. Alergol. Pol. 65, 621–627 (1997)

[7] Świder, K., Jędrzejec, B.: A Query-Driven Exploration of Association Rule Models in PMML. In: Tadeusiewicz, R., Ligęza, A., Szymkat, M. (eds.) Proc. of the 5th Conference Computer Methods and Systems – CMS 2005, Kraków, Poland, pp. 409–414 (2005)

[8] Świder, K., Jędrzejec, B., Wysocki, M.: A Query-Driven Exploration of Discovered Association Rules. Studies in Computational Intelligence, pp. 275–290. Springer, Heidelberg (2007) (in printing)

[9] Obtułowicz, K.: Choroby alergiczne młodzieży w okresie dojrzewania. Medycyna wieku młodzieńczego. Klinika i postępowanie w chorobach przewlekłych. Wydawnictwo Medyczne, Kraków, pp. 55–78 (2001)

[10] PMML, Predictive Model Markup Language (PMML) Project Page (2003), `http://sourceforge.net/projects/pmml`

[11] Stelmach, W., Korzeniowska, A., Piechota, M., et al.: Preliminary results of prophylactic program of allergic diseases in children in Łódź district. Pneumonol. Alergol. Pol. 70, 561–565 (2002)

[12] Strachan, D.: Worldwide variations in the prevalence of symptoms of allergic rhinoconiunctivitis in children: the International Study of Asthma and Allergies in Childhood (ISAAC). Pediatr. Alergy. Immunol., 161–176 (1997)

Medical Diagnosis with Type-2 Fuzzy Decision Trees

Łukasz Bartczuk and Danuta Rutkowska

Departament of Computer Engineering,
Częstochowa University of Technology, Częstochowa, Poland
bartczuk@kik.pcz.czest.pl, drutko@kik.pcz.czest.pl

Abstract. In this paper, we propose type-2 fuzzy decision trees in application to medical diagnosis. This means that attribute values employed in the tree structures may be characterized by type-2 fuzzy sets. Three medical benchmark data sets, available on the Internet, have been used to illustrate results of diagnosis obtained by this method.

Keywords: Type-2 fuzzy sets, decision trees, medical diagnosis.

1 Introduction

Decision trees are commonly used in artificial intelligence, as knowledge representation as well as an approach to classification, and appreciated for their clarity and high accuracy.

The well-known ID3 algorithm [18]-[21], proposed by Quinlan for creating decision trees, has been combined by other researchers with fuzzy sets introduced by Zadeh [23]. In this way, fuzzy decision trees have been considered and built by means of Fuzzy ID3 algorithm developed by Janikow [11]. More research on creating fuzzy decision trees and their applications to classification problems have been done by different authors [1], [2], [3], [17], [24], [28].

The main motivation to introduce fuzzy set theory and fuzzy logic by Zadeh [29], [30], was a necessity for describing phenomena and concepts that were uncertain or imprecisely defined. In the fuzzy set theory, a single object can belong to many sets with different membership grades — real numbers from [0,1] interval. Membership functions that represent fuzzy sets, and take values from this interval, provide a formal description of such concepts like e.g. "low temperature", "high blood pressure".

In a classification problem, that can be solved by a decision tree, we have a set of examples, called a training set, where each example includes an object described by a set of attributes. Each object belongs to a class from a set of classes. The attributes take values that can be symbolic (like in the classic ID3 algorithm) or numerical (like in decision trees created e.g. by the C4.5 algorithm [20]) or fuzzy (in the case of fuzzy decision trees).

Medical diagnosis can be treated as the classification problem, where objects are patients with symptoms described as attribute values, and classes correspond to diagnosis according to medical doctors' classification.

E. Kącki, M. Rudnicki, J. Stempczyńska (Eds.): Computers in Medical Activity, AISC 65, pp. 11–21.
springerlink.com

A fuzzy decision tree is a generalization of the classic (crisp) decision tree [7], [11]. Each node of the fuzzy tree is associated with a fuzzy set of examples and labeled by an attribute. Each branch from the node is assigned to a fuzzy set defined on the domain of the attribute. Each leaf is labeled by a set of classes with different membership grades instead of one class (like in crisp decision trees).

In the fuzzy approach, a shape of each membership function may be crucial to the performance of the classifier. The membership functions can be defined by experts or determined by means of a special algorithm based on the data (training set). In both cases additional levels of uncertainty may appear. Using opinions of many experts, each of them may propose different membership functions for the same fuzzy set. It can happen because like Mendel noticed "words can mean different things to different people" [13], [14]. When the algorithm is employed for generating the membership functions from the data, we can encounter the same situation because results of such an algorithm highly depend on the data and other factors, e.g. parameters of the algorithm.

Thus, we should take into account the uncertainty concerning the membership grades (values of the membership functions). Therefore, we apply the so-called type-2 fuzzy sets that are characterized by fuzzy membership grades, introduced by Zadeh [30]. This means that the membership grades are not crisp values but fuzzy sets defined on [0,1] interval. As a special, simpler case, we can consider the type-2 fuzzy sets with interval membership grades [12]-[16], [18], [23].

In this paper, fuzzy decision trees are combined with type-2 fuzzy sets. Thus, we propose the so-called type-2 fuzzy decision trees, in application to medical diagnosis as a classification problem with uncertainty and vague data. Some simulation results illustrate performance of the proposed algorithm on selected medical diagnosis problems.

This paper is organized as follows: the next section describes basic concepts of type-2 fuzzy sets. The third section presents the algorithm proposed for creating the fuzzy decision tree of type-2 and inference process based on the tree. Experimental results are illustrated in Section 4, and final conclusions are included in Section 5.

2 Type-2 Fuzzy Sets

A type-2 fuzzy set, $\tilde{A}$, in the universe of discourse, X, may be represented as a set of ordered pairs [12]-[15], [18], [23]

$$\tilde{A} = \{(x, \mu_{\tilde{A}}(x)), x \in X\} \tag{1}$$

where $\mu_{\tilde{A}}(x)$ is a fuzzy grade of membership defined as follows

$$\mu_{\tilde{A}}(x) = \int_{J_x} \frac{f_x(u)}{u} \tag{2}$$

In this equation, like in the definition of classic (type-1) fuzzy set [29], the integral sign does not denote integration, but the collection of all points $x \in X$. The arithmetic division sign has also different meaning. The function $f_x(u)$, defined as $f_x : [0,1] \rightarrow [0,1]$, is called the secondary membership function, and $J_x \in [0,1]$ determines the domain of this function.

Thus, the type-2 fuzzy set, $\tilde{A}$, can be expressed by means of the fuzzy set notation [29], in the form

$$\tilde{A} = \int_{x \in X} \mu_{\tilde{A}}(x)/x = \int_{x \in X} \left(\int_{u \in J_x} f_x(u)/u \right) \Big/ x \tag{3}$$

According to the definition of classic (type-1) fuzzy set [29], a fuzzy set, A', in X, is characterized by a membership function, $\mu_{A'}(x)$, which associates with each point $x \in X$ a real number in the interval $[0,1]$ representing the grade of membership of x in A'. The type-2 fuzzy set is defined by a fuzzy membership function, the grade (that is, fuzzy grade) of which is a fuzzy set (type-1) in the unit interval $[0,1]$, rather than a point in $[0,1]$. Thus, while membership functions of classic (type-1) fuzzy sets range over the interval $[0,1]$, membership functions of the type-2 fuzzy sets range over type-1 fuzzy sets. The concept of type-2 fuzzy sets was introduced by Zadeh [30]. These definitions can also be found e.g. in [22].

Basic operations on fuzzy sets, such as union, intersection, etc. have been defined as generalizations of corresponding operations for crisp (non-fuzzy) sets, by use of functions called triangular norms (*T*-norm, and *T*-conorm known as *S*-norm); for details see e.g. [22]. The minimum and maximum, applied by Zadeh [29] to define the intersection and union of fuzzy sets (type-1), are special cases of the *T*-norm and *S*-norm, respectively.

With regard to the type-2 fuzzy sets, the operations may be defined by the Zadeh Extension Principle [29], [30], [31]. However, this approach implies very high computational cost, but it can be significantly reduced if simpler (e.g. interval) shape of the secondary membership function is assumed. In such a case, the fuzzy grade of membership is expressed as follows [12]-[15], [18], [23]

$$\mu_{\tilde{A}}(x) = \int_{u \in J_x} f_x(u)/u = \int_{u \in J_x} 1/u \tag{4}$$

This value can also be represented by minimum and maximum points in which function $f_x(u)$ has non-zero values

$$\mu_{\tilde{A}}(x) = [\inf(J_x), \sup(J_x)] = [\underline{\mu_{\tilde{A}}(x)}, \overline{\mu_{\tilde{A}}(x)}] \tag{5}$$

When the above notation is used, the so-called extended *T*-norm and *S*-norm functions can be employed to define the intersection and union operations, respectively, on the type-2 fuzzy sets. The following equations express the extended *T*-norm (denoted $\tilde{T}$-norm) and extended *S*-norm (denoted $\tilde{S}$-norm)

$$\mu_{\tilde{A}}(x) \overset{\tilde{T}}{*} \mu_{\tilde{B}}(x) = \left[\underline{\mu_{\tilde{A}}(x)} \overset{T}{*} \underline{\mu_{\tilde{B}}(x)}, \overline{\mu_{\tilde{A}}(x)} \overset{T}{*} \overline{\mu_{\tilde{B}}(x)} \right] \tag{6}$$

$$\mu_{\tilde{A}}(x) \overset{\tilde{S}}{*} \mu_{\tilde{B}}(x) = \left[\underline{\mu_{\tilde{A}}(x)} \overset{S}{*} \underline{\mu_{\tilde{B}}(x)}, \overline{\mu_{\tilde{A}}(x)} \overset{S}{*} \overline{\mu_{\tilde{B}}(x)} \right] \tag{7}$$

where T and S are classic *T*-norm and *S*-norm, that can be min and max functions, respectively.

Some examples of type-2 fuzzy sets are portrayed in Section 4, in Fig. 1, for medical data. Fuzzy relations that correspond to the rules represented by type-2 fuzzy decision trees, are expressed by use of the extended *T*-norm and *S*-norm functions. According to the concept of fuzzy relations, introduced by Zadeh [29], a fuzzy relation can be viewed as a multi-dimensional fuzzy set. The definition of fuzzy relations (type-1) can be found e.g. in [22]. In this paper, in Section 3, fuzzy relations of type-2 are considered with regard to type-2 fuzzy decision trees, with the special case of the interval secondary membership functions of type-2 fuzzy sets.

3 Type-2 Fuzzy Decision Trees

Tree structures are very popular in many fields of computer science. Decision trees can be applied to data mining and decision support. Crisp decision trees [19]-[21], as well as fuzzy decision trees [1], [2], [11], [17], are created by recursive procedures that allow to construct a tree structure from data set E and attribute set A. Every attribute A^{k}, $k = 1,...,|\mathrm{A}|$, contains $|\mathrm{A}^{k}|$ values a_{m}^{k}, $m = 1,...,|\mathrm{A}^{k}|$, which may be characterized by a symbol, crisp set, fuzzy set or type-2 fuzzy set. Every object from data set E can be considered as a pair $e_i = (\mathbf{x}_i, y_i)$ where $\mathbf{x}_i = [x_1,...,x_n]$ is an n-dimensional vector of input values, and y_i is a label (value of decision attribute A^{D}).

Every node of a tree contains a subset E^{N} of the data set, while the root node includes all objects from set E. The homogeneity of E^{N} subset is measured by information content and it should be increased in every child node.

One of the most popular method for creating crisp decision trees is the ID3 algorithm proposed by Quinlan [19]. In paper [11] Janikow describes an extension of this algorithm that allows to build fuzzy decision trees. Another version of the ID3 algorithm for creating fuzzy decision trees when values of attributes are characterized by interval type-2 fuzzy sets, is presented in paper [3]. Details concerning this algorithm are described in the next subsection.

3.1 Type-2 Fuzzy ID3 Algorithm

Now we present the method proposed in order to split the tree node N in order to construct the tree structure. This approach is based on the Fuzzy-ID3 algorithm introduced by Janikow [11].

Let us assume that $\mu_{N}(e_i)$ means the membership of object e_i in the type-2 fuzzy set created for node N. This set is defined using the join operation of all interval type-2 fuzzy sets that are included in the path from the root node to the N node, and can be computed according to Equation (6).

In step 1, examples count P_j^{N} and examples frequency Q_j^{N}, $j = 1,...,|\mathrm{A}^{D}|$, are computed. The first value is the sum of the objects' membership $R_j^{(N|e_i)}$ in the type-2 fuzzy relation between fuzzy sets defined for node N and decision $\tilde{a}_j^{D}$. These values can be obtained as follows

$$P_j^N = \left[\underline{P_j^N}, \overline{P_j^N}\right] = \left[\sum_{i=1}^{|E^N|} \underline{R_j^{(N|e_i)}}, \sum_{i=1}^{|E^N|} \overline{R_j^{(N|e_i)}}\right] \tag{8}$$

where $\underline{R_j^{(N|e_i)}}$ and $\overline{R_j^{(N|e_i)}}$ denote, respectively, lower and upper values of fuzzy grade of membership of data object e_i in the type-2 fuzzy relation, defined as

$$R_j^{(N|e_i)} = \left[\underline{R_j^{(N|e_i)}}, \overline{R_j^{(N|e_i)}}\right] = \left[f\left(\underline{\mu_N(e_i)}, \underline{\mu_{\tilde{a}_j^D}(y_i)}\right), f\left(\overline{\mu_N(e_i)}, \overline{\mu_{\tilde{a}_j^D}(y_i)}\right)\right] \tag{9}$$

where f is a fuzzy relation (of type-1).

In typical classification problems, value $\mu_{\tilde{a}_j^D}(y_i)$ equals to [1,1] what simplifies Equation (9) to the following form

$$R_j^{(N|e_i)} = \left[\underline{R_j^{(N|e_i)}}, \overline{R_j^{(N|e_i)}}\right] = \left[\underline{\mu_N(e_i)}, \overline{\mu_N(e_i)}\right] \tag{10}$$

The examples frequency $Q_j^N = \left[\underline{Q_j^N}, \overline{Q_j^N}\right]$ may be expressed by formulas

$$\underline{Q_j^N} = \frac{\underline{P_j^N}}{\underline{P_j^N} + \sum_{\substack{o=1\\ o\neq j}}^{|A^D|} \overline{P_j^N}}, \quad \overline{Q_j^N} = \frac{\overline{P_j^N}}{\overline{P_j^N} + \sum_{\substack{o=1\\ o\neq j}}^{|A^D|} \underline{P_j^N}} \tag{11}$$

In step 2, the total examples count P^N in node N should be obtained by

$$P^N = \left[\underline{P^N}, \overline{P^N}\right] = \left[\sum_{j=1}^{|A^D|} \underline{P_j^N}, \sum_{j=1}^{|A^D|} \overline{P_j^N}\right] \tag{12}$$

This value will be applied to compute the weighted entropy in potential child nodes.

In step 3, in order to determine the value of entropy I^N, we should find the minimum and maximum values of the following function

$$Y(q_1, \ldots, q_{|A^D|}) = -\sum_{j=1}^{|A^D|} q_j \log_2 q_j$$

with additional assumptions $\sum_{j=1}^{|A^D|} q_j = 1$ and $q_j \in Q_j^N$.

The analytical solution that allows to compute the minimum and maximum values of function Y is difficult to find, so the authors proposed two heuristic algorithms to determine these values.

In step 4, for each attribute not included in the path from the root node to N node, the information gain should be computed, based on the weighted entropy. In the Fuzzy ID3 algorithm, this value is calculated by use of the following expression [11]

$$I^{(N|A^k)} = \sum_{m=1}^{|A^k|} P^{(N|a_m^k)} I^{(N|a_m^k)} \Big/ \sum_{m=1}^{|A^k|} P^{(N|a_m^k)} \tag{13}$$

where $P^{(N|a_m^k)}$ and $I^{(N|a_m^k)}$ denote the total examples count and the entropy in the node (child of node N) that contains value a_m^k , respectively.

In the proposed algorithm, values $P^{(N|\tilde{a}_m^k)}$ and $I^{(N|\tilde{a}_m^k)}$ are intervals. Therefore, in order to use Equation (13), the minimum and maximum values of the following function

$$Y\left(p_1,\ldots,p_{|A^k|},t_j,\ldots,t_{|A^k|}\right) = \sum_{m=1}^{|A^k|} p_m t_m \Big/ \sum_{m=1}^{|A^k|} p_m \tag{14}$$

for $t_m \in I^{(N|\tilde{a}_m^k)}$, $p_m \in P^{(N|\tilde{a}_m^k)}$, should be obtained by means of the Karnik-Mendel algorithm described in [12], [15].

The information gain can be computed as follows

$$G^{A^k} = \left[\underline{G}^{A^k}, \overline{G}^{A^k}\right] = \left[\underline{I}^{N} - \overline{I}^{(N|A^k)}, \overline{I}^{N} - \underline{I}^{(N|A^k)}\right] \tag{15}$$

In step 5, the attribute with the highest value of the information gain must be chosen. Because this is the interval value, as a comparison operation, one of the methods employed to compare fuzzy numbers [1], [5], [6], [8], [9], [25]-[27] can be used. However, it is difficult to find the optimal method for comparing fuzzy numbers that can be suitable in the proposed algorithm. Of course, the choice of the best method depends on the problem.

In step 6, the node N should be split using the chosen attribute, with the highest information gain value.

In step 7, for each new created node the stopping criterion must be checked. The most popular stopping criterions are

- all attributes are included in the path from the root node to N node
- all objects in data set E^N have the same decision label
- the maximum number of nodes have to be reached
- the information gain for any attribute does not reach the minimum value.

When one or more of the above stopping criterions are met, the node becomes a leaf and the decision for which the examples frequency reaches the biggest value is assigned to him. In other cases, the node must be further split according to the described algorithm.

3.2 Inference Process Using Type-2 Fuzzy Decision Tree

A decision tree can be considered as a set of decision rules. Every rule corresponds to exactly one leaf of the tree and may be written in the following form

$$R^l : \textbf{IF}\, x_1 \textbf{ IS } \tilde{a}_l^1 \textbf{ AND...AND} x_s \textbf{ IS } \tilde{a}_l^s \textbf{ THEN} y \textbf{ IS } \tilde{a}_l^D, \quad l = 1,...,|L| \tag{16}$$

where: $|L|$ – number of rules (leaves), s – length of rule; $1 \le s \le |A|$.

The degree of fulfillment of antecedent part of the rule may be computed using any kind of the extended T-norm

$$\mu_{A^l}(\mathbf{x}) = \mu_{\tilde{a}_l^1}(x_1) \overset{\tilde{T}}{*} \mu_{\tilde{a}_l^2}(x_2) \overset{\tilde{T}}{*} \ldots \overset{\tilde{T}}{*} \mu_{\tilde{a}_l^s}(x_s) \tag{17}$$

Every rule represents some fuzzy relations which, for simplicity, can be defined using some extended T-norms, so the degree of satisfaction of the antecedent to the consequent (which is often referred as the degree of satisfaction of the consequent) may be written as follows

$$\mu_{\tilde{R}^l}(y) = \mu_{A^l}(\mathbf{x}) \overset{\tilde{T}}{*} \mu_{\tilde{a}_l^D}(y) \tag{18}$$

Equation (18) expresses typical and the simplest approach to compute the degree of satisfaction of the consequent. In this method, all leaves are treated in the same way. In paper [11], Janikow noticed that leaves that contain small number of objects from the data set may have negative influence on the inference process. He suggested that every rule generated by a decision tree should be weighted by examples count P_κ^l. However, this value is often bigger than one, so this approach can generate supernatural fuzzy sets (the fuzzy sets for which the biggest value of fuzzy grade of membership is bigger than one). In paper [3], authors proposed to use the normalized examples count ψ_l for which the lower and upper values can be expressed by the following equations

$$\underline{\psi_l} = \frac{\underline{P_{\kappa_l}^l}}{\underline{P_{\kappa_l}^l} + \sum_{\substack{i=1 \\ i \ne l}}^{|L|} \overline{P_{\kappa_l}^i}}, \qquad \overline{\psi_l} = \frac{\overline{P_{\kappa_l}^l}}{\overline{P_{\kappa_l}^l} + \sum_{\substack{i=1 \\ i \ne l}}^{|L|} \underline{P_{\kappa_l}^i}} \tag{19}$$

where: κ_l - decision assigned to l^{th} leaf.

By use of the normalized examples count ψ_l, Equation (18) can be rewritten in the following form

$$\begin{aligned} \mu_{\tilde{R}^l}(y) &= \left[\mu_{A^l}(\mathbf{x}) \overset{\tilde{T}}{*} \mu_{\tilde{a}_l^D}(y) \right] \cdot \psi_l = \left[\underline{\mu_{A^l}(\mathbf{x})} \overset{T}{*} \underline{\mu_{\tilde{a}_l^D}(y)}, \overline{\mu_{A^l}(\mathbf{x})} \overset{T}{*} \overline{\mu_{\tilde{a}_l^D}(y)} \right] \cdot \psi_l \\ &= \left[\underline{\mu_{A^l}(\mathbf{x})} \overset{T}{*} \underline{\mu_{\tilde{a}_l^D}(y)} \cdot \underline{\psi_l}, \overline{\mu_{A^l}(\mathbf{x})} \overset{T}{*} \overline{\mu_{\tilde{a}_l^D}(y)} \cdot \overline{\psi_l} \right] \end{aligned} \tag{20}$$

The last step in the inference process is defuzzification. In type-2 fuzzy systems this step consists of two stages: type reduction and defuzzification. One of the most popular method of the type reduction is the height method. In order to compute the reduced fuzzy set $C_{\tilde{R}'}$ this method uses only one point y_l' for each set $\mu_{\tilde{R}^l}(y)$ in which the function of upper memberships reaches its maximum. The reduced set is expressed as follows

$$C_{\tilde{R}'} = \int_{u_{C_1}^1 \in J_{y_1}^1} \cdots \int_{u_{C_{|L|}}^{|L|} \in J_{y_{|L|}}^{|L|}} 1 \Big/ \left(\sum_{l=1}^{|L|} y_l' u_{C_l}^l \Big/ \sum_{l=1}^{|L|} u_{C_l}^l \right) \tag{21}$$

where: $C_{\tilde{R}'}$ - reduced fuzzy set, $J_{y_1'}^1, \ldots J_{y_{|L|}'}^{|L|}$ - the domain of fuzzy membership grade $\mu_{\tilde{R}^l}(y)$ $l = 1, \ldots, |L|$.

The type reduction is realized according to Equation (21), and may be a very computational intensive task. In paper [13], Karnik and Mendel proposed an iterative algorithm to complete this task. In this paper, this algorithm is also employed to compute the value of the weighted entropy. The result of the type reduction step is an interval fuzzy value. In order to get a real number y', the defuzzification process must be applied. In case of the interval fuzzy sets, crisp value y' can be computed by following equation

$$y' = \left(\underline{C}_{\tilde{R}'} + \overline{C}_{\tilde{R}'} \right) / 2 \tag{22}$$

4 Experimental Results

In order to illustrate performance of the proposed algorithm in medical diagnosis problems, three benchmark data from UCI machine-learning repository [4] have been used. These data sets concern heart disease, breast cancer, and Pima Indians diabetes.

4.1 Medical Data Description

The heart disease data set was collected by the Cleveland Clinic Foundation. The data consist of 303 cases, where 164 cases represent the normal condition and 139 heart disease. There are 13 input variables and one output. In order to make the problem simpler, the output is reduced from five to two values. There are five continuous-value variables and the rest are categorized variables. The complete data set consists of six rows with missing values which have been deleted.

The breast cancer data set was prepared by the University of Wisconsin Hospitals. The data consist of 699 cases; where 458 cases represent the benign class and 241 cases represent the malignant class. There are 10 input numerical variables taking values from interval [1÷10]. The complete data set consists of 16 instances with missing values which are removed as in the case of the heart disease data set.

The Pima Indians diabetes data set is a result of medical examinations of 768 women from the Pima Indians tribe living near Phoenix in Arizona. The data consist of 500 cases representing the normal condition and 268 cases of the diabetes disease.

4.2 Results from Type-2 Fuzzy Decision Trees

Every data set, described in Section 4.1, was split into two disjoint subsets: the training set that consisted of 70 % of all cases and the testing set consisting of 30% of the cases (data items, examples). The examples were chosen randomly to both training and testing sets. The training data set was applied in order to build the tree as well as to generate type-2 fuzzy sets for all attributes. The testing data set was employed to check performance of the created decision tree.

The type-2 fuzzy sets have been generated by use of the uncertain fuzzy clustering algorithm presented in [9], [10]. In this algorithm, an additional grade of uncertainty is associated with the fuzzifier m, because like the authors explained, it may be difficult to determine an appropriate fuzzifier value for the data sets that contain clusters of different volume or density. In Fig. 1, the fuzzy sets created for the Wisconsin breast cancer data are illustrated.

After generating the type-2 fuzzy sets, the tree was build. In the case of the Wisconsin breast cancer data, in all experiments the proposed algorithm used only three attributes: Uniformity of Cell Shape, Uniformity of Cell Size, Bare Nuclei.

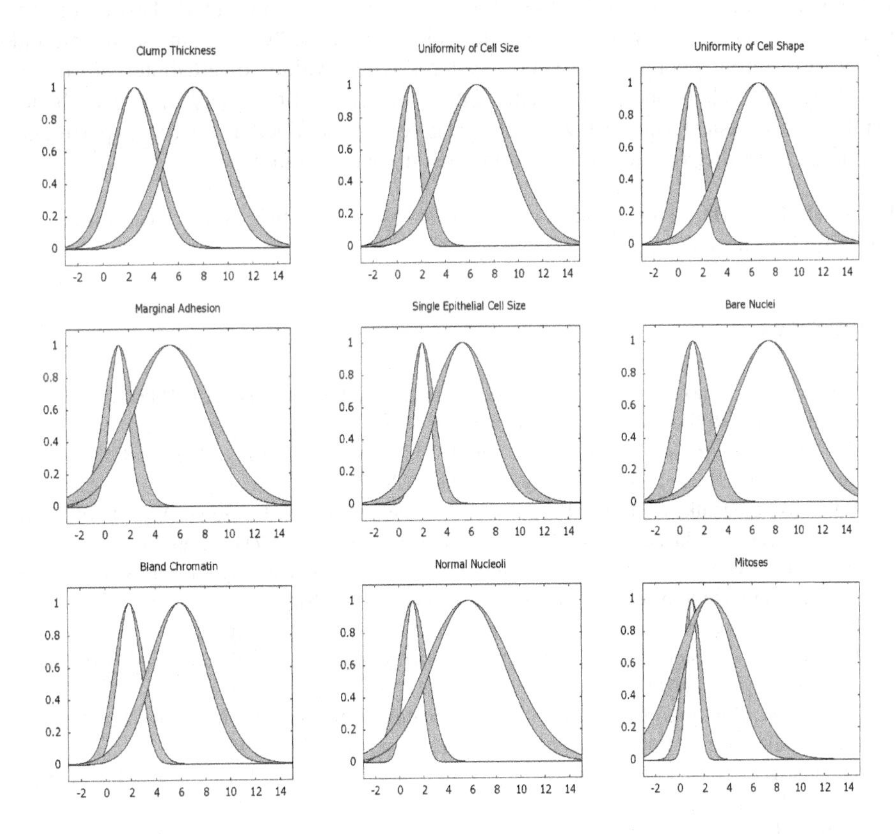

Fig. 1. The type-2 fuzzy sets generated for Wisconsin Breast Cancer data by Uncertain Fuzzy Clustering Algorithm

Table 1. Average results of experiments

Database	Training set	Testing set
Heart disease data	82.59%±1%	82%
Wisconsin breast cancer data	96%	95.5%±1.54
Pima Indians diabetes data	76.34%±1.2%	76.49%

For all data sets employed, every experiment was repeated ten times. The average results are shown in Table 1, where the percentage of correct diagnosis for training and testing set is presented for the three medical data sets. The training and testing success is quite good comparing with results obtained for other methods applied to these benchmark data sets.

5 Conclusions

In this paper, a new algorithm for creating decision trees is presented. This algorithm allows to use type-2 fuzzy sets as attribute values. Because "words can mean different things to different people", in experts systems where values of attributes are determined by more than one expert, application of type-2 fuzzy sets may give better results than classic (type-1) fuzzy sets. The results obtained from the experiments encourage to further research on this approach in medical diagnosis.

Acknowledgments. This work is supported by the Polish State Committee for Scientific Research (Grant N518 035 31/3292).

References

1. Adamo, J.M.: Fuzzy decision trees. Fuzzy Sets and Systems 4, 207–219 (1980)
2. Bartczuk, Ł., Rutkowska, D.: A new version of the fuzzy-ID3 algorithm. In: Rutkowski, L., Tadeusiewicz, R., Zadeh, L.A., Żurada, J.M. (eds.) ICAISC 2006. LNCS (LNAI), vol. 4029, pp. 1060–1070. Springer, Heidelberg (2006)
3. Bartczuk, Ł., Rutkowska, D.: Fuzzy decision trees of type-2. In: Some Aspects of Computer Science. EXIT Academic Publishing House, Warsaw (2007) (in Polish)
4. Blake, C., Keogh, E., Merz, C.: UCI repository of machine learning databases. University of California, Dept. of Computer Science, Irvine, CA (1998), `http://www.ics.uci.edu/~mlearn/MLRepository.html`
5. Canfora, G., Troiano, L.: Fuzzy ordering of fuzzy numbers. In: Proc. Fuzz-IEEE, Budapest, pp. 669–674 (2004)
6. Chang, W.: Ranking of fuzzy utilities with triangular membership functions. In: Proc. Intern. Conference on Policy Analysis and Systems, pp. 263–272 (1981)
7. Dong, M.: Look-ahead based fuzzy decision tree induction. IEEE Trans. Fuzzy Systems 9(3), 461–468 (2001)
8. Dubois, D., Prade, H.: Fuzzy Sets and Systems: Theory and Applications. Academic Press, San Diego (1980)

9. Hwang, C., Rhee, F.: Uncertain fuzzy clustering: interval type-2 fuzzy approach to C-means. IEEE Trans. Fuzzy Systems 15(1), 107–120 (2007)
10. Rhee, F.: Uncertain Fuzzy clustering: insights and recommendations. IEEE Comp. Intelligence Magazine 2(1), 44–56 (2007)
11. Janikow, C.Z.: Fuzzy decision trees: issues and methods. IEEE Trans. Systems Man Cybern. 28(3), 1–14 (1998)
12. Liang, Q., Mendel, J.M.: Interval type-2 fuzzy logic systems: theory and design. IEEE Trans. Fuzzy Systems 8, 535–550 (2000)
13. Mendel, J.M.: Uncertain Rule-Based Fuzzy Logic Systems - Introduction and New Directions. Prentice Hall PTR, Englewood Cliffs (2001)
14. Mendel, J.M.: Computing with words, when words can mean different things to different people. In: Proc. Intern. ICSC Congress on Computational Intelligence, Rochester, New York (1999)
15. Mendel, J.M., John, R.I.: Type-2 fuzzy sets made simple. IEEE Trans. Fuzzy Systems 10, 117–127 (2002)
16. Moore, R.E.: Interval Analysis. Prentice-Hall, Englewood Cliffs (1966)
17. Olaru, C., Wehenkel, L.: A complete fuzzy decision tree technique. Fuzzy Sets and Systems 138, 221–254 (2003)
18. Piegat, A.: Modeling and Fuzzy Control. EXIT Academic Publishing House, Warsaw (1999) (in Polish)
19. Quinlan, J.R.: Induction of decision trees. Machine Learning 1, 81–106 (1986)
20. Quinlan, J.R.: C4.5: Programs for Machine Learning. Morgan Kaufmann Publishers, Inc., Los Altos (1993)
21. Quinlan, J.R.: Learning with continuous classes. In: Proc. 5th Australian Joint Conference on Artificial Intelligence, pp. 343–348. World Scientific, Singapore (1992)
22. Rutkowska, D.: Neuro-Fuzzy Architectures and Hybrid Learning. Physica-Verlag, Springer-Verlag Company, Heidelberg (2002)
23. Rutkowski, L.: Methods and Techniques of Artificial Intelligence. PWN, Warsaw (2005) (in Polish)
24. Wang, X., Borgelt, C.: Information measures in fuzzy decision trees. In: Proc. IEEE Intern. Conference on Fuzzy Systems, Budapest, vol. 1, pp. 85–90 (2004)
25. Yager, R.R.: Ranking fuzzy subsets over the unit interval. In: Proc. CDC, pp. 1435–1437 (1978)
26. Yager, R.R.: On choosing between fuzzy subsets. Kybernetes 9, 151–154 (1980)
27. Yager, R.R.: Procedure for ordering fuzzy sets of the unit interval. Inform. Sci. 24, 143–161 (1981)
28. Yuan, Y., Shaw, M.J.: Induction of fuzzy decision trees. Fuzzy Sets and Systems 69, 125–139 (1995)
29. Zadeh, L.A.: Fuzzy sets. Information and Control 8, 338–353 (1965)
30. Zadeh, L.A.: The concept of a linguistic variable and its application to approximate reasoning. Information Science, Part I 8, 199–249, Part II 8, 301–357, Part III 9, 43–80 (1975)
31. Zimmermann, H.-J.: Fuzzy Set Theory. Kluwer Academic Publishers, Boston (1994)

Ranked Modeling of Causal Sequences of Diseases for the Purpose of Early Diagnosis*

Leon Bobrowski[1,2], Tomasz Łukaszuk[1], and Hanna Wasyluk[3]

[1] Faculty of Computer Science, Białystok Technical University
[2] Institute of Biocybernetics and Biomedical Engineering, PAS, Warsaw, Poland
[3] Medical Center of Postgraduate Education, Warsaw

Abstract. Medical knowledge in the form of causal sequences of diseases can be used in designing ranked models. Considered ranked models are based on linear transformation of multivariate feature vectors on a line that preserves in a best possible way a causal order between diseases. Clinical data sets from particular diseases supplied with a causal order within pairs of these diseases may be used in the definition of the convex and piecewise linear (*CPL*) criterion function. The linear ranked transformations can be designed through minimization of the *CPL* criterion functions.

Keywords: causal order between diseases, ranked linear transformations, convex and piecewise linear (*CPL*) criterion functions, linear separability of data sets, causal sequence of liver diseases.

1 Introduction

Medical knowledge in the form of a causal sequence of particular diseases ω_k ($k = 1,\ldots, K$) could be available in some cases. The causal sequence of liver diseases is a good example of such a situation [1]. Clinical databases allow to form *reference* (*learning*) sets C_k for such diseases that are linked in the causal sequence. Patients $O_j(k)$ allocated by medical doctors to the disease ω_k are represented in the form of feature vectors $\mathbf{x}_j(k)$ with the same number n of numerical components (features) or as points in n-dimensional feature space. Each learning sets C_k should be formed by a sufficiently large number of the feature vectors $\mathbf{x}_j(k)$ allocated to the disease ω_k.

Methods of exploratory data analysis or pattern recognition give the possibility of discovering regularities in multivariate data sets or in large databases [2], [3]. Enhancing trends in temporal databases is a particularly interesting problem with many important applications. The regression analysis methods plays a prominent role in data exploration and can be used for trends enhancing and modeling [4].

* This work was partially supported by the KBN grant 3T11F01130, by the grant 16/St/2007 from the Institute of Biocybernetics and Biomedical Engineering PAS, and by the grant W/II/1/2007 from the Białystok University of Technology.

E. Kącki, M. Rudnicki, J. Stempczyńska (Eds.): Computers in Medical Activity, AISC 65, pp. 23–31.
springerlink.com

The regression models describe a dependence of one feature on a selected set of other features and can be used for the purpose of prognosis. The ranked regression models can also serve a similar purpose [5], [6], [7]. The ranked regression models are particularly useful when values of the dependent feature cannot be measured precisely or directly and additional information about feature vectors is available only in the form of ranked relations within selected pairs of these vectors. Such ranked relations can be treated as a priori knowledge about linear sequential patterns hidden in data. In this context, inducing the linear ranked model from the ranked pairs can be treated as a pattern recognition problem. The induced ranked model can also be used for prognosis or decision support purposes.

The method of inducing linear ranked models from a set of feature vectors and ranked relations within selected pairs of these vectors was proposed [5] [6]. This method was based on the minimization of convex and piecewise-linear (*CPL*) criterion functions. Properties of this approach in the context of modeling of causal sequences of diseases are analyzed in the presented paper. These considerations are illustrated on the example of feature vectors from hepathological database of the system *Hepar* and additional medical knowledge in the form of a causal sequence of liver diseases were used in designing ranked linear transformation [1].

2 Ranked Relations between Feature Vectors Based on a Causal Sequence of Diseases

In some cases medical knowledge allows to form a *causal sequence* among regarded diseases ω_k ($k = 1,\ldots, K$):

$$\omega_1 \rightarrow \omega_2 \rightarrow \ldots\ldots \rightarrow \omega_K \tag{1}$$

The symbol "$\omega_i \rightarrow \omega_{i+1}$"in the above sequence means that the given patient disease ω_{i+1} resulted from the disease ω_i, or ω_{i+1} is a consequence of the disease ω_i ($i = 1,\ldots, K\text{-}1$). In other words, the disease ω_{i+1} is more *advanced* than ω_i in the process of the disease development in given patient.

Let us assume that a clinical database contains descriptions of m patients $O_j(k)$ ($j = 1,\ldots,m$) labeled in accordance with their clinical diagnosis ω_k ($k = 1,\ldots, K$). Each patient $O_j(k)$ is represented by n-dimensional feature vector $\mathbf{x}_j(k) = \mathbf{x}_j = [x_{j1},\ldots,x_{jn}]^T$. The vectors $\mathbf{x}_j$ belong to the *feature space* $F[n]$ ($\mathbf{x}_j \in F[n]$). The component x_{ji} ($i = 1,\ldots, n$) of the vector $\mathbf{x}_j$ is a numerical result of the i-th examination (*feature*) x_i of a given patient O_j ($j = 1,\ldots,m$). The feature vectors $\mathbf{x}_j$ can be of a mixed type, and represent different types of features (measurements) x_i of a given patient O_j (for example: $x_{ji} \in \{0,1\}$ or $x_{ji} \in R$).

The labeled feature vector $\mathbf{x}_j(k)$ represents such a patient $O_j(k)$, that has been assigned by medical doctors to the k-th disease ω_k. The learning set C_k contains m_k labeled feature vectors $\mathbf{x}_j(k)$:

$$C_k = \{\ \mathbf{x}_j(k) \colon j \in J_k\ \} \tag{2}$$

where J_k is the set of indices j of m_k feature vectors $\mathbf{x}_j(k)$ labeled to the class ω_k.

The causal sequence (1) determines the below sequence of the learning sets C_k (2):

$$C_1 \rightarrow C_2 \rightarrow \ldots\ldots \rightarrow C_K \tag{3}$$

The causal sequence (1) allows also to determine the below *ranked relation* "$\prec$" between the feature vectors $\mathbf{x}_j(k)$ ($\mathbf{x}_j(k) \in C_k$) representing patients $O_j(k)$ assigned to particular diseases ω_k:

$$\mathbf{x}_j(k) \prec \mathbf{x}_{j'}(k') \Leftrightarrow \mathbf{x}_{j'}(k') \text{ is a more risky than } \mathbf{x}_j(k) \tag{4}$$

We can remark that the feature vectors $\mathbf{x}_{j'}(k')$ from the learning set $C_{k'}$ (1) are *more risky than* the vectors $\mathbf{x}_j(k)$ from the learning set C_k if and only if the disease ω_k appears earlier than $\omega_{k'}$ in the causal sequence (1).

$$(\forall k, k' \in \{1, \ldots, K\})\ (\forall \mathbf{x}_j(k) \in C_k) \text{ and } (\forall \mathbf{x}_{j'}(k') \in C_{k'}) \quad \text{if } \omega_k \rightarrow \omega_{k'} \text{ then } \mathbf{x}_j(k) \prec \mathbf{x}_{j'}(k') \tag{5}$$

3 Ranked Linear Transformations

Let us consider a linear transformation $y = \mathbf{w}^T\mathbf{x}$ of n-dimensional feature vectors $\mathbf{x}_j$ ($\mathbf{x}_j \in R^n$) on the points y_j of the line R^1 ($y_j \in R^1$):

$$(\forall j \in \{1, \ldots\ldots, m\}) \quad y_j = \mathbf{w}^T\mathbf{x}_j \tag{6}$$

where $\mathbf{w} = [w_1, \ldots\ldots, w_n]^T \in R^n$ is the weight vector.

We are considering a linear transformation (*ranked line*) $y = (\mathbf{w}^*)^T\mathbf{x}$ (6) which preserves the relation "$\prec$" (5) as precisely as possible. It means that the below implication is fulfilled in the ideal case:

$$(\exists \mathbf{w}^* \in R^n)\ (\forall k, k' \in \{1, \ldots, K\})\ (\forall \mathbf{x}_j(k) \in C_k) \text{ and } (\forall \mathbf{x}_{j'}(k') \in C_{k'}) \quad \text{if } \omega_k \rightarrow \omega_{k'} \text{ then } (\mathbf{w}^*)^T\mathbf{x}_j(k) < (\mathbf{w}^*)^T\mathbf{x}_{j'}(k') \tag{7}$$

The problem of there being an optimal weight vector $\mathbf{w}^*$ which assures the implication (7) can be linked to the linear separability of the positive set C^+ and the negative set C^- of the differential vectors $\mathbf{r}_{jj'} = (\mathbf{x}_{j'} - \mathbf{x}_j)$ [5]:

$$\begin{aligned} C^+ &= \{\mathbf{r}_{jj'} = (\mathbf{x}_{j'} - \mathbf{x}_j) : j < j' \text{ and } \mathbf{x}_j(k) \prec \mathbf{x}_{j'}(k')\} \\ C^- &= \{\mathbf{r}_{jj'} = (\mathbf{x}_{j'} - \mathbf{x}_j) : j < j' \text{ and } \mathbf{x}_{j'}(k') \prec \mathbf{x}_j(k)\} \end{aligned} \tag{8}$$

Definition 1: The positive set C^+ and the negative set C^- of are linearly separable if and only if there exists such a weight vector $\mathbf{w}'$ that the below inequalities hold

$$\begin{aligned} &(\exists \mathbf{w}')\ (\forall \mathbf{r}_{jj'} \in C^+)\ (\mathbf{w}')^T\mathbf{r}_{jj'} > 0 \\ &(\forall \mathbf{r}_{jj'} \in C^-)\ (\mathbf{w}')^T\mathbf{r}_{jj'} < 0 \end{aligned} \tag{9}$$

The weight vector $\mathbf{w}'$ defines the hyperplane $H(\mathbf{w}')$ in the feature space:

$$H(\mathbf{w}') = \{\mathbf{x}: (\mathbf{w}')^T\mathbf{x} = 0\} \tag{10}$$

The hyperplane $H(\mathbf{w}')$ passes through the point $\mathbf{0}$ in in the feature space. If the inequalities (9) hold, then the hyperplane $H(\mathbf{w}')$ separates the sets C^+ and C^- (9). This means that all elements $\mathbf{r}_{jj'}$ of the set C^+ are located on the positive side of the hyperplane $H(\mathbf{w}')$ and all elements $\mathbf{r}_{jj'}$ of the set C^- are located on the negative side of this hyperplane.

The below *Lemma* can be proved [5]:

Lemma 1: The linear transformation $y = (\mathbf{w}')^T\mathbf{x}$ (6) preserves all the ranked relations "$\prec$" (5) if and only if the hyperplane $H(\mathbf{w}')$ separates the sets C^+ and C^- (9).

The line $y = (\mathbf{w}')^T\mathbf{x}$ (6) is *completely ranked* if and only if the hyperplane $H(\mathbf{w}')$ separates the sets C^+ and C^- (9).

4 Designing Ranked Transformations through Minimization of the CPL Criterion Function

It is known that the minimisation of the convex and piecewise linear (*CPL*) criterion function $\Phi(\mathbf{w})$ similar to the perceptron criterion function allows to find such a hyperplane $H(\mathbf{w}^*)$ (10) which separates two sets in the best possible manner [1]. In order to define an adequate *CPL* criterion function $\Phi(\mathbf{w})$ let us introduce the positive $\varphi_{jj'}^+(\mathbf{w})$ and the negative $\varphi_{jj'}^-(\mathbf{w})$ penalty functions [7]:

$(\forall \mathbf{r}_{jj'} \in C^+)$

$$\varphi_{jj'}^+(\mathbf{w}) = \begin{cases} 1 - \mathbf{w}^T\mathbf{r}_{jj'} & \text{if } \mathbf{w}^T\mathbf{r}_{jj'} \le 1 \\ 0 & \text{if } \mathbf{w}^T\mathbf{r}_{jj'} > 1 \end{cases} \tag{11}$$

and

$(\forall \mathbf{r}_{jj'} \in C^-)$

$$\varphi_{jj'}^-(\mathbf{w}) = \begin{cases} 1 + \mathbf{w}^T\mathbf{r}_{jj'} & \text{if } \mathbf{w}^T\mathbf{r}_{jj'} \ge -1 \\ 0 & \text{if } \mathbf{w}^T\mathbf{r}_{jj'} < -1 \end{cases} \tag{12}$$

The criterion function $\Phi(\mathbf{w})$ is the sum of the penalty functions $\varphi_{jj'}^+(\mathbf{w})$ and $\varphi_{jj'}^-(\mathbf{w})$:

$$\Phi(\mathbf{w}) = \sum_{(j,j')\in J^+} \gamma_{jj'}\varphi_{jj'}^+(\mathbf{w}) + \sum_{(j,j')\in J^-} \gamma_{jj'}\varphi_{jj'}^-(\mathbf{w}) \tag{13}$$

where $\gamma_{jj'}$ ($\gamma_{jj'} > 0$) is a positive parameter (*price*) related to the differential vectors $\mathbf{r}_{jj'} = \mathbf{x}_{j'} - \mathbf{x}_j$ from the positive set C^+ ($(j,j') \in J_p^+$) or from the negative set C^- (8) ($(j,j') \in J_p^-$).

$\Phi(w)$ (13) is the convex and piecewise linear (*CPL*) criterion function as the sum of such type of penalty functions as $\phi_{jj'}^{+}(w)$ and $\phi_{jj'}^{-}(w)$ The basis exchange algorithms, like linear programming, allow one to find the minimum of such a function efficiently, even in the case of large multidimensional data sets C^{+} and C^{-} (8) [9]:

$$\Phi^{*} = \Phi(\mathbf{w}^{*}) = \min_{\mathbf{w}} \Phi(\mathbf{w}) \geq 0 \tag{14}$$

The below *Lemma* can be proved [5]:

Lemma 2: The minimal value $\Phi(\mathbf{w}^{*})$ (14) of the criterion function $\Phi(\mathbf{w})$ is equal to zero if and only if the line $y = (\mathbf{w}^{*})^{T}\mathbf{x}$ (6) preserves all the implications "$\lessdot$" (7).

5 Example: Causal Sequence of Liver Diseases

The database of the system *Hepar* contains descriptions of patients with variety of chronic liver diseases ω_k ($k = 1,\ldots, K$) [8]. The feature vectors $\mathbf{x}_j(k)$ in the database of *Hepar* are of the mixed, qualitative-quantitative type. They contain both symptoms and signs ($x_i \in \{0,1\}$) as well as the numerical results of laboratory tests ($x_i \in R$). About 200 different features x_i describe one case of a patient in this system. For the purpose of these computations, each patient has been described by the feature vector $\mathbf{x}_j(k)$ composed of 62 features x_i chosen as a standard by medical doctors. The following $K = 7$ groups of patients C_k (15) have been extracted from the *Hepar* database:

C_1. *Non hepatitis patients* - 16 patients
C_2. *Hepatitis acuta* - 8 patients
C_3. *Hepatitis persistens* - 44 patients
C_4. *Hepatitis chronica active* - 95 patients
C_5. *Cirrhosis hepatitis compensate* - 38 patients (15)
C_6. *Cirrhosis decompensate* - 60 patients
C_7. *Carcinoma hepatis* - 11 patients

Total: 272 patients

In accordance with medical knowledge, the learning sets C_k (15) have been formed as the causal sequence (3) with $K = 7$. The ranked relation "$\lessdot$" (5) between feature vectors $\mathbf{x}_j(k)$ ($\mathbf{x}_j(k) \in C_k$) and $\mathbf{x}_{j'}(k')$ ($\mathbf{x}_{j'}(k') \in C_{k'}$) has been defined on this basis. This ranked relation allowed to define the the positive set C^{+} (8) and the negative set C^{-} of the differential vectors $\mathbf{r}_{jj'} = (\mathbf{x}_{j'} - \mathbf{x}_j)$. The sets C^{+} and C^{-} have been used in the definition of the convex and piecewise linear (*CPL*) criterion function $\Phi(\mathbf{w})$ (13). The optimal parameter vector $\mathbf{w}^*$ (14) constituting the minimum of the function $\Phi(\mathbf{w})$ (13) defines the ranked linear model $y = (\mathbf{w}^*)^T\mathbf{x}$ (6) that can be used among others for prognosis purposes:

$$y_j(k) = (\mathbf{w}^*)^T\mathbf{x}_j(k) \tag{16}$$

The feature selection allows to determine the most important features x_i influencing the future of a given patient $\mathbf{x}_0$ and to neglect the unimportant features x_i. The feature selection problem can be also based on the minimization of the convex and piecewise linear (*CPL*) criterion function $\Phi(\mathbf{w})$ (13) [6].

The causal sequence (3) of diseases ω_k (the learning sets C_k (15)) is preserved in a great part by the ranked model (16). Elements $\mathbf{x}_j(k)$ of each learning set C_k (15) are transformed in accordance with the equation (16) on the points $y_j(k)$ of the ranked line. In result, the sets C_k' of the numbers $y_j(k)$ (16) can be defined (2):

$$C_k' = \{y_j(k): j \in J_k\} \tag{17}$$

The sets C_k' can be characterized by mean values μ_k and variances σ_k^2, where

$$\mu_k = \frac{\sum_j y_j(k)}{m_k} \quad (j \in J_k\} \tag{18}$$

and

$$\sigma_k^2 = \frac{\sum_j (y_j(k) - \mu_k)^2}{m_k} \quad (j \in J_k\} \tag{19}$$

The results of computations based on the model (17) of data sets C_k (15) are summarized in the below Table 1:

Table 1. The mean values μ_k and variances σ_k^2 of the sets C_k' (17)

Data sets C_k' (33)	Number of patients m_k	Mean value μ_k	Variance σ_k^2 (σ_k)
C_1'	16	-1,02	0,46 (0,68)
C_2'	8	-0,58	0,57 (0,76)
C_3'	44	0,12	1,1 (1,05)
C_4'	95	0,89	1,46 (1,21)
C_5'	38	2,11	2 (1,41)
C_6'	60	3,02	2,2 (1,48)
C_7'	11	3,78	0,62 (0,79)

Let us consider an additional linear scaling $y' = \alpha\, y + \beta$ of the model $y = (\mathbf{w}^*)^T \mathbf{x}$ (16) in order to improve the interpretability of its prognostic applications.

$$y'_j(k) = \alpha\ (\mathbf{w}^*)^T \mathbf{x}_j(k) + \beta \tag{20}$$

where α and β are the scaling parameters.

We can remark that the ranked implications do not depend on the linear scaling of the model. This means that

$$(\forall \alpha > 0)(\forall \beta) \quad (\mathbf{w}^*)^T \mathbf{x}_j < (\mathbf{w}^*)^T \mathbf{x}_{j'} \Rightarrow \alpha(\mathbf{w}^*)^T \mathbf{x}_j + \beta < \alpha(\mathbf{w}^*)^T \mathbf{x}_{j'} + \beta \tag{21}$$

The parameters α and β have been fixed through minimization of the sum $Q(\alpha, \beta)$ of the differences $|k - \alpha(\mathbf{w}^*)^T \mathbf{x}_j(k) + \beta|$ for all the sets C_k (15) and all the feature vector $\mathbf{x}_j(k)$.

$$Q(\alpha, \beta) = \sum_{k=1,..,K} \sum_{j \in I_k} |k - \alpha(\mathbf{w}^*)^T \mathbf{x}_j(k) + \beta| \tag{22}$$

where I_k is the set of indices j of the feature vectors $\mathbf{x}_j(k)$ from the set C_k (15).

Let us remark that $Q(\alpha, \beta)$ is the convex and piecewise linear (*CPL*) function. The basis exchange algorithms also allow to find efficiently the parameters α^* and β^* constituting the minimum of the function $Q(\alpha, \beta)$. Some results of the scaled model evaluation are shown in the Table 2 and on the Fig. 1.

Table 2. The mean values μ_k' and variances $\sigma_k'^2$ of the sets C_k' (17) obtained from the ranked model (16) after scaling (20) with the optimal parameters α^* and β^*

Data sets C_k' (33)	Number of patients m_k	Mean value μ_k'	Variance $\sigma_k'^2$ (σ_k')
C_1'	16	1,41	0,64 (0,8)
C_2'	8	1,93	0,79 (0,89)
C_3'	44	2,75	1,51 (1,23)
C_4'	95	3,65	1,99 (1,41)
C_5'	38	5,08	2,74 (1,65)
C_6'	60	6,14	3,02 (1,74)
C_7'	11	7,03	0,85 (0,92)

The linear ranked model $y = \alpha^*(\mathbf{w}^*)^T\mathbf{x} + \beta^*$ can be used in the diagnosis support of a new patient $\mathbf{x}_0$. The location of the point $y_0 = \alpha^*(\mathbf{w}^*)^T\mathbf{x}_0 + \beta^*$ on the ranked line (16) constitutes a valuable characteristic of the patient $\mathbf{x}_0$ and his perspectives. In the case the scaled model (Fig. 1), we can expect that the point y_0 representing a new patient $\mathbf{x}_0$ with the k-th disease ω_k will be situated near the index k.

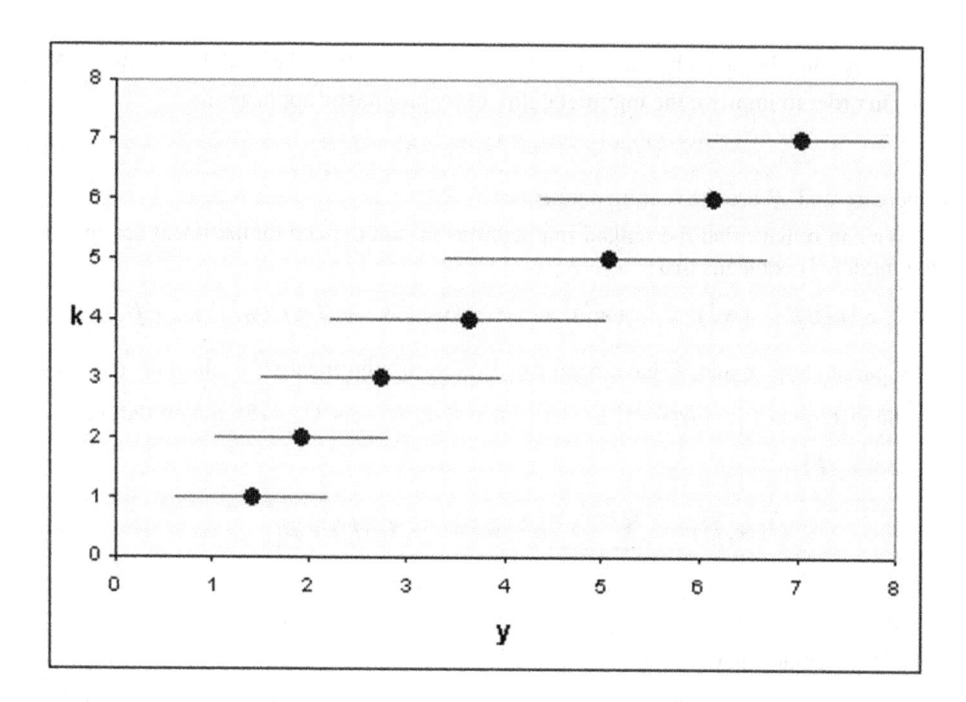

Fig. 1. Graphical presentation the mean values μ_k' and variances $\sigma_k'^2$ of the sets C_k' (17) obtained from the ranked model (18) after scaling (20) with the optimal parameters α^* and β^*

6 Concluding Remarks

The medical knowledge in the form of a causal sequence of diseases ω_k that are represented by learning sets C_k of labeled feature vectors $\mathbf{x}_j(k)$ ($k = 1,\ldots, K$) allows for designing ranked models. Such models can be based on linear transformations $y_j(k) = (\mathbf{w}^*)^T\mathbf{x}_j(k)$ (16) of n-dimensional feature vectors $\mathbf{x}_j(k)$ on the points $y_j(k)$ of the ranked line which preserves in the best possible manner the order relations "$\prec$" (5) between vectors $\mathbf{x}_j(k)$. The ranked model can be used for the purpose of prognosis, in particular for risk prognosis of new patients. An initial part of the ranked line contains mainly the points $y_j(k)$ related to the first diseases ω_k in the causal sequence () and the final part of the line contains mainly the points $y_j(k)$ representing patients $O_j(k)$ from the last, typically the most dangerous diseases in the sequence (1). The location $y_0 = (\mathbf{w}^*)^T\mathbf{x}_0(k)$ of a new patient O_0 on the ranked line can be used for the purpose of initial diagnosis or risk evaluation for this patient. The screening procedures for the search of potentially ill patients eligible for further investigations and therapy could be based on the above ranked model.

The feature selection problem allows to determine the most important features x_i influencing significantly the future of a given patient, and to neglect unimportant features. The feature selection problem can be solved through the minimization of a modified CPL criterion function $\Phi(\mathbf{w})$ (13) [6], [7].

Bibliography

1. Bobrowski, L., Łukaszuk, T., Wasyluk, H.: Ranked modeling of liver diseases sequence. European Journal of Biomedical Informatics (2007) (to be published)
2. Duda, O.R., Hart, P.E., Stork, D.G.: Pattern Classification. J. Wiley, New York (2001)
3. Fukunaga, K.: Introduction to Statistical Pattern Recognition. Academic Press, London (1972)
4. Johnson, R.A., Wichern, D.W.: Applied Multivariate Statistical Analysis. Prentice-Hall Inc., Englewood Cliffs (1991)
5. Bobrowski, L.: Ranked modelling with feature selection based on the CPL criterion functions. In: Perner, P., Imiya, A. (eds.) MLDM 2005. LNCS (LNAI), vol. 3587, pp. 218–227. Springer, Heidelberg (2005)
6. Bobrowski, L., Łukaszuk, T.: Ranked linear modeling in survival analysis. In: Bobrowski, L., Doroszewski, J., Victor, N. (eds.) Lecture Notes of the ICB Seminars: Statistics and Clinical Practice, pp. 61–67. IBIB PAN, Warsaw (2005)
7. Bobrowski, L.: Eksploracja danych oparta na wypukłych i odcinkowo-liniowych funkcjach kryterialnych (Data mining based on convex and piecewise linear (CPL) criterion functions). Białystok Technical University (2005) (in Polish)
8. Bobrowski, L., Wasyluk, H.: Diagnosis support rules of the Hepar system. In: Petel, V.L., Rogers, R., Haux, R. (eds.) MEDINFO 2001, pp. 1309–1313. IOS Press, Amsterdam (2001)
9. Bobrowski, L.: Design of piecewise linear classifiers from formal neurons by some basis exchange technique. Pattern Recognition 24(9), 863–870 (1991)

A Comparative Analysis of SPECT Images of the Left and Right Cerebral Hemispheres in Patients with Diagnosed Epileptic Symptoms

Małgorzata Przytulska[1], Juliusz L. Kulikowski[2], and Adam Bajera[3]

[1,2] IBIB PAN ul. Ks. Trojdena 4, 02-109 Warszawa
gosia@ibib.waw.pl, jlkulik@ibib.waw.pl
[3] Zakład Medycyny Nuklearnej AM, ul. S. Banacha 1, 02-097 Warszawa
abajera@amwaw.edu.p

Abstract. The aim of his work was examination of asymmetries in activity of the left and right cerebral hemispheres as well as localization and contouring of the regions of reduced or increased activity on the basis of single photon emission computer tomography (SPECT) images. Advantage of this technique lies in possibility of brain activity map acquisition at the time of radiotracer injection during seizures though the image registration is done one hour after seizure. The SPECT imaging method makes possible a more accurate spatial localization of seizure source than analysis of EEG signals. Simultaneous EEG signal registration allows to qualify exactly the moment of seizure onset when radiotracer injection could be done to register an unequivocal image. The mean and standard deviation of normalized intensities inside the contoured areas of images were calculated.

1 Materials

The scintigraphic examinations of cerebral perfusion in 6 patients were performed in the Department of Nuclear Medicine (headed by Prof. L. Królicki) of the Medical Academy of Warsaw. From each patient after delivering them the HMPAO Tc99m isotope in interictal phase several transverse cerebral images have been acquired. In the below-shown series of images they have been ordered from the basis to the top of the examined brain; left side of an image corresponds to the right side of the brain and vice versa. An increased/reduced cerebral perfusion corresponds to a higher/lower isotope density and is manifested by an increased/ reduced image luminance registered in an 8-bits scale and normalized to the maximum (255 steps) luminance level. Images of 128x128 pixels size were registered. Below, several examples of medical description of the corresponding cases are given a sequence of scintigraphic images of cerebral lesions (data delivered by the team headed by prof. L. Królicki, Hospital of the Medical Academy of Warsaw).

E. Kącki, M. Rudnicki, J. Stempczyńska (Eds.): Computers in Medical Activity, AISC 65, pp. 33–40.
springerlink.com

Table 1. Kind of perfusion and localization of the brain region by medical assessment

Patent number (slices number)	Medical description	Kind of perfusion	Localization on the image	Brain region
1 (16)	Examination shows a reduced perfusion in the area of both frontal lobes (on the left side rather) and a single focus in the frontal lobe base on the left side.	Reduced	Right upper	Left frontal lobe
2 (15)	Examination shows within the temporal lobe, on the left side, reduced perfusion area that may correspond to an epileptic focus.	Disabled	Right	Left temporal lobe
3 (15)	Examination has shown a wide area of reduced perfusion on the left temporal side that may correspond to epileptic focus.	Reduced	Right	Left temporal lobe
4 (14)	Examinations have shown a focus of perfusion impairment in the right side of the retrotemporal area which may correspond to an epileptic focus. Moreover, a general perfusion impairment in both hemispheres can be observed.	Disabled	Left upper	Right frontal temporal lobe
5 (15)	Examination has shown a perfusion impairment focus in the pole area of right frontal temporal lobe which may correspond to an epileptic focus	Disabled	Left upper	Right frontal temporal lobe
6 (11)	Numerous movement artifacts make the image interpretation difficult. Examination has shown a focus of increased perfusion on the right side of temporal lobe which may correspond to an epileptic focus. Moreover, a perfusion impairment in the left hemisphere is visible.	Increased	Left	Right temporal lobe (numerous movement artifacts)

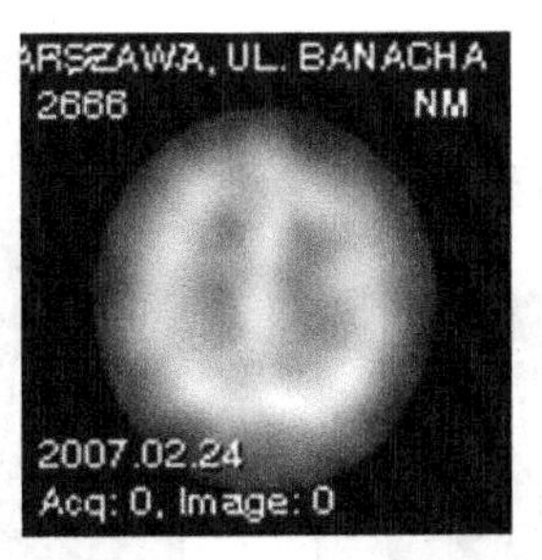

Fig. 1. Original image

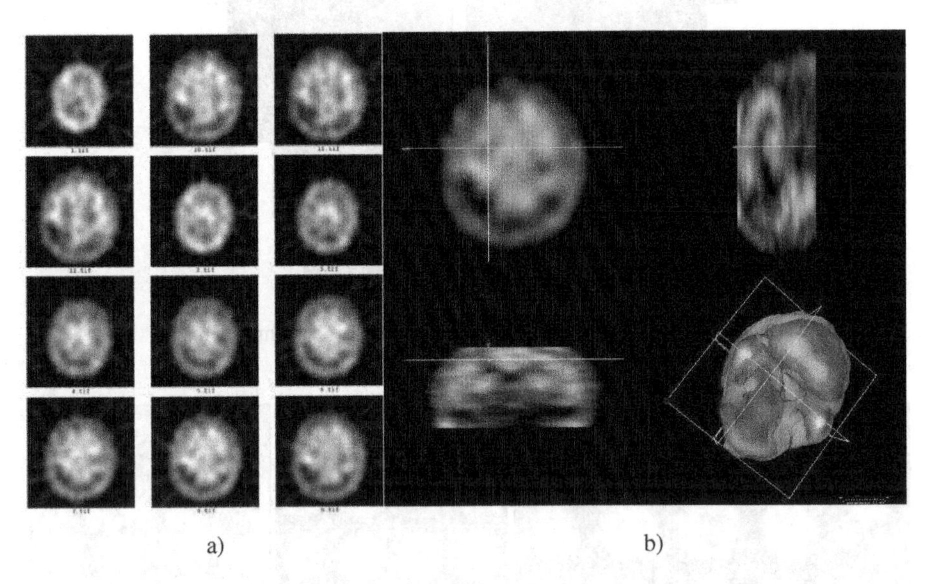

Fig. 2. Original image (a), images after 3D reconstruction (b)

2 The Method

In order to evaluate the effectiveness of various methods a comparative analysis of the images of the left and right cerebral hemispheres by using independent methods was performed: comparison of the mean and standard deviation values,

The mean:

$$\mu = \sum_{i-0}^{N-1} ip(i) \tag{1}$$

the standard deviation:

$$\sigma^2 = \sum_{i=0}^{N-1} (i-\mu)^2 \, p(i) \tag{2}$$

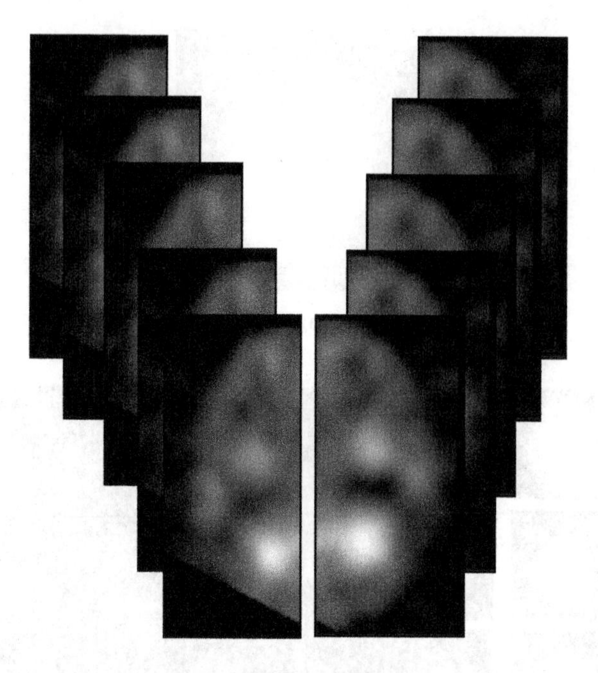

Fig. 3. Image division into the right a) and left b) hemispheres

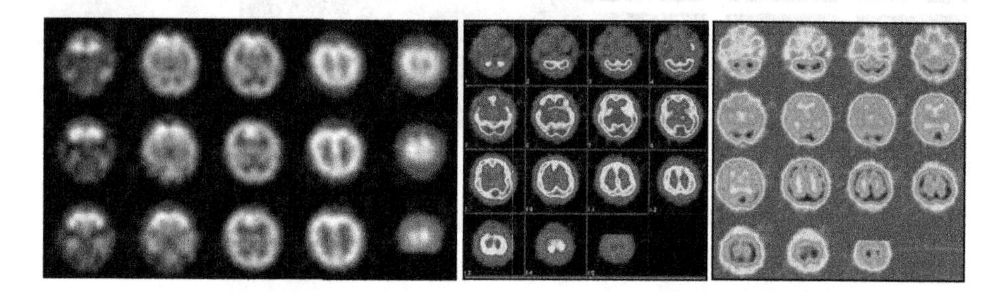

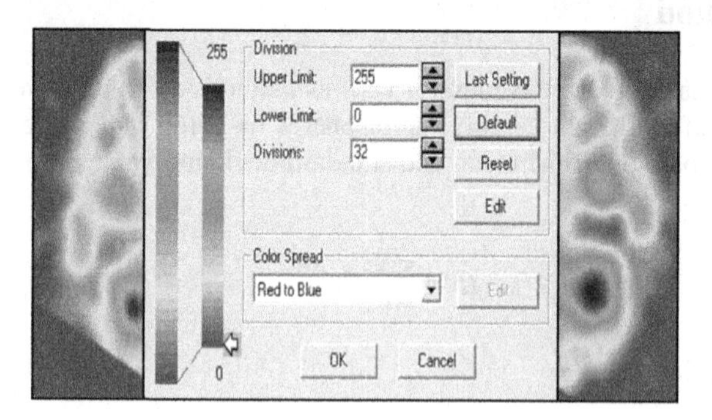

Fig. 4. Rescaling of images in pseudocolors

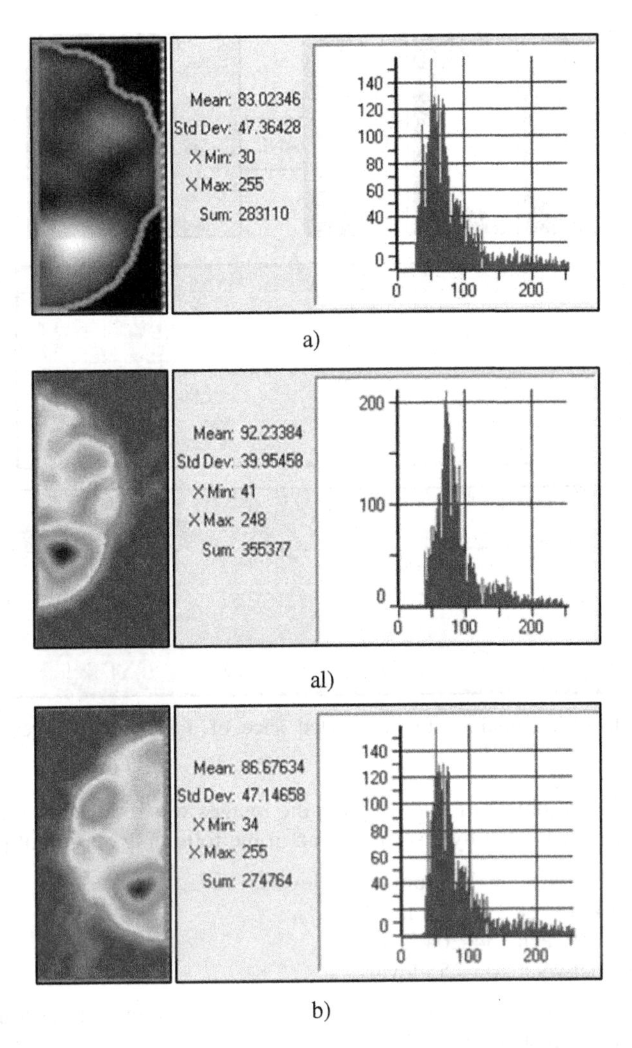

Fig. 5. Calculation of the mean and standard deviation of brightness in the contours of the left a), al) and right b) cerebral hemispheres. There are shown examples of images, measured parameters and histograms of luminance.

where i denotes the luminance level and $p(i)$ is a relative frequency the given luminance level occurs in the examined area.

The images were processed and analyzed using standard Image Pro Plus (Media Cybernetics) and Microsoft Excel software packages [1]. Each image was geometrically divided into the left and right parts (Fig. 1). For a direct visual assessment of monochromatic images they also were visualized in pseudocolors, as shown in Fig. 3. Then the left and right cerebral hemispheres were automatically contoured and the mean and standard deviation of normalized luminance inside the contoured areas of images were calculated (Fig. 4). At the next step the surrounding background, outside

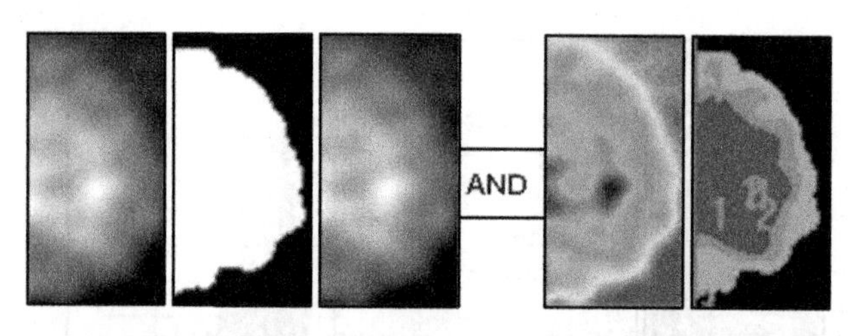

Obj.# (Rge)	Area	Density (mean)	Density (max)
1 (4)	702	110.63960	123
3 (3)	1	125	125
1 (3)	27	127.66666	134
2 (3)	428	136.66121	152
1 (2)	905	183.83205	203
1 (1)	111	218.54955	244
2 (1)	117	226.34187	255

Range	Objects	% Objects	% Area	% Density (mean)	% Density (max)
1	2	28.571428	9.9519863	39.416584	40.372169
2	1	14.285714	39.502399	16.287191	16.423948
3	3	42.857143	19.903973	34.493755	33.252426
4	1	14.285714	30.641642	9.8024712	9.9514561

Fig. 6. Example of calculations for a selected slice of a series of images (left cerebral hemisphere)

a mask selecting the object of interest from the images was reduced to the 0 level and the images were segmented by discrimination of the following classes of pixels:

1st class: pixels between 96-124 luminance levels,
2nd class: pixels between 125-153 levels,
3rd class: pixels between 154-204 levels,
4th class: pixels between 205-255 levels.

The threshold levels between the classes were chosen by taking into account the shape of luminance levels histograms.

For each segment the area measure, mean and maximum luminance as well as the percentage of each of the parameters with respect to this one in the entire area of the given class were calculated, as illustrated in Fig. 5.

3 Results

The comparative analysis was performed in 6 patients for which mean values and standard deviations of luminance on the left and right cerebral hemispheres were measured. In order to make the results independent on the mean brightness level the results were normalized by calculation of the rate of the difference to the sum of mean luminance levels in the hemispheres. The regions of reduced/increased perfusion were localized on the basis of the above-described image segmentation method. The results of calculations (in the two patients mentioned above) are shown in Fig. 6. The horizontal axes indicate the numbers of consecutive slices.

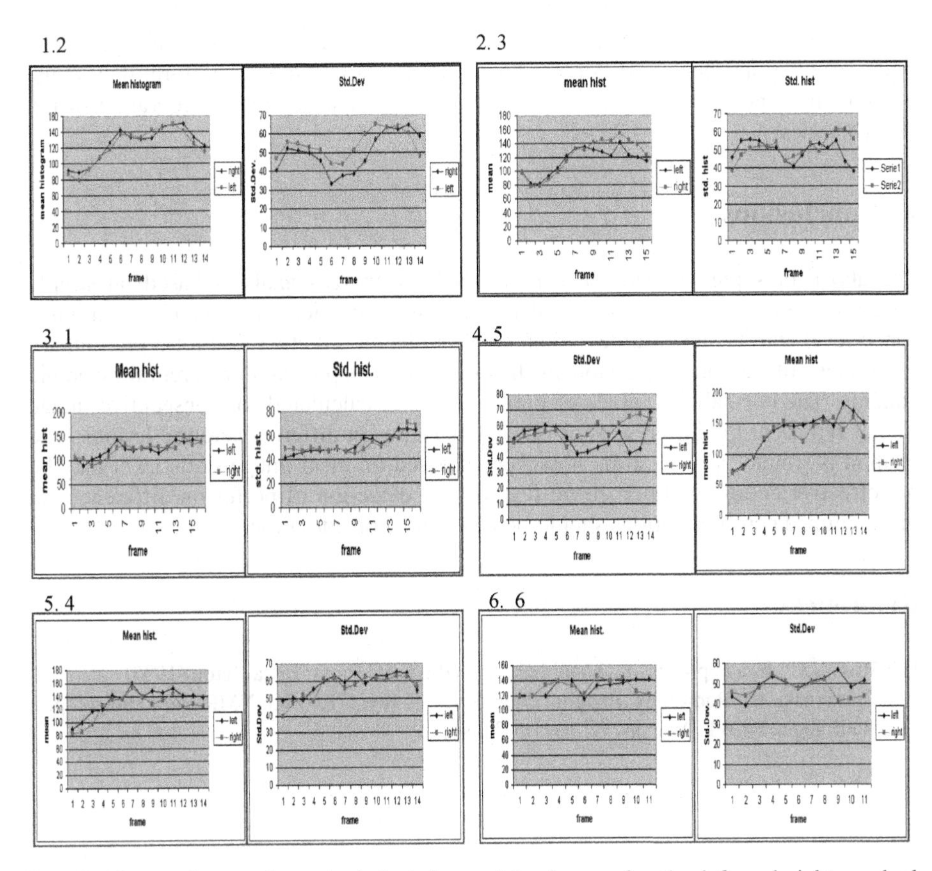

Fig. 7. Mean values and standard deviations of luminance for the left and right cerebral hemispheres in 6 patients

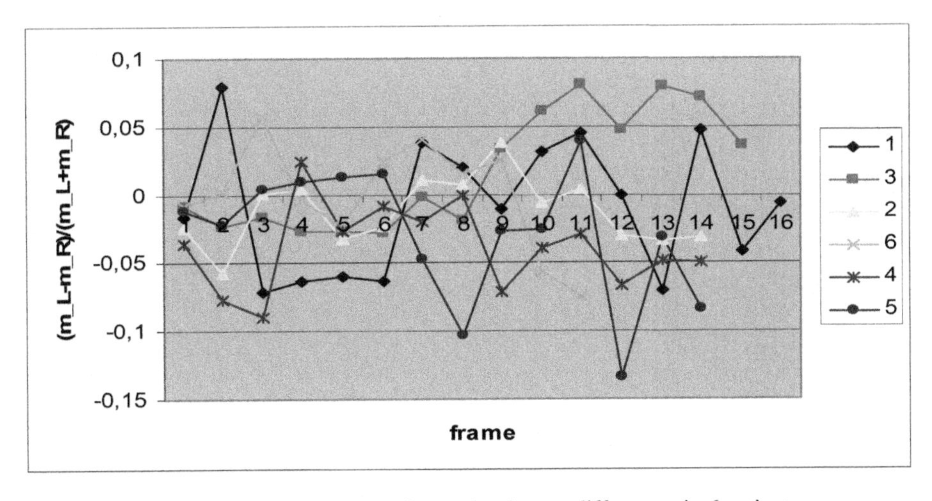

Fig. 8. Normalized values of mean luminance differences in 6 patients

The normalized values of mean luminance in 6 patients are shown in Fig. 7. The frames correspond here to different levels of cerebral lesion. Therefore, they make possible an inspection and rough assessment of +a 3D structure of cerebral perfusion abnormalities.

4 Conclusions

The above presented method of cerebral SPECT images analysis based on simple image processing methods and calculation of basic statistical parameters: mean luminance level and its standard deviation, seems to be an effective tool for a preliminary assessment of cerebral perfusion in diagnosis of epileptic and/or cerebral ischemic patients. The normalized values of luminance level calculated for consecutive image frames represent the differences of isotopic densities in different cerebral lesions. The method is simple in realization, however, as based on local image statistics it may be not effective enough if finer image features for detection of perfusion differences in the examined cerebral regions should be taken into consideration.

References

[1] Russ, J.C.: Image processing handbook, 2nd edn. CRC Press, Boca Raton (1995)
[2] Pruszyński, B.: Radiology. Imaging diagnostics: X-ray, CT, USG, NMR and radioisotopes. Radiologia. PZWL, Warsaw (2006) (in Polish)

Rough Set Theory in the Classification of Diagnoses

Elisabeth Rakus-Andersson

Blekinge Institute of Technology/Department of Mathematics and Science,
S-37179 Karlskrona, Sweden
Elisabeth.Andersson@bth.se

Abstract. Rough sets, surrounded by two approximation sets filled with sure and possible members constitute perfect mathematical tools of the classification of some objects. In this work we adopt the rough technique to verify diagnostic decisions concerning a sample of patients whose symptoms are typical of a considered diagnosis. The objective is to extract the patients who surely suffer from the diagnosis, to indicate the patients who are free from it, and even to make decisions in undefined diagnostic cases. By applying selected logical decision rules, we also discuss a possibility of reducing of symptom sets to their minimal collections preserving the previous results in order to minimize a number of numerical calculations.

1 Introduction

Rough set theory is a new mathematical approach to intelligent data analysis and data mining [1-11, 13-15].

Rough set philosophy is founded on the assumption that some information is associated with every object of the considered universe set. The objects characterized by the same information are indiscernible (similar) in view of the available information about them. The indiscernibility relation generated for similar objects is the mathematical basis of rough set theory. Any set of similar objects, being the equivalence class of the similarity relation, is called an elementary set. Any union of some elementary sets (equivalence classes) is a crisp set (a precise set). Such union of elementary sets, which has boundary-line cases, i.e., objects that cannot be classified with certainty, constitutes a rough set (an imprecise, vague set).

With any rough set, a pair of precise sets – called a lower and an upper approximation of the rough set – is associated. The lower approximation consists of all objects that are surely included in the set, and the upper approximation contains all objects that possibly belong to the set. A difference between the upper and the lower approximation constitutes the boundary region of the rough set. Approximations are two basic operations in the rough set theory.

We utilize this technique to classify some patients who are supposed to suffer from the same diagnosis. The presence of the diagnosis is primarily confirmed, denied or undefined in the patients. We intend to verify the predetermined hypotheses by stating sets of patients assigned to classes of the considered diagnosis surely or possibly and,

E. Kącki, M. Rudnicki, J. Stempczyńska (Eds.): Computers in Medical Activity, AISC 65, pp. 41–51.
springerlink.com

by the way, we also want to find patients who are attached to a class that does not confirm the diagnosis presence.

In Section 2 we first discuss the theoretical aspect of adaptation of rough set axioms to the medical task to prove the clues in a clinical exercise afterwards. We also would like to diminish a number of clinical data concerning symptoms, treated here as conditional attributes of the model, without depriving the data of its decisive character. A selection of minimal samplings of symptoms possessing full power in decision-making is accomplished in Section 3. Section 4 provides a reader with some summarized conclusions.

2 Rough Set Theory in the Diagnostic Classification of Patients

Let us first introduce the theoretical background of rough sets and let us then prove their usefulness via presenting a practical problem concerning medical diagnosing. All conceptions and annotations will be accommodated to a medical model to make it easier at the stage of practical interpretation.

2.1 Theoretical Assumptions of the Classification Model

We start with an information system constructed as a data decision table whose columns are labelled by attributes. Objects of interest label the table rows, and entries of the table are attribute values.

In a scenario of the diagnostic discussion already sketched in the introduction and interpreted as a classification of objects assigned to a certain diagnosis, we adopt the set of patients $P = \{P_1, \ldots, P_m\}$ possessing objects P_i, $i = 1, \ldots, m$, as a *universe set* P. The set of *condition attributes* S is established as a set of symptoms $S = \{S_1, \ldots, S_n\}$ [8, 13]. With every attribute $S_j \in S$, $j = 1, \ldots, n$, we associate a set $V_{S_j} = \{x_{S_j}^1, x_{S_j}^2, \ldots, x_{S_j}^{t(S_j)}\}$ of its values, called the *domain* of S_j. In the diagnostic problem the set V_{S_j} will contain either linguistic terms or values of the membership degrees of S_j expressed by codes that correspond to the intensity grades of S_j. Any subset $B = \{S_{j_1}, \ldots, S_{j_p}\}$, $p \leq n$, of S, consisting of some selected symptoms $S_1, \ldots, S_n$, determines a binary relation $I(B)$ on P, which will be called an *indiscernibility* relation. The relation $I(B)$ is defined by an inclusion operation

$$(P_i, P_l) \in I(B) \text{ if } S_{j_k}(P_i) = S_{j_k}(P_l) \tag{1}$$

for each $S_{j_k} \in B \subseteq S$, $i, l = 1, \ldots, m$, $j = 1, \ldots, n$, $k = 1, \ldots, p$, where $S_{j_k}(P_i)$ denotes the value $x_{S_{j_k}}^c$, $c = 1, \ldots, t(S_{j_k})$, of attribute S_{j_k} for the element P_i.

The relation $I(B)$ is *reflexive* because $(P_i, P_i) \in I(B) \leftrightarrow S_{j_k}(P_i) = S_{j_k}(P_i)$ for each $P_i \in P$.

Since $(P_i, P_l) \in I(B) \leftrightarrow S_{j_k}(P_i) = S_{j_k}(P_l) \leftrightarrow S_{j_k}(P_l) = S_{j_k}(P_i) \leftrightarrow (P_l, P_i) \in I(B)$ for P_i, $P_l \in I(B)$, then $I(B)$ will be a *symmetric* relation, too.

Finally, the assumptions made for pairs $(P_i, P_l) \in I(B)$ and $(P_l, P_r) \in I(B)$, for P_i, P_l, $P_r \in P$, imply $S_{j_k}(P_i) = S_{j_k}(P_r) \leftrightarrow (P_i, P_r) \in I(B)$. $I(B)$ thus is a *transitive* relation.

The sign "$\leftrightarrow$" is interpreted as "which is equivalent to".

For the reason of such properties as reflexivity, symmetry and transitivity $I(B)$ is recognized as an equivalence relation.

We make a partition of the set P, with respect to B, by means of the relation $I(B)$ to obtain equivalence classes $IB(P_i)$ defined by

$$IB(P_i) = \{P_l : (P_i, P_l) \in I(B)\} \tag{2}$$

for each i, $l = 1, \ldots, m$.

The classes $IB(P_i)$ are additionally called elementary sets. We realize that these sets contain the objects P_i that are identical, i.e., in the considered case, they gather patients who suffer from presence of the same symptoms characterized by the same intensity.

The symptoms S_{j_k} $k = 1, \ldots, p$, constitute the condition attributes in the diagnostic model of classification. Besides these, we also consider a decision attribute – the diagnosis D_1 that is initially recognized with a different status in the patients from set P. D_1 has a set of values determined as "*yes*" if it has been found in the patient, "*no*" if the patient seems to be free from it and "*unknown*" when a decision about the presence of the diagnosis cannot be clearly formulated.

By resuming the assumptions made so far we can come to a conclusion that the contents of the classification table, giving rise to the indiscernibility relation $I(B)$, corresponds to a *triple* (P, B, D_1) in the model of diagnoses. The patients P_i are placed in the first column of the table; the three values of D_1 appear in the last column while the rest of the table positions are filled with the values of condition attributes S_{j_k}, i.e. codes assigned to S_{j_k}.

The aim of the classification, accomplished by $I(B)$ or rather its equivalence classes, is to divide the patients belonging to P in three groups. These three groups are: a group of patients who surely are ill with D_1, a sample of patients who may suffer from D_1 and a collection of patients who do not have diagnosis D_1.

Let us create a set $P_{yes} \subseteq P$ in accordance with the following definition

$$P_{yes} = \{P_i : D_1 \text{ has decision "} yes \text{" assigned in the table}\} \tag{3}$$

for $i = 1, \ldots, m$.

We now state two sets surrounded $P_{yes} \subseteq P$ that are treated as its lower and upper approximations.

The lower approximation $B_*(P_{yes})$ of P_{yes} is built by the inclusion operator as

$$B_*(P_{yes}) = \{P_i : IB(P_i) \subseteq P_{yes}\} \tag{4}$$

and is apprehended to be a set of these P_i that have D_1 assigned with a full security.

The other set, the upper approximation $B^*(P_{yes})$ of P_{yes}, is designed by

$$B^*(P_{yes}) = \{P_i : IB(P_i) \cap P_{yes} \neq 0\} \tag{5}$$

and is accepted as a sampling of those objects P_i that possibly are members of the D_1-class possessing the attribute "*yes*" (D_1 = "*yes*").

The set P_{yes} is thus bounded by two sets in compliance with the inclusion $B_*(P_{yes}) \subseteq P_{yes} \subseteq B^*(P_{yes})$ and referred to the approximation sets as rough or inexact with respect to B.

Even a boundary set

$$B_{border}(P_{yes}) = B^*(P_{yes}) - B_*(P_{yes}) \tag{6}$$

contains some useful information about attendance of the objects that are uncertain members of the class D_1 = "*yes*".

To measure a grade of membership uncertainty in the D_1 = "*yes*" class for each P_i, we recommend applying a formula

$$\mu_{D_1="yes"}(P_i) = \frac{|P_{yes} \cap IB(P_i)|}{|IB(P_i)|}, \tag{7}$$

in which the symbol "$|\ |$" denotes the cardinality of a set (the number of elements belonging to a set).

A selection of the B-subset of S should be made with the special care to assure good classification results, i.e., we wish to avoid making too great differences between the contents and cardinalities of approximated sets. We can measure a coefficient α_B called *the accuracy of approximation* in conformity with

$$\alpha_B(P_{yes}) = \frac{|B_*(P_{yes})|}{|B^*(P_{yes})|} \tag{8}$$

to state the grade of roughness of the set P_{yes}.

2.2 The Practical Explanation of the Patients' Allocation within Diagnostic Classes

We demonstrate the utility of rough sets in the diagnosis classification process by studying steps of the following example.

Example 1

A physician has listed 10 symptoms that are the elements of the set of symptoms S = {S_1 – "*hereditary inclination*", S_2 – "*ECG changes in resting position*", S_3 – "*smoking*", S_4 – "*lack of physical activity*", S_5 – "*pain in chest*", S_6 –"*breathlessness*", S_7 – "*feeling of sickness*", S_8 – "*hypertension*", S_9 – "*increased level of LDL-cholesterol*", S_{10} – "*obesity*"}. These are associated with three diagnoses D_1 = "*high risk of cardiovascular diseases*", D_2 = "*coronary heart disease*" and D_3 = "*myocardial infarct*".

Let us select set $B \subseteq S$ as $B = \{S_3, S_4, S_8, S_9, S_{10}\}$. Set B contains the most significant symptoms for diagnosis D_1.

We now prepare sets of values corresponding to the selected symptoms.

The symptoms S_3 and S_4 are compound qualitative parameters measured by means of a questionnaire while S_8, S_9 and S_{10} are the quantitative indicators. By using the adaptive techniques for biological parameters S_3, S_4, S_8, S_9 and S_{10} to convert them to fuzzy sets S_j, j = 3, 4, 8, 9, 10, with corresponding membership degrees $\mu_{S_j}(P_i)$ [12, 13] we furnish the symptoms with numerical representatives coming from the continuous interval [0, 1]. In order to vary some intensity grades of the symptoms' appearance as discrete characteristic quantities, we construct the following codes associated with the membership values $\mu_{S_j}(P_i)$, j = 3, 4, 8, 9, 10, belonging to subintervals of [0, 1]. We assign the code 0 to $\mu_{S_j}(P_i) \in [0, 0.25)$, 1 – to $\mu_{S_j}(P_i) \in [0.25, 0.5)$, 2 – to $\mu_{S_j}(P_i) \in [0.5, 0.75)$ and, finally, 3 – to $\mu_{S_j}(P_i) \in [0.75, 1]$. The codes generate sets $V_{S_j} = \{0,1,2,3\}$, j = 3, 4, 8, 9, 10.

Assume that $P = \{P_1, P_2, P_3, P_4, P_5, P_6\}$. The patients P_1, P_2 and P_5 are supposed to suffer from D_1, P_3 and P_6 have D_2 assigned, and the diagnosis concerning P_4 is unknown. We decide the members of set $P_{yes} = \{P_1, P_2, P_5\}$. To regard P_{yes} as rough, we should find its lower and upper approximation. In this way we also count on classifying the unknown object P_4.

We now fill the entries of Table 1 known as (P, B, D_1) that constitutes a basis for establishing an indiscernibility relation $I(B)$.

The relation $I(B)$ consists of the pairs (P_i, P_l), i, l = 1, …, 6, containing patients who, when comparing rows i and l, have all symptom codes equal.

We list $I(B)$ as $I(B) = \{(P_1, P_1), (P_2, P_2), (P_3, P_3), (P_4, P_4), (P_5, P_5), (P_6, P_6), (P_2, P_4), (P_4, P_2)\}$.

The elementary sets of $I(B)$ or its equivalence classes are given as the sets $IB(P_1) = \{P_1\}$, $IB(P_2) = \{P_2, P_4\}$, $IB(P_3) = \{P_3\}$, $IB(P_4) = \{P_2, P_4\}$, $IB(P_5) = \{P_5\}$, $IB(P_6) = \{P_6\}$.

The lower approximation of P_{yes} is established as the set $B_*(P_{yes}) = \{P_1, P_5\}$ while P_{yes}'s upper approximation is obtained as $B^*(P_{yes}) = \{P_1, P_2, P_4, P_5\}$.

The boundary set $B_{border}(P_{yes}) = \{P_2, P_4\}$.

Table 1. The table (P, B, D_1) in diagnosis classification

Patients	Codes characteristic of symptoms					Decision about D_1
	S_3	S_4	S_8	S_9	S_{10}	
P_1	1	3	2	1	2	*yes*
P_2	2	3	3	2	1	*yes*
P_3	0	2	1	1	1	*no*
P_4	2	3	3	2	1	*unknown*
P_5	3	3	2	2	2	*yes*
P_6	0	1	1	2	3	*no*

The membership degrees, whose sizes confirm the patients' membership in the D_1 = "*yes*" class, have been evaluated as

$$\mu_{D_1="yes"}(P_1)=1,\quad \mu_{D_1="yes"}(P_2)=\frac{1}{2},\quad \mu_{D_1="yes"}(P_3)=0,\quad \mu_{D_1="yes"}(P_4)=\frac{1}{2},$$
$$\mu_{D_1="yes"}(P_5)=1,\quad \mu_{D_1="yes"}(P_6)=0.$$

We can assume that P_1 and P_5 have D_1 with a one hundred percent confidence, while P_2 and P_4 may suffer from D_1 to a certain grade. We can also notice that P_4 affects a status of P_2 negatively, and on the contrary, we can see that P_2 upgrades an importance of P_4 as a member in the D_1 = "*yes*"-class.

The accuracy approximation coefficient $\alpha_B(P_{yes})=\frac{1}{2}$ measures the grade of imprecision of the set P_{yes} in the meaning of its roughness when comparing to a crisp set.

3 The Selection of Reducts from a Set of Conditional Attributes

The indiscernibility relation reduces the data by identifying the equivalence classes since only one element of the equivalence class is entailed to represent the entire class.

On the other hand, we sometimes observe the presence of superfluous data brought in the decision table (P, B, D_1) by some needless attributes belonging to $B \subset S$. To remove the unnecessary conditional attributes from S (or, particularly, from its subset B) and, at the same time, to preserve the induction of the same approximation sets of P_{yes} we try to extract collections of B's subsets being *minimal* sets. The sets are called *reducts* and they warrant that the essence of information will be mantained [3, 4, 5, 6, 14].

3.1 The Generation of Reducts by Dependency Rules

Let us still consider the set of patients $P = \{P_1, \ldots, P_m\}$ and the set of symptoms $S = \{S_1, \ldots, S_n\}$. For each symptom S_j, $j = 1, \ldots, n$, we adopt the set $V_{S_j}=\{x^1_{S_j}, x^2_{S_j}, \ldots, x^{t(S_j)}_{S_j}\}$ of its values.

For any subset $B=\{S_{j_1}, \ldots, S_{j_p}\}$, $p \le n$, of S we can determine an $p \times p$ discernibility relation $M^P_{D_1}(B)$ of pairs (P_i, P_l), i, $l = 1, \ldots, m$, with associated entries e_{il} introduced by the definition

$$e_{il}=\{S_{j_k}\in B : S_{j_k}(P_i)\neq S_{j_k}(P_l)\}. \tag{9}$$

Hence, in each cell of matrix $M^P_{D_1}(B)$ we sample these symptoms that take different values of codes for two compared patients.

Further, a discernibility function $f^P_{D_1}(B)$ is a function defined by

$$f^P_{D_1}(B)=\wedge\{\vee(e_{il}):1\le i,l\le m, i<l, e_{ij}\neq 0\}. \tag{10}$$

where $\vee(e_{il})$ is the logical disjunction of the symptoms $S_{j_k} \in e_{il}$, while $\wedge$ stands for the logical conjunction of listed disjunctions.

A dependency rule is a disjunctive normal form of (10). This emerges combinations of symptoms belonging to B that satisfy the common expectation, namely, these samplings should maintain the previous results obtained for the entire B. It means, with other words, that we expect to get the same lower and upper approximation of set P_{yes} even if the approximation is generated by reduced collections of symptoms. Thus, a principal task in the method of dependency rule generation is to compute reducts relative to a particular kind of information system.

Let us add a decision D_1 to sets P and B in the further development of the *reduct information system*. D_1 is characterized by the set of values already mentioned as d_1 = "*yes*", d_2 = "*no*" and d_3 = "*unknown*". The set $V_{D_1} = \{d_1, d_2, d_3\}$ represents three different decision classes. We now divide the decision table (P, B, D_1) into three tables (P^b, B, $D_1 = d_b$), $b = 1, 2, 3$, due to three decision attributes d_1, d_2, d_3.

Let us note that we refer to the set of patients $P^b = \{P^b_{i_1}, \ldots, P^b_{i_h}\}$, $h \le m$, gathering the objects of P associated with the decision attribute d_b, $b = 1, 2, 3$. For each d_b-decision we state a discernibility matrix $M^{P^b}_{d_b}(B)$ with the entries $e_{i_x l_y}$ in conformity with

$$e_{i_x l_y} = \{S_{j_k} \in B : S_{j_k}(P^b_{i_x}) \neq S_{j_k}(P^b_{l_y})\} \tag{11}$$

for $x, y = 1, \ldots, h$.

For the sets P^b and the decisions d_b the discernibility function $f^{P^b}_{d_b}(B)$ is defined as

$$f^{P^b}_{d_b}(B) = \wedge\{\vee(e_{i_x l_y}) : 1 \le i_x, l_y \le m, 1 \le x, y \le h \le m, i_x < l_y, e_{i_x j_y} \neq 0\} \tag{12}$$

where $\vee(e_{i_x l_y})$ is a disjunction of all members of $e_{i_x l_y}$. Afterwards, by using logical laws for conjunctions and disjunctions (especially commutative, associative, distributive and absorption laws) we convert $f^{P^b}_{d_b}(B)$ to its disjunctive normal form (*d.n.f*) known as a dependency rule for obtaining reducts. The disjunction now will be an outer function tying together the brackets having conjunction of symptoms as an inner function. The contents of each bracket, in which the symptoms S_{j_k} are joined by conjunction $\wedge$, provides us with a new sample of symptoms that are the conditional attributes of a decision table assimilated only to them. The table (P, *a reduct of* B, D_1), in turn, collects fundamental data to build an indiscernibility relation that should provide us with the original approximation sets determined for set B. In this way we exclude symptoms of less importance for the classification of D_1 without making changes in final classification results.

3.2 The Action of Reducts in an Example

We return to Ex. 1 to use its data in the further investigations concerning the classification of patients on the basis of reducts.

Table 2. The table $(P^1, B, D_1 = d_1)$

Patients	Codes characteristic of symptoms					$D_1 = d_1$
	S_3	S_4	S_8	S_9	S_{10}	
P_1	1	3	2	1	2	*yes*
P_2	2	3	3	2	1	*yes*
P_5	3	3	2	2	2	*yes*

Example 2

We recall set $B \subseteq S$ stated as $B = \{S_3, S_4, S_8, S_9, S_{10}\}$. In conformity with three values of the decision attribute D_1 equal to d_1 = "*yes*", d_2 = "*no*" and d_3 = "*unknown*" we can split Table 1 in three tables.

Let us only extract a table associated with d_1 = "*yes*" because the acceptance of D_1 is the most essential decision in the considered classification. We thus reorganize Table 1 as Table 2 by deleting all rows of Table 1 that are not marked by the decision "*yes*". The set $P^1 = \{P_1, P_2, P_5\}$.

The discernibility matrix $M_{d_1}^{P^1}(B)$, established on the basis of Table 2 and determined for pairs of P_1, P_2 and P_5 due to (11), contains entries filled with the symptoms whose values differ from each other for two compared patients. Thus, $M_{d_1}^{P^1}(B)$ takes a form of Table 3 below.

Table 3. The matrix $M_{d_1}^{P^1}(B)$

Patients	P_1	P_2	P_5
P_1		S_3, S_8, S_9, S_{10}	S_3, S_9
P_2			S_3, S_8, S_{10}
P_5			

In accordance with (12) we derive the formula of the discernibility function $f_{d_1}^{P^1}(B)$ as

$$f_{d_1}^{P^1}(B) = (S_3 \vee S_8 \vee S_9 \vee S_{10}) \wedge (S_3 \vee S_9) \wedge (S_3 \vee S_8 \vee S_{10}).$$

We adopt the logical laws for the conjunction and the disjunction to expand $f_{d_1}^{P^1}(B)$ in the *d.n.f.*-form. Hence

$$\begin{aligned} f_{d_1}^{P^1}(B) &= (S_3 \vee S_8 \vee S_9 \vee S_{10}) \wedge (S_3 \vee S_9) \wedge (S_3 \vee S_8 \vee S_{10}) \\ &= [[(S_3 \vee S_9) \vee (S_8 \vee S_{10})] \wedge (S_3 \vee S_9)] \wedge (S_3 \vee S_8 \vee S_{10}) \\ &= (S_3 \vee S_9) \wedge [S_3 \vee (S_8 \vee S_{10})] = S_3 \vee [S_9 \wedge (S_8 \vee S_{10})] \\ &= S_3 \vee (S_8 \wedge S_9) \vee (S_9 \wedge S_{10}) \end{aligned}$$

Table 4. The table (P, $B^1_{d_1}$, D_1) in diagnosis classification

Patients	Codes characteristic of symptoms					Decision about D_1
	S_3	deleted data	deleted data	deleted data	deleted data	
P_1	1					*yes*
P_2	2					*yes*
P_3	0					*no*
P_4	2					*unknown*
P_5	3					*yes*
P_6	0					*no*

The disjunctive normal form of $f_{d_1}^{P1}(B)$ generates reducts of set B, i.e., the sets $B^1_{d_1} = \{S_3\}$, $B^2_{d_1} = \{S_8, S_9\}$ and $B^3_{d_1} = \{S_9, S_{10}\}$. These configurations of symptoms should replace the contents of set B in the decision table without inserting different information about the rough set P_{yes}.

Let us prove set $B^1_{d_1} = \{S_3\}$ as a set of new condition attributes. Then, Table 4 yielding a new appearance of Table 1 is stated for only S_3.

$I(B^1_{d_1})$ = {(P_1, P_1), (P_2, P_2), (P_3, P_3), (P_4, P_4), (P_5, P_5), (P_6, P_6), (P_2, P_4), (P_4, P_2), (P_3, P_6), (P_6, P_3)}. The elementary sets of $I(B^1_{d_1})$ are determined as $IB^1_{d_1}(P_1) = \{P_1\}$, $IB^1_{d_1}(P_2) = \{P_2, P_4\}$, $IB^1_{d_1}(P_3) = \{P_3, P_6\}$, $IB^1_{d_1}(P_4) = \{P_2, P_4\}$, $IB^1_{d_1}(P_5) = \{P_5\}$, $IB^1_{d_1}(P_6) = \{P_3, P_6\}$.

The lower approximation of $P_{yes} = \{P_1, P_2, P_5\}$ is still equal to $B^1_{d_1*}(P_{yes}) = \{P_1, P_5\}$ and its upper approximation is a set $B^{1\,*}_{d_1}(P_{yes}) = \{P_1, P_2, P_4, P_5\}$. The approximation sets surrounding P_{yes} are exactly the same as obtained by means of B.

We test the next set of symptoms $B^2_{d_1} = \{S_8, S_9\}$ in the classification of D_1. Table 5 contains the rearranged data influenced by new condition attributes.

Table 5. The table (P, $B^2_{d_1}$, D_1) in diagnosis classification

Patients	Codes characteristic of symptoms					Decision about D_1
	deleted data	deleted data	S_8	S_9	deleted data	
P_1			2	1		*yes*
P_2			3	2		*yes*
P_3			1	1		*no*
P_4			3	2		*unknown*
P_5			2	2		*yes*
P_6			1	2		*no*

Table 6. The table (P, $B^3_{d_1}$, D_1) in diagnosis classification

Patients	Codes characteristic of symptoms					Decision about D_1
	deleted data	deleted data	deleted data	S_9	S_{10}	
P_1				1	2	*yes*
P_2				2	1	*yes*
P_3				1	1	*no*
P_4				2	1	*unknown*
P_5				2	2	*yes*
P_6				2	3	*no*

Since $I(B^2_{d_1})$ = {(P_1, P_1), (P_2, P_2), (P_3, P_3), (P_4, P_4), (P_5, P_5), (P_6, P_6), (P_2, P_4), (P_4, P_2)} is exactly the same as $I(B)$ from Ex. 1 then the partition of P and the approximating sets are not expected to change. This confirms that the application of set $B^2_{d_1}$, truncated when comparing to B, preserves the effects brought by B and reduces the number of performed operations in the process of the attribute comparison.

At last we set $B^3_{d_1} = \{S_9, S_{10}\}$ as condition attributes of the classification. The modified Table 1 appears as Table 6.

Even though we have cut off some symptoms from B, the indiscernibility relation $I(B^3_{d_1})$ = {(P_1, P_1), (P_2, P_2), (P_3, P_3), (P_4, P_4), (P_5, P_5), (P_6, P_6), (P_2, P_4), (P_4, P_2)} decided for $B^3_{d_1} = \{S_9, S_{10}\}$ is still invariable when comparing to B's results. This means that P_{yes} will be located as rough in the same neighborhood of two approximation sets.

4 Concluding Remarks

The decision-makers, who have prepared a database concerning some clinical symptoms observed in a sample of patients, have been furnished with a mathematical apparatus known as rough sets.

To accomplish a classification of patients, due to a decision criterion accepted as the presence of a considered diagnosis, the technique engaging conditional and decision attributes has been used in order to verify and correct the initial diagnostic hypotheses. The obtained rough classification emerges patients who surely suffer from the diagnosis as well as patients who may be ill. These objects of the patients' population are members of two approximation sets called the lower approximation and the upper approximation, respectively.

The classification has also allowed the decision-makers to exclude the category of patients who have been free from the illness in spite of heightened values of the observed symptoms. Even an undefined case of a patient, in which the decision was not made before, has found its solution since the patient has been allocated in the group of possibly ill population members.

To avoid performing too many numerical operations on the patients' reports concerning documented symptoms we have made a successful trial of introducing reduced groups of symptoms provided that the genuine results will be preserved. This has been accomplished by means of dependency rules referred to symptoms.

In the end, we emphasize that rough set theory provides us with very thorough and reliable results of categorizing of objects and thus, we should often use the theory assumptions to check and clarify decisions made in different medical models.

References

[1] Bazan, J., Nguyen, H.S., Szczuka, M.: A View on Rough Set Concept Approximations. Fundamenta Informaticae 59, 107–118 (2004)

[2] Jensen, R., Shen, Q.: Semantics-Preserving Dimensionality Reduction: Rough and Fuzzy-Rough Based Approaches. IEEE Transactions on Knowledge and Data Engineering 16(12), 1457–1471 (2004)

[3] Lin, T.Y., Chen, R.: Finding Reducts in Very Large Databases. In: Proc. Joint Conf. Information Science Research, pp. 350–362 (1997)

[4] Pal, S.K., Skowron, A. (eds.): Rough Fuzzy Hybridization: New trends in Decision Making. Springer, Singapore (1999)

[5] Pal, S.K., Mitra, P.: Multi-layer Perception, Fuzzy Sets and Classification. IEEE Trans. Neural Networks 3, 683–697 (1992)

[6] Pal, S.K., Mitra, P.: Case Generation Using Rough Sets with Fuzzy Representation. IEEE Transactions on Knowledge and Data Engineering 16(3), 292–300 (2004)

[7] Pawlak, Z.: Rough Sets. Int. J. Computer and Information Science 11, 341–356 (1982)

[8] Pawlak, Z.: On Rough Sets. Bulletin of the EATCS 24, 94–108 (1984)

[9] Pawlak, Z.: Rough Sets. Theoretical Aspects of Reasoning about Data. Kluwer Academic, Dordrecht (1991)

[10] Pawlak, Z.: Vagueness – a Rough Set View. Structures in Logic and Computer Science, 106–117 (1997)

[11] Pawlak, Z.: Decision Networks. In: Tsumoto, S., Słowiński, R., Komorowski, J., Grzymała-Busse, J.W. (eds.) RSCTC 2004. LNCS (LNAI), vol. 3066, pp. 1–7. Springer, Heidelberg (2004)

[12] Rakus, E.: Fuzzy Set Theory Assisting Medical Diagnosis and Appreciation of Drug Effectiveness. Doctor's dissertation, Medical Academy of Łódź (1991) (in Polish)

[13] Rakus-Andersson, E.: Fuzzy and Rough Techniques in Medical Diagnosis and Medication. Springer, Heidelberg (2007)

[14] Skowron, A., Rauszer, C.: The Discernibility Matrices and Functions in Information Systems, Intelligent Decision Support. In: Skowron, A. (ed.) Handbook of Applications and Advances of the Rough Set Theory, pp. 331–362. Kluwer Academic, Dordrecht (1992)

[15] Yao, J.T., Yao, Y.Y.: Induction of Classification Rules by Granular Computing. In: Proc. of the Third International Conference on Rough Sets and Current Trends in Computing (TSCTC 2002), pp. 331–338. Springer, London (2002)

Computer Program for Aiding in Wireless Endoscopic Video Interpretation

Piotr M. Szczypiński

Institute of Electronics, Technical University of Łódź
Wólczańska 211/215, 90-924 Łódź, Poland
piotr.szczypinski@p.lodz.pl

Abstract. The MoDeRi program for aiding in wireless capsule endoscopy (WCE) video interpretation is presented. It implements the model of deformable rings (MDR), which is a dedicated technique applied to extract certain information from the video. The MDR performs a motion analysis of the video, produces a map of the gastro-intestinal system, estimates a longitudinal velocity of the capsule and detects strong mixing contractions. The extracted data allows for quick identification of gross pathologies and serves as a reference to the video fragments. It was found that certain characteristics that indicate areas of bleeding, ulceration and obscuring froth could be recognized within maps. Moreover, the MoDeRi program adaptively adjusts the video frame-rate, while playing the video, to optimize the interpretation process. Preliminary studies have proven usefulness of the MoDeRi program.

1 Introduction

Wireless capsule endoscopy (WCE) [3, 4], is a relatively new technique that facilitates the imaging of the human gastrointestinal system including small intestine. The WCE system consists of a pill-shaped capsule (Fig. 1) with built-in video camera, light-emitting diodes, video signal transmitter and battery, as well as a video signal receiver-recorder device.

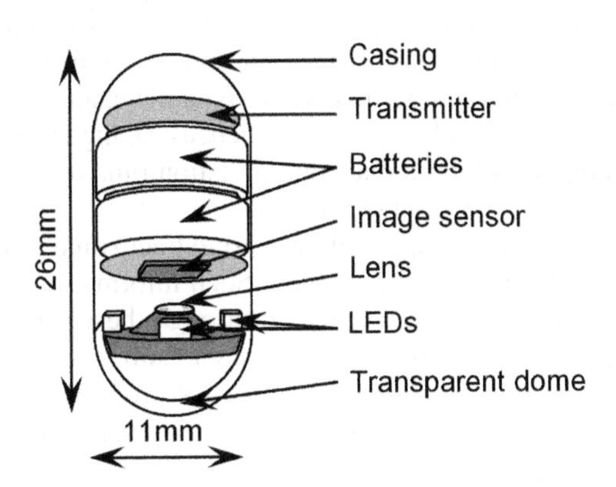

Fig. 1. Wireless capsule endoscope

E. Kącki, M. Rudnicki, J. Stempczyńska (Eds.): Computers in Medical Activity, AISC 65, pp. 53–61.
springerlink.com

The wireless capsule endoscope used in this study produces images of the internal lumen of the GI tract, covering a circular 140° field of view. The battery provides energy sufficient for approximately 8 hours of operation. The generated video frames are color images, each one with a 256×256 pixels dimension. The field of view covers a 240 pixels diameter circular area in the center of a frame.

A patient under investigation ingests the capsule, which then passes through the gastrointestinal (GI) tract. The capsule transmits video data at a rate of two frames per second for approximately 8 hours. The transmitted images are received and recorded by an external receiver-recorder device. A trained clinician then investigates the recorded WCE's video. It is a tedious task that usually takes more than an hour. The video interpretation involves viewing the video and searching for abnormal-looking entities like bleedings, erosions, ulcers, polyps and narrow sections of the bowel.

When the capsule goes through the small bowel it is propelled by peristaltic movements. Due to contractions, which are separated by refraction phases, the motion of the capsule is usually a little jumpy. The capsule maybe almost motionless in refraction phase and then it moves quickly during migrating contractions. Folded walls of digestive tract and strong mixing contractions may also cause the capsule to turn or even flip around. However, since the shape of the capsule is elongated and the GI tract is akin to a collapsed tube, most of the time the wireless capsule endoscope aligns in a direction parallel to the GI tract. The video produced by the wireless endoscope reminds a view that can be seen from a car passing through a tunnel. The tunnel walls converge in perspective at the vanishing point, and as we drive they shift outward from that point (when we look forward).

There are several approaches to aid in WCE video interpretation. First it may be useful to divide video into segments [9, 10] that show different fragments of gastrointestinal system. Thus, the clinician interpreting video would focus on this video segment which show fragment of the highest interest, e.g. the small intestine, without looking at other segments, e.g. stomach, duodenum or colon. The other approach is to categorize frames into normal and abnormal classes to focus the clinician's attention on abnormal looking images only. Unfortunately, the techniques that have been used for such segmentation and classification often produce erroneous or inexact results and cannot be accepted in clinical practice.

The WCE video includes fragments that show dynamic change in image content (during contractions) as well as almost motionless fragments (obtained during refraction phase). The other concept to aid in video interpretation [6] is to control the video playback frame rare to present frames that show dynamic change in image content for a longer time, and play motionless video sequences at higher frame rates. It was claimed that such approach would reduce interpretation time by fast forwarding video fragments insignificant for medical interpretation.

Yet, the other idea to aid in interpretation is to extract some information from the video frames that would supplement the video. Such information presented in a form of a graph or a color bar would guide clinician through the video. The application of such an idea is a color bar in commercially available software for WCE video interpretation. The bar represents variations in average color of consecutive video frames. By pointing at chosen location on the bar, the clinician may initiate the video playback starting at the corresponding frame.

This paper presents a computer system for preprocessing the WCE video and for aiding in the video interpretation. The system implements the Model of Deformable Rings (MDR) technique [5, 8, 11, 12] for video preprocessing. The model analyses the image motion and roughly estimates velocity of the capsule endoscope, it detects video fragments corresponding with contraction phases and it scans video for texture of the GI internal surface. After the video preprocessing the system switches to interpretation mode. In interpretation mode the system works as a unique video player, which supplements video with a map of internal GI surface, plots of velocity estimation and automatically controls video frame rate (fast-forwarding motionless fragments and slowing the playback down at fragments that exhibit contractions or significant changes in image content).

2 Model of Deformable Rings

The WCE video processing with MDR involve tracking motion of digestive system walls by elastic matching image information of consecutive video frames. The model measures the average speed of these movements toward and outward from the center of the video frame. It collects data on texture of the digestive system interior surface in a form of image bitmap or a map of the GI tract. The MDR is generally a tool for WCE egomotion estimation, which in addition scans video data for texture of the GI tract internal surface.

The MDR is a member of the deformable models family [1, 2]. It is composed of interconnected nodes arranged to form several concentric rings (Fig. 2) with their centers located near the center of the image frame. MDR does not entirely follow the motion present within the video. Rather it focuses on the motion component along radial directions originating in the center of the image frame that correspond with the forward or backward motion of the endoscope. In case of other motion component, which may correspond with mixing contractions, the model deforms and by degree of this deformation indicates the strength of contractions.

Essentially, the model works as follows: The nodes store image portions (image blocks) of a current image frame. The center of each block located close to the current location of corresponding node. As the image frame changes to the subsequent one, nodes are shifted toward locations the image resembles the stored fragments. The motion vector is estimated here with block matching technique, which searches for the minimum value of the mean absolute difference (MAD) function [12].

Since nodes search the image independently, individual nodes would "go their own way," and as the result the MDR arrangement would adversely change. To preserve the arrangement of nodes the internal tensions are modeled between neighboring nodes. Therefore, on one hand nodes push toward the locations they found and on the other the excessive relocation is prevented by tension modeling.

In the MDR the innovative technique for tension computation was applied. For each p, q node an n-neighborhood is defined. The n-neighborhood is a set of all MDR nodes connected with the node by n or less number of connecting lines, and it includes the node itself. The averaged transformation of a neighborhood from its initial, undeformed shape and location is computed. The transformation is defined by a translation vector $\mathbf{T}_{p,q}$ and a scaling, rotation and shear matrix $\mathbf{J}_{p,q}$. The tension vector for

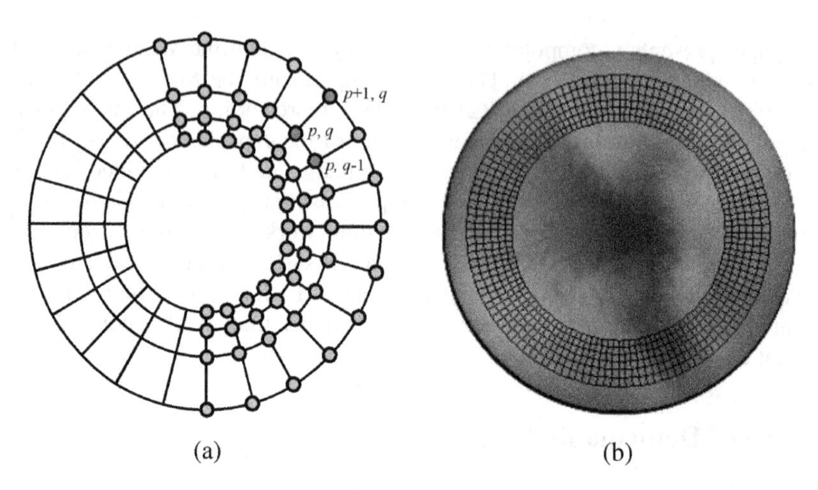

Fig. 2. MDR structure: a) initial form of MDR structure with node indexing style, and b) the model superimposed on a WCE video frame

node *p, q* is computed as difference between the transformed coordinates from its initial location in undeformed model and the node's actual location. The details of the tension computation implementation are published in [8].

The final location of each node is found iteratively, after obtaining balance between the two factors (the motion estimate and the tension). The total deformation of the model is computed as sum of tensions within every node. The deformation coefficient is later used to detect mixing contraction events. After that, image characteristics are again stored within the nodes' memories and the process repeats. It continues until the last frame of the video sequence is reached.

While the MDR follows the video content it shrinks during backward motion, or grows during forward motion. The degree of such model growing or shrinking is used to estimate the WCE speed within the GI tract [5, 8, 11].To prevent the model from excessive expansion or from shrinking, limits on the model size are set. If the model is bigger then the upper limit, the outer ring of a model is erased and a new inner ring is created. If it is smaller then the lower limit, the inner ring is erased and a new outer one is added. In either case, the image content is sampled along the outer ring to form a row of pixels. All such rows collected during the video processing are put together to form a map of the internal GI tract surface.

3 The MDR Optimization

There are a number of parameters that can be tuned in MDR to get more reliable preprocessing results. The model's initial size, number of nodes, strength of image influence, size of image block for motion estimation, strength and span of tensions are adjustable. The efficiency of the MDR was optimized by appropriate setup of its parameters.

The MDR was tested on selected fragments of natural WCE video and on artificially generated videos [12]. The artificial videos, created with 3D graphics rendering software, demonstrate motion of a strictly specified type. The camera virtually moved within a texturized rigid cylinder that simulated the small intestine surface. The MDR was used to preprocess artificial videos and to produce quantitative description of detected motion (like camera advance and rotation). The set of parameters was selected, for which the generated results were the closest to the motion actually demonstrated in the videos. In addition, the MDR with the chosen set of parameters was verified on natural WCE videos. The [12] publication presents details of the MDR optimization experiment and lists the most effective, selected parameters.

4 The MoDeRi Program Functionality

The MoDeRi program was implemented in C++ for *Windows* system platforms. The program consists of four modules. The first module is a graphical user interface (GUI), which implements controls for a video player, a map viewer, a plot viewer and text editor. The other modules are video processing modules implemented by means of *Microsoft® Direct Show* ™ technology. These are: the MDR processing module, the video decoder and the video frame multiplier. These modules are responsible for video data processing and necessary conversions.

The interpretation of a new WCE video with MoDeRi program requires preprocessing (Fig. 3). Therefore, after loading the video into the video player module, the program prompts to start preprocessing with the MDR module. The preprocessing of 8-hours video takes up to 40 minutes (with Pentium IV 3GHz processor). As a result is obtained a data file that holds a bitmap image of the GI tract surface, transient estimates of the capsule's velocity, deformation and other properties of the model attained during the preprocessing.

After the video has been preprocessed the program switches to the interpretation mode. In the interpretation mode, there are several tools available, intended for speeding up the interpretation process.

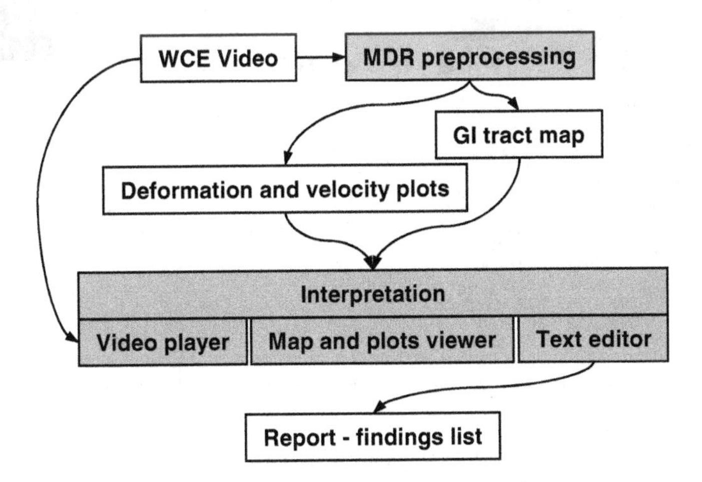

Fig. 3. Flowchart of data processing in MoDeRi program

The program combines a map and velocity graph visualization module with a video player (Fig. 4). The map enables the clinician to quickly get an overview of the entire

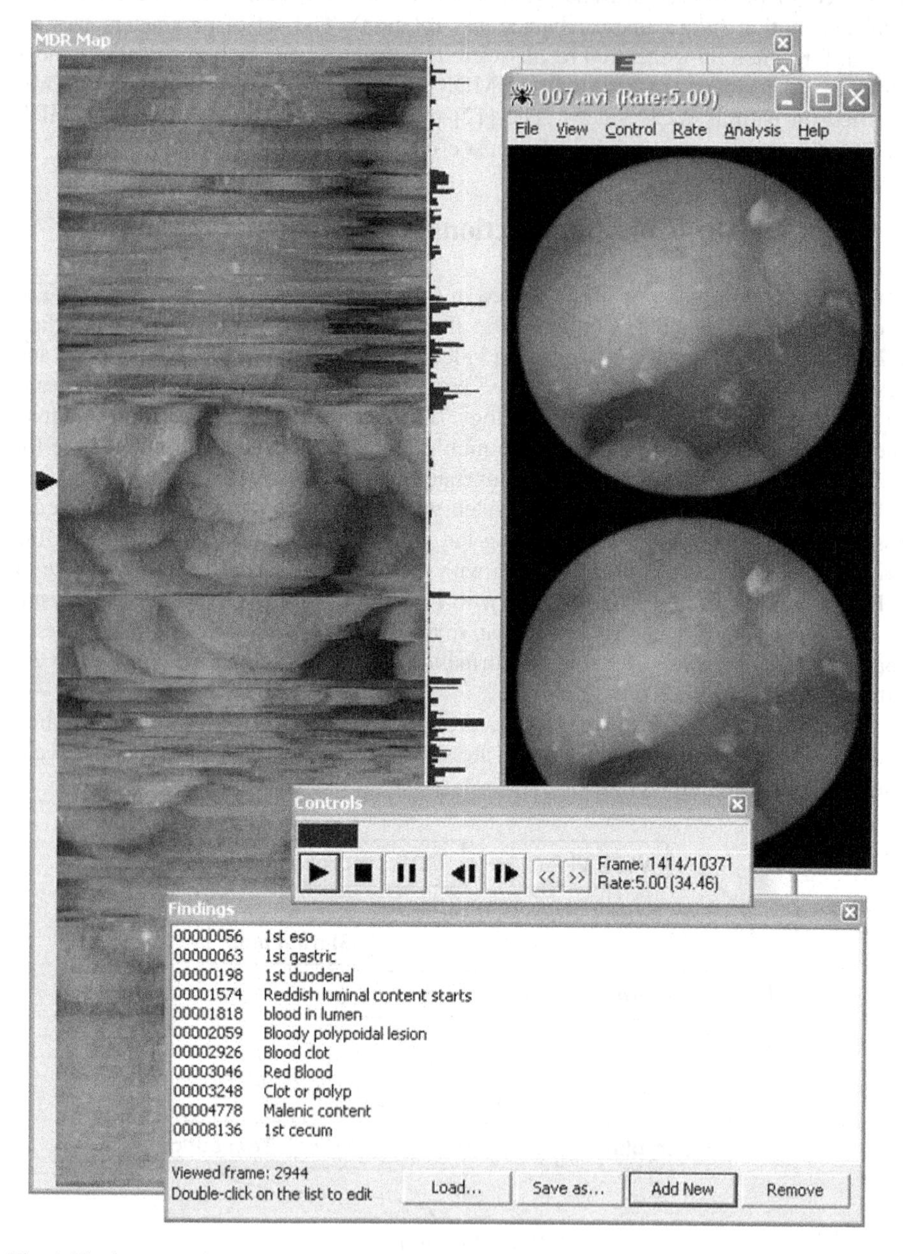

Fig. 4. The interpretation mode of MoDeRi program; the GUI consists of map viewer, video player (here concurrent presentation of two consecutive frames), controls window and findings list

recording in terms of completeness and the recording quality. It also facilitates the identification of abnormal areas and focuses the efforts on selected areas. By clicking on the map, the corresponding fragment of the video is invoked and immediately presented within the video player window. Furthermore, while playing the video, a marker advances, pointing at the corresponding position on the map. The map is scrolled as the video advances, to show a relevant section. Thus, the MDR map is applied as a reference to the video data.

Moreover, the video is supplemented with a plot of the capsule's velocity. The very low values of velocity may indicate narrow sections of the bowel due to disease or any other abnormal-looking entities.

The motion of the capsule presented by video data is irregular, characterized by quick changes of image information during the contractions and very slow changes of image information during the refraction phase. From the clinician point of view more important for the interpretation are these video fragments which present quick changes of image information. Thus, the video frame-rate may be controlled manually or automatically. If it is automatically controlled, then it is adjusted according to the deformation coefficient and the estimated velocity. The program fast-forwards video fragments which present a little variation in image content, it is when both the deformation and the velocity are small. It immediately slows down when the velocity or deformation factor indicate that the capsule rushed forward or was turned by mixing contractions. Thus, the essential fragments of video are played at low frame-rates, not to overlook any focal abnormalities.

When playing the video, the program may show one or several consecutive frames of video concurrently. The option for viewing several frames at the same time was implemented after the *GivenImaging® Rapid Reader™4*, which is commercially available software for WCE video interpretation. The several frames are presented on the screen side-by-side. Therefore, each frame is seen for a longer time, which results in interpretation efficiency increase.

When the clinician spots any abnormality (finding), he or she should note the frame number and write a short depiction of the abnormality. The program includes a simple text editor, which lets the user to store a short description of a finding. It automatically complements this with the necessary technical data on the video file and frame number. Then, it presents a list of findings with their descriptions. When the user selects an item from the list the corresponding video frame is presented. In consequence, the final result of the WCE interpretation is a report, which includes list of findings with their descriptions and illustrations.

5 The Program Evaluation

The MDR was tested extensively with the database consisted of over 30 video recordings. Twenty of them were used for preliminary tests, adjustment of the model parameters and training. The other ten were used for comparison of interpretation efficiency with and without use of MDR preprocessing.

It was found that certain characteristics that indicate areas of bleeding, ulceration, obscuring froth could be accurately recognized within maps (Fig. 5). Therefore, the maps can be glanced through for quick identification of such abnormal areas. Also, by means of the capsule velocity estimation, areas of capsule retention can be detected, which indicate narrow sections of gastrointestinal tract.

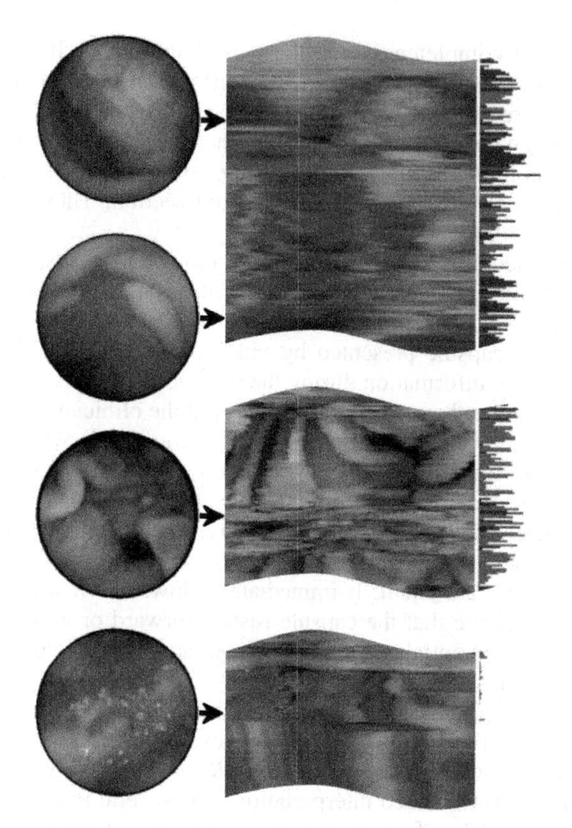

Fig. 5. Example map fragments with corresponding video frames and velocity plots: ulcer due to Crohn's disease, bleeding area, focal erosion and area of capsule retention

The obtained results show the time spent on interpretation may be reduced by several percent in specific cases. Some other results demonstrate the number of discovered pathologies and gastrointestinal landmarks is higher in case the MDR map was applied. The detailed research data, results of these tests and final conclusions will be published in forthcoming paper.

Acknowledgments

This work was supported by the National Institute of Standards and Technology, Gaithersburg, U.S.A. The video data were supplied by the Asian Institute of Gastroenterology, Hyderabad, India.

References

[1] Kass, M., Witkin, A., Terzopoulos, D.: Snakes: Active contour models. Int. J. of Computer Vision 1(4), 321–331 (1988)

[2] Szczypiński, P.M.: Rozprawa doktorska: Modele deformowalne do ilościowej analizy i rozpoznawania obiektów w obrazach cyfrowych. Politechnika Łódzka (2000), `http://www.eletel.p.lodz.pl/~pms/`

[3] Iddan, G., Meron, G., Glukhowsky, A., Swain, P.: Wireless capsule endoscopy. Nature, 405–417 (2000)
[4] Adler, D.G., Gostout, C.J.: Wireless capsule endoscopy. Hospital Physician, 16–22 (May 2003)
[5] Szczypinski, P.M., Sriram, P.V.J., Sriram, R.D., Reddy, D.N.: Model of Deformable Rings for Aiding the Wireless Capsule Endoscopy Video Interpretation and Reporting. In: ICCVG 2004, Warsaw, Poland, pp. 167–172. Springer, Heidelberg (2004)
[6] Vilarinao, F., Kuncheva, L.I., Radeva, P.: ROC Curves and Video Analysis Optimization in Intestinal Capsule Endoscopy. Pattern Recognition Letters, 875–881 (2005)
[7] Coimbra, M., Campos, P., Silva Cunha, J.P.: Extracting clinical infromation from endoscopic capsule exams Using MPEG-7 Visual Descriptors. In: EWIMT 2005, pp. 105–110 (2005)
[8] Szczypinski, P.M., Sriram, P.V.J., Sriram, R.D., Reddy, D.N.: Przetwarzanie i wspomaganie interpretacji danych z endoskopu bezprzewodowego za pomocą modelu deformowalnych pierścieni. Zeszyty Naukowe Elektronika, Instytut Elektroniki PŁ 10, 129–147 (2005)
[9] Coimbra, M., Kustra, J., Campos, P., Silva Cunha, J.P.: Combining color with spatial and temporal position of the endoscopic capsule for improved topographic classification and segmentation. In: Proc. of SAMT 2006, Athens, Greece (2006)
[10] Mackiewicz, M., Berens, J., Fisher, M., Bell, G.D.: Colour and texture based gastrointestinal tissue discrimination. In: Proc. IEEE International Conference on Acoustics, Speech and Signal Processing, ICASSP, Toulouse, France, May 2006, vol. II, pp. 597–600 (2006)
[11] Szczypiński, P.M.: Przetwarzanie danych video z endoskopu bezprzewodowego za pomocą modelu deformowalnych pierścieni. In: Sympozjum TPO 2006, Serock, pp. 232–243 (2006)
[12] Szczypinski, P.M.: Selecting a Motion Estimation Method for a Model of Deformable Rings. In: Proc. ICSES 2006, Lodz, Poland, pp. 297–300 (2006)

Segmentation of Biomedical Images Using Network of Synchronized Oscillators

Michal Strzelecki and Hyoungsuk Kim

Institute of Electronics, Technical University of Lodz, 211/215 Wolczanska,
90-924 Lodz, Poland
mstrzel@p.lodz.pl
Division of Electronics and Information Engineering, Chonbuk National University,
561-756 Jeonju, Korea
hskim@chonbuk.ac.kr

Abstract. This paper is focused on segmentation of biomedical images, including textured ones. A segmentation method which is based on network of synchronised oscillators is presented. This technique is able to provide analysis of image regions or volumes, this means that it can be applied both for two dimensional and three dimensional images. The proposed method was tested on several biomedical images acquired based on different modalities. Principles of operation of oscillator network are described and discussed. Obtained segmentation results for sample 2D and 3D biomedical images were presented and compared to multilayer perceptron network (MLP) image segmentation technique.

1 Introduction

Automation of medical diagnosis often requires automatic analysis of biomedical images. Usually, such images contain a large variety of different textures. Visual texture is a rich source of image information, but its definition is rather descriptive than formal. Texture is considered as complex visual patterns, composed of spatially organized entities that have characteristic brightness, color, shape, size. This local sub-patterns are characterized by given coarseness, fineness, regularity, smoothness etc [1]. Texture is also homogeneous for human visual system. These textures reflect cross-sections or projections of different human tissues or organs. Thus, there is a strong need to develop image texture processing techniques, firstly to obtain new information, directly not available for human eyes [2,3]. Secondly, these techniques are essential in automatic and semi-automatic systems for medical diagnosis support [4].

This work focuses on biomedical image segmentation techniques, where image is divided into disjoint homogeneous regions. This is a preliminary step which allows further image analysis, like identification or classification of analyzed human tissues.

Segmentation method presented in this paper implements network of synchronized oscillators of the Terman-Wang type [5]. This recently developed tool that is based on temporal correlation theory attempts to explain scene recognition as it would be performed by a human brain. This theory assumes that different groups of neural cells encode different properties of homogeneous image regions (e.g. shape, colour, texture).

E. Kącki, M. Rudnicki, J. Stempczyńska (Eds.): Computers in Medical Activity, AISC 65, pp. 63–72.
springerlink.com

Monitoring of temporal activity of cell groups allows detection of such image regions and consequently, leads to scene segmentation. Synchronized oscillator network (SON) was successfully used for segmentation of Brodatz textures, biomedical images, and also textured images [6]. The advantage of this network is its adaptation to local image changes (related both to the image intensity and texture), which in turn ensures correct segmentation of a noisy and blurred image fragments. Another advantage is that synchronized oscillators do not require any training process, unlike the artificial neural networks. In consequence, this leads to shorter analysis time. Finally, such a network can be manufactured as a VLSI chip, for very fast image segmentation [7].

This paper is organized as follows: Section 2 describes basic steps in image processing and analysis. Section 3 presents operation principles of oscillator network. Extension of the SON concept to the three-dimensional case for segmentation of 3D images is also presented. Segmentation results obtained by means of SON and multilayer perceptron network are compared and discussed in Section 4. Finally, Section 5 concludes this paper.

2 Image Preprocessing and Analysis

Basic steps of textured images processing and analysis are presented in Fig. 1. First, image acquisition takes place, it can be performed using different scanners (like for example CT, MRI, echocardiography). Then, digitally stored image is preprocessed in order to improve its quality and/or to eliminate noise and distortions.

Next, in case of textured images, a set of texture features (parameters) is evaluated. These features are mathematical descriptors, which are used for texture characterization in further analysis steps.

Among three major approaches to texture feature estimation, i.e. statistical, structural and signal processing, the first one seems to be the most comprehensive and efficient for description of majority of textured images, especially for medical ones. In this approach, features represent the texture indirectly by the non-deterministic properties that govern the distributions and relationships between the gray levels of an image. Examples of such statistical features can be divided into three groups:

1. Features calculated directly in image domain. In this group the most popular are the features estimated based on the following matrices:

- Co-occurrence matrix. It contains co-occurrence probabilities $p[i,j]$ of pixel pair with grey level i and j respectively, forgiven direction and interpixel distance. This matrix was originally proposed in [8], features calculated based on this matrix belong to most common used for texture discrimination;
- Run length matrix. Its elements $R[i,j]$ represent the number of occurrence of pixel set of j length and brightness equal to i;
- Gradient matrix. The image gradient matrix is initially determined with an appropriate filter with a mask of usual size 3x3 or 5x5 pixels;

2. Model-based features, which attempt to interpret an image texture by use of some mathematical model. The parameters of the model are estimated and then used for

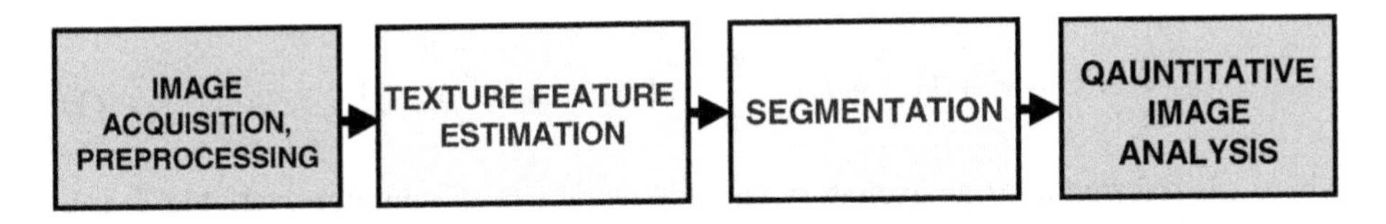

Fig. 1. A block diagram of textured image processing and analysis

image analysis. As en example, autoregressive model can be considered. This statistical model is based on the assumption that the brightness of a given image pixel depends on a weighted sum of neighboring pixels. Number of parameters depends on the model size.
3. Transform-based features represent an image in a space whose co-ordinate system has an interpretation that is closely related to the characteristics of a texture (such as frequency or size). The most popular are Gabor or discrete wavelet transformations. Then, energy of ROI sub-images in such transform coefficients space is estimated and used for texture description.

Feature vectors computed for analyzed image textures may include up to several hundred features per individual region of interest. Such a big number of features is rather not suitable for statistical analysis. Thus, techniques for reduction of feature vector dimensionality by selecting its most discriminative elements are needed. There are several methods for feature selection, like Fisher criterion, another one based on minimization of classification error and correlation coefficient, or mutual information coefficient [9].

Further feature analysis may be related to different feature reduction approach, called feature extraction or projection. In this case, the original feature space is transformed into a different space of lower dimensionality. This provides a set of new features, reduced in size if compared to the original one. The sample feature extraction techniques are principal component analysis (PCA), linear discriminant analysis (LDA), and nonlinear discriminant analysis (NDA).

Finally, suboptimal feature set obtained as a result of feature selection and/or reduction techniques can be applied for description of analyzed textures.

Image segmentation techniques cover a very large number of different approaches, like neural networks (several architectures), Bayes estimation (based on MRF image models) or k-means clustering (unsupervised approach) to mention just a few. Among them, network of synchronized oscillators is a promising technique, with application also to textured images [15].

After segmentation, quantitative or qualitative image analysis can be performed comprising for example image classification or estimation of geometrical parameters of segmented objects and regions.

3 Network of Synchronised Oscillators

To implement the image segmentation technique based on temporary correlation theory, an oscillator network was proposed. Each network oscillator is defined by two differential equations [5,10]:

$$\frac{dx}{dt} = 3x - x^3 + 2 - y + I_T \qquad \frac{dy}{dt} = \varepsilon[\gamma(1 + \tanh(\frac{x}{\beta})) - y] \tag{1}$$

where x is referred to as an excitatory variable while y is an inhibitory variable. I_T is a total stimulation of an oscillator and ε, γ, β are parameters. The x-nullcline is cubic curve while the y-nullcline is a sigmoid function as shown in Fig. 2a. If $I_T > 0$, then equation (1) possesses periodic solution, represented by bold black line shown in Fig. 2a. The operating point moves along this line, from the left branch (LB - it represents so-called silent phase), then jumps from the left knee (LK) to right branch (RB - it represents so-called active phase), next reaches the right knee (RK) and jumps again to the left branch. Waveform of an active oscillator is presented in Fig. 2b. If $I_T \leq 0$, the oscillator is inactive (produces no oscillation). Oscillators defined by (1) are connected to form a two-dimensional network. In the simplest case, each oscillator is connected only to its four nearest neighbours (2-domensional case) or to 26 neighbours (3-domensional case). Larger neighbourhood sizes are also possible. Sample networks are shown in Fig. 2c,d. Network dimensions are equal to dimensions of the analyzed image and each oscillator represents a single image pixel. Each oscillator in the network is connected with so-called global inhibitor (GI in Fig. 1b), which receives information from oscillators and in turn eventually can inhibit the whole network. Generally, the total oscillator stimulation I_T is given by the equation: (2) [5,10]:

$$I_T = \sum_{k \in N(i)} W_{ik} H(x_k - \theta_x) - W_z GI \tag{2}$$

where W_{ik} are synaptic dynamic weights connecting oscillator i and k. Number of these weights depends on neighbourhood size $N(i)$. In the case presented in Fig. 2c, $N(i)$ contains six nearest neighbours of ith oscillator for 2D case and 26 for 3D extension (except for oscillators located on network boundaries).

Due to these local excitatory connections an active oscillator spreads its activity over the whole oscillator group, which represent image object. This provides synchronisation of this group. θ_X is a threshold, above which oscillator k becomes active. H is a Heaviside function, it is equal to one if its argument is higher then zero and zero otherwise. W_z is a weight of inhibitor GI, it is equal one if at least one network oscillator is in active phase ($x>0$) and it is equal to zero otherwise. The role of global inhibitor is to provide desynchronization of oscillator groups representing different objects from this one which is actually being under synchronisation. Global inhibitor will not affect any synchronised oscillator group because the sum in (2) has greater value then W_z.

The weight W_{ik} connecting two neighbour oscillators which represent image pixels i and k is defined by formula (3):

$$W_{ik} = \frac{N_o L}{|f_i - f_k| + 1} \tag{3}$$

where f_i, f_k are a grey levels of pixels i and k respectively, N_o is a number of active oscillators of in neighbourhood $N(i)$ and L is a number of image grey levels. Hence,

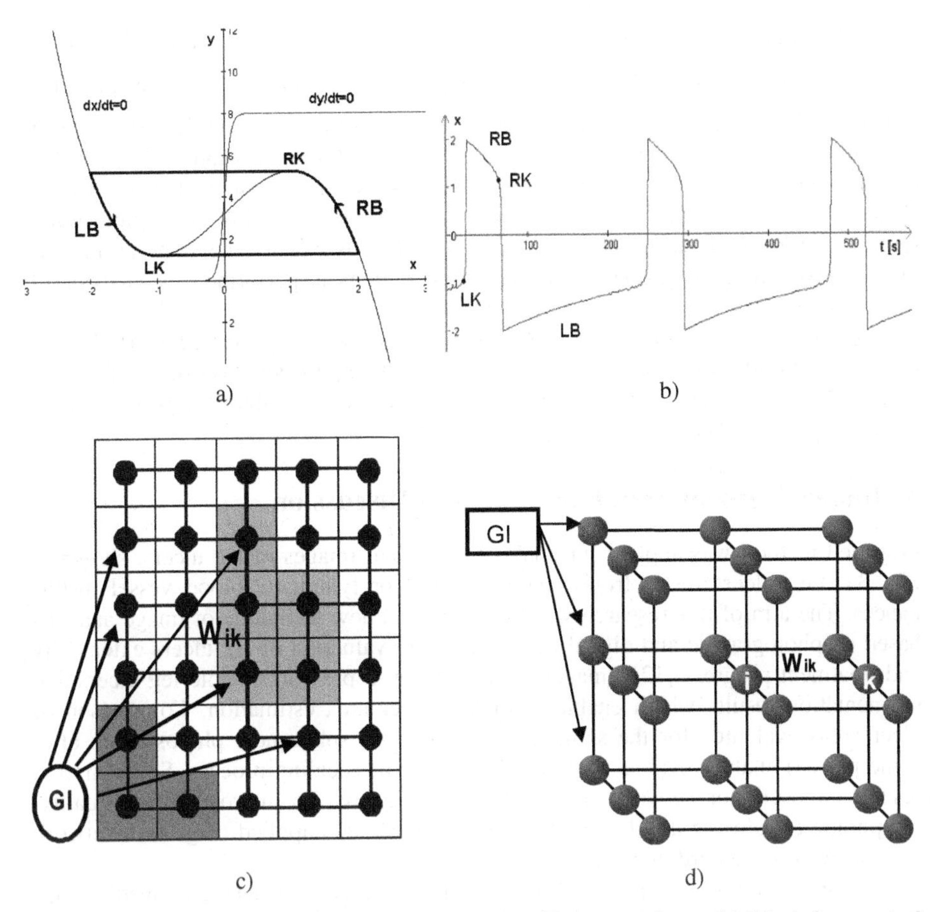

Fig. 2. Nullclines and trajectory of eq. (1) (a) and oscillator waveform *x(t)* (b). A fragment of oscillator network for 2-dimenasional (c) and 3-dimensional case (d). Each oscillator is connected with its neighbors using positive weights W_{ik}. GI means the global inhibitor, connected to each network oscillator.

weights are high for homogeneous regions and low for region boundaries. Because excitation of any oscillator depends on the sum of weights of its neighbours, all oscillators in the homogeneous region oscillate in synchrony. Different oscillators groups represent each region. Oscillators activation is switching sequentially between groups in such a way, that at a given time only one group (representing given region) is synchronously oscillating.

In case of segmentation of texture images, network weights are set according to equation (3) [10]:

$$W_{ij} = \frac{A\sqrt{\sum_{k=1}^{s} f_i^k \sum_{k=1}^{s} \bar{f}_{N(i)}^k}}{\varepsilon + \sum_{k=1}^{s} | f_i^k - f_j^k |} \tag{4}$$

where A is a number of active oscillators in neighborhood $N(i)$, f_i^k, f_j^k correspond to k-th texture feature evaluated for oscillators i and j respectively, $\bar{f}_{N(i)}^k$ is a mean value of feature f^k calculated for active oscillators in neighborhood $N(i)$ and s is the number of texture parameters. These parameters are evaluated for some windows centered at pixels i and j. They are selected to ensure good separation of analyzed textures. Hence, weights are high for homogeneous texture regions and low for region representing texture boundaries. Thus, network operation is exactly the same as in case of gray-level images. Segmentation of texture regions is performed by analysis of oscillators outputs.

A segmentation algorithm using oscillator network was presented in [11]. It is based on simplified oscillator model and does not require solution of (1) for each oscillator; it can be also easily adapted to 3D network. This algorithm was used for segmentation of different biomedical images [10].

4 Image Segmentation Examples and Discussion

Proposed method was applied for analysis of optical images of leg ulcers, shown in Fig. 3a. Leg ulcers result from venous, arterial or lymphatic blood vessel disturbances. The aim of this research was to elaborate a new technique of image analysis based on photographic and digital image data for evaluation of leg ulcers extensivity and treatment progress [12]. Images shown in Fig. 3 presents sample leg ulcers and segmentation results which enable automatic ulcer area estimation. Comparison of ulcer areas evaluated for the same patient (based on subsequent photos taken after some period) enables evaluation the efficiency of the healing process. Segmentation results for oscillator network are presented in Fig. 3b. To improve image quality, morphological closing and boundary object removal was applied (Fig. 3c). Network weights were set according to equation (3) in this case.

Described method was also tested on sample magnetic resonance biomedical images, representing human foot cross-section, containing heel and metatarsus bones.

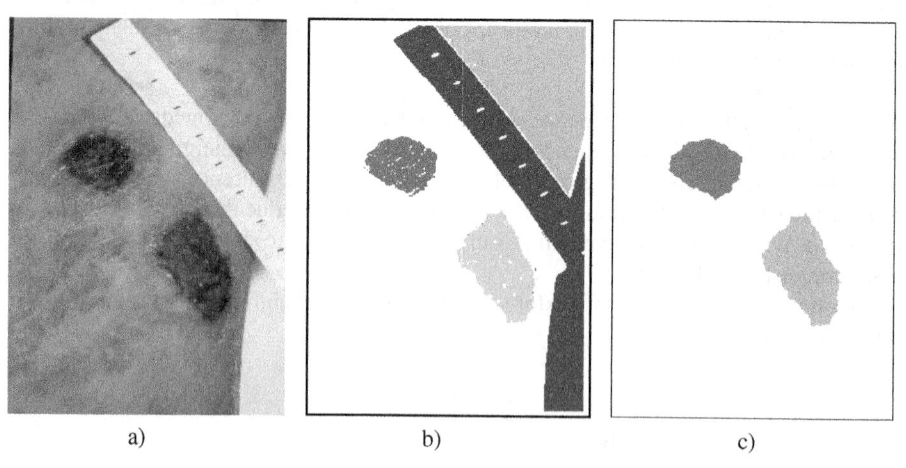

Fig. 3. Optical image of leg ulcers (a), segmentation result using SON (b), morphological closing and boundary object removal (c)

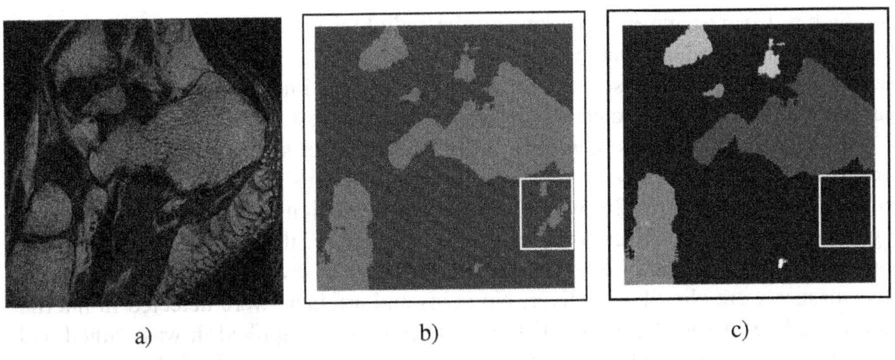

a) b) c)

Fig. 4. Sample MRI image of human foot cross-section (a), segmentation results using multilayer perceptron (b) synchronised oscillator network (c)

These images were recorded in German Cancer Research Centre, Heidelberg, Germany using a 1.5T Siemens scanner. An example image of size 512×512 is shown in Fig. 4a. Segmentation of these images is aimed at detection of foot and heel bones (marked by white lines) from other tissues and image background. The extracted region is interpreted by physicians to evaluate bone microarchitecture in osteoporosis diagnosis. As texture features, the Gaussian-Markov random field (GMFR) model parameters were assumed. It was demonstrated in [13] that GMRF model fit very well to this class of textures. Thus the GMRF parameters were estimated for each image point (a vector of 15 parameters). Then NDA analysis was performed, as in case of echocardiograms. Two new nonlinear features were used to form oscillator network weights. Three following segmentation tools were tested on the same texture feature set: multilayer perceptron network and oscillator network. Segmentation results are shown in Figs. 4b,c respectively. The results for perceptron and oscillator network programmed for region detection are similar. Generally, the bones were correctly extracted from the image background. A number of segmentation errors is visible at bone boundary. Another type of error can be observed in image background, where some tissue regions were identified as bone by multilayer perceptron (lower right part of Figs 4b,c marked by white rectangle). In case of oscillator network this fragment was correctly recognised. The better performance of oscillator network can be explained by local interaction between oscillators, which are activated based on active neighbours. Suppose that uniform region contains a point or small group of points, which differ in some way from this region. Then, during network operation on this region, active oscillators assigned to it will surround these points. Thus, the oscillator weights connected to these points will increase because of increasing factor A in (4). As a consequence, these oscillators can be activated assigning the distinctive points to the uniform region. Oscillator network provides bone object labelling that can be useful for further processing.

The SON based segmentation method was finally applied for segmentation of 3D liver images obtained using magnetic resonance tomography (Philips Medical System). These images were recorded in the University of Rennes, France. Image size was equal to 192x192x80 voxels, with resolution 2.08x2.08x2.0 mm/voxel, and 12 bits per voxel. Sample axially oriented cirrhotic liver cross-sections are presented in

Fig. 5a,b,c. Liver shape was marked by the radiologist using dotted line. The long-range objective of this research is to check, if morphological changes which occur in liver (caused by liver diseases) are reflected in their MR images. The objective of this particular analysis was to detect a liver region from the rest of the image.

Two segmentation methods were used to perform liver segmentation. The first approach implemented oscillator network. Network weights were set according to (3) and neighbourhood $N(i)$=26 was assumed Segmentation results are presented in Fig. 5d,e,f, where only liver tissue is shown. Generally, the liver area was detected correctly, some segmentation errors are visible close to liver boundary, where some other tissues were classifies as liver. No veins and artefacts were detected in internal part of the liver tissue. Next, the MLP neural network was applied. It was trained with training set containing 64 gray level samples drawn randomly from both liver and background regions. This network had 8 neurons in the hidden layer and two neurons in the output layer, corresponding to two classes. The number of network neurons limited to maintain appropriate relation between network weights and number of samples in training set (42/128<1/3). For network training, a b11 software was used

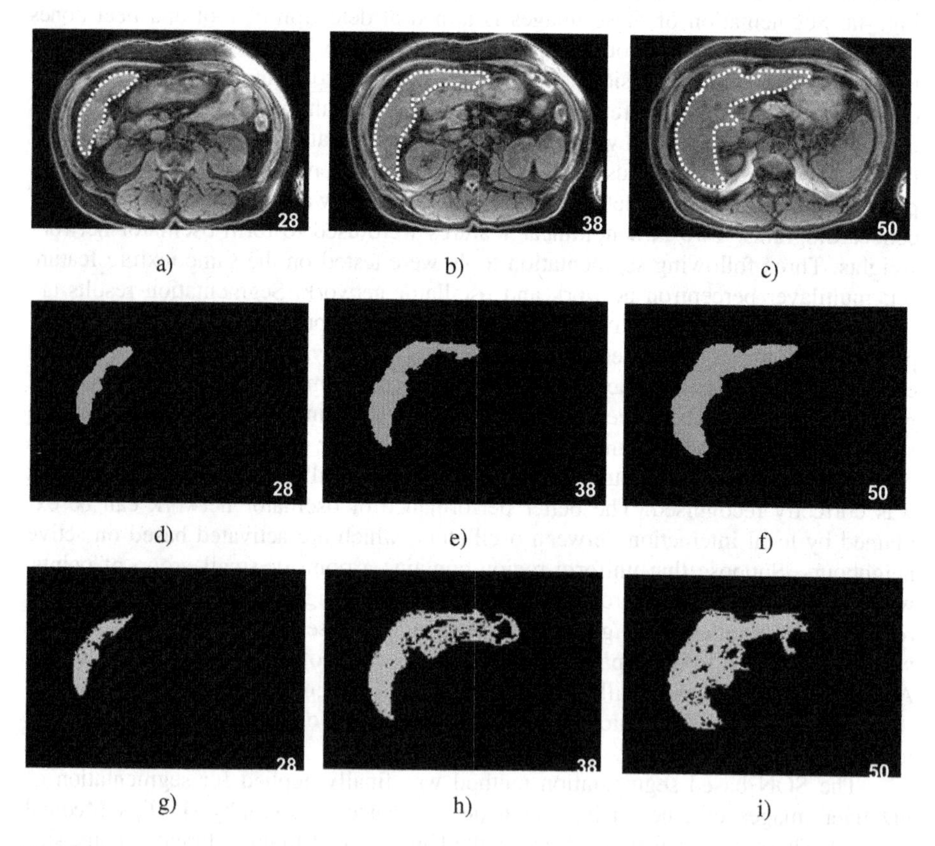

Fig. 5. Sample cross-sections of MR cirrhotic human liver images extracted from 3D data (a,b,c). Segmentation results using network of synchronized oscillators (d,e,f) and multilayer perceptron (g,h,i). Numbers indicate the slice number.

[14]. Segmentation results are presented in Fig. 5g,h,i (also in this case, the detected liver region is displayed only). They are worst when compared to SON, because other organs and tissues in liver neighborhood were also classified as a liver. In almost all slices liver veins and some artifacts were also detected.

As can be seen from Fig. 5, oscillator network provides a better segmentation results when compared to these obtained for the multilayer perceptron. It corresponds with a shape marked by the expert. In case of MLP some other organs and tissues were misclassified, while the oscillator network was able to classify them properly. This is caused by different weight setting for two considered segmentation techniques: in the case of MLP, weights are evaluated during learning process and then remain constant during image segmentation. Thus, image classification performed by this network and consequently, segmentation results depend on training set selection. Gray level distribution in the whole image may differ from this present in test set used for network training. In consequence, several image fragments might be wrongly segmented by the MLP. In the case of oscillator network, its weights depend on the difference between the gray levels of neighbor image pixels. Thus, if gray levels for some part of liver region differ from their neighbors, network weights can adapt to these changes. Due to this ability, sufficient high weight values (according to eq. (3)) to exceed oscillator activation threshold I_T in eq. (2) are obtained. Consequently, the analyzed region will be correctly classified as a liver. This phenomenon explains correct segmentation of images shown in Fig. 5d,e,f. Furthermore, SON is computationally very simpler (no image preprocessing, feature extraction and iterative calculations are required) and relatively fast. Analysis of images from Fig. 5 using SON took 4.6s using Pentium IV 2.6 GHz computer (3.5s in case of MLP).

5 Conclusion

In this paper the image segmentation based on the network of synchronized oscillators was presented. The proposed segmentation technique provides reliable segmentation results for analysed biomedical images, including textured ones. Also, it was demonstrated that:

- SON provides quite accurate segmentation results when compared to MLP
- The advantage of the proposed method is its resistance to changes of visual image information and also to noise and artifacts, often present in biomedical images
- The proposed technique is simple and computationally feasible, no image preprocessing, network training (as in case of MLP) or iterative calculations (as for cellular network) are required
- SON can be extended to 3D image segmentation

Further research will focus on application of oscillator network to segmentation of 3D textured images.

Acknowledgements

This research was supported by the MIC (Ministry of Information and Communication), Korea, Under the ITFSIP (IT Foreign Specialist Inviting Program) supervised by the IITA (Institute of Information Technology Advancement).

This work was performed within the framework of COST B21 European project: "Physiological Modeling of MR Image Formation".

References

[1] Hajek, M., Dezertova, M., Materka, A., Lerski, R. (eds.): Texture analysis for Magnetic Resonance Imaging. Med4 Publishing, Prague (2006)
[2] Lerski, R., Straughan, R., Shad, L., Boyce, D., Bluml, S., Zuna, I.: MR Image Texture Analysis – An Approach to Tissue Characterisation. Magnetic Resonance Imaging 11, 873–887 (1993)
[3] Zieliński, K., Strzelecki, M.: Compuyerised analysis of biomedical images. PWN, Warszawa (2002) (in Polish)
[4] Yu, S., Guan, L.: A CAD System for the Automatic Detection of Clustered Microcalcifications in Digitized Mammogram Films. IEEE Trans. on Medical Imaging 19, 115–126 (2000)
[5] Wang, D.: Emergent Synchrony in Locally Coupled Neural Oscillators. IEEE Trans. on Neural Networks 4, 941–948 (1995)
[6] Shareef, N., Wang, D., Yagel, R.: Segmentation of Medical Images Using LEGION. IEEE Trans. on Med. Imag. 18, 74–91 (1999)
[7] Kowalski, J., Strzelecki, M., Majewski, P.: CMOS VLSI Chip of Network of Synchronised Oscillators: Functional Tests Results. In: Proc. of IEEE Workshop on Signal Processing 2006, Poznan, Poland, September 29, pp. 71–76 (2006)
[8] Haralick, R., Shanmugan, K., Dinstain, I.: Textural Features for Image Classification. IEEE Transactions on Systems, Man and Cybernetics 3, 610–622 (1973)
[9] Jain, A.K., Duin, R.P., Mao, J.: Statistical pattern recognition: a review. IEEE Transactions on Pattern Analysis and Machine Intelligence 22, 4–37 (2000)
[10] Çesmeli, E., Wang, D.: Texture Segmentation Using Gaussian-Markov Random Fields and Neural Oscillator Networks. IEEE Trans. on Neural Networks 12, 394–404 (2001)
[11] Linsay, P., Wang, D.: Fast numerical integration of relaxation oscillator networks based on singular limit solutions. IEEE Trans. on Neural Networks 9, 523–532 (1998)
[12] Zalewska- Janowska, A., Strzelecki, M., Kwiecień, A.: Ocena rozległości owrzodzeń podudzi z wykorzystaniem metod komputerowej analizy obrazu. Postępy Dermatologii i Alergologii XXI, 291–295 (2004)
[13] Strzelecki, M.: Segmentation of MRI trabecular-bone images using network of synchronised oscillators. Machine Graphics & Vision 11, 77–100 (2002)
[14] Materka, A., Klepaczko, A.: On-line b11 User's Manual, file b11.chm, Lodz (2007), http://www.eletel.p.lodz.pl/merchant/mazda/order1_en.epl
[15] Strzelecki, M.: Segmentacja tekstury obrazu z wykorzystaniem neuronowych sieci oscylacyjnych i metod statystycznych, Zeszyty Naukowe nr 946, wydawnictwo Politechniki Łódzkiej, Łódź (2004)

MaZda – The Software Package for Textural Analysis of Biomedical Images

Piotr M. Szczypiński, Michał Strzelecki, Andrzej Materka, and Artur Klepaczko

Institute of Electronics, Technical University of Łódź
Wólczańska 211/215, 90-924 Łódź, Poland
piotr.szczypinski@p.lodz.pl

Abstract. A MaZda software package for 2D and 3D image texture analysis is presented. The software was written to compute a variety of textural features within arbitrarily shaped regions of interest. It also includes procedures for statistical analysis of computed feature sets, to aid in image classification and image content recognition. The software was used for research within framework of COST B11 and COST B21 multi-center international projects and it has proven to be an efficient tool for quantitative analysis of magnetic resonance images (MRI) – an aid to more accurate and objective medical diagnosis.

1 Introduction

The texture as perceived by humans is a visualization of complex patterns composed of spatially organized, repeated subpatterns, which have characteristic somewhat uniform appearance [27]. The local subpatterns within an image are perceived to demonstrate specific brightness, color size, roughness, directivity, randomness, smoothness, granulation, etc. The texture may carry substantial information about the structure of physical objects. Thus, the textural image analysis is an important issue in image processing and understanding.

Although image texture is easily perceived by humans, we still lack a strict definition what exactly the texture is. Therefore, the process of texture analysis is in many cases somewhat intuitive, and results of such analysis are rarely predictable. To aid in textural analysis computer programs, such as MaZda, may be beneficial. The MaZda software was already utilized [19, 23] in many areas including MRI measurement protocol optimization, various medical studies, food quality studies, et caetera.

At the beginning of 1998, the European COST B11 project started. One of the objectives of the project was development of quantitative textural analysis methods of magnetic resonance images. At that time there was no commercially available software capable of quantitative analysis of texture within freely selected regions of interest (ROI) and interpretation of computed results. MaZda was the first program created to satisfy this objective. In fact, its development started two years before, as it was a program for texture analysis in mammogram images. The early version of MaZda computed textural features derived from co-occurrence matrix, which is Macierz Zdarzen in Polish. Hence the name of the software is an abbreviation of Macierz

E. Kącki, M. Rudnicki, J. Stempczyńska (Eds.): Computers in Medical Activity, AISC 65, pp. 73–84.
springerlink.com

Zdarzen. In 1998, several procedures implemented in NMRWin program developed at the German Cancer Research Center were adapted and implemented in MaZda. Later, in 1999, procedures for statistical and discriminative analysis of feature vectors were developed. Throughout the last ten years MaZda was continuously enhanced and expanded with further functionality including color and 3D image analysis, 2D and 3D image segmentation, data classification, analysis automation and others.

The program code has been written in C++ and Delphi™ with use of OpenGL libraries. It has been compiled for computers that use Microsoft Windows® 9x/NT/2000/XP operating systems. The package includes two executable files named MaZda (image processing and computation of textural features) and b11 (for statistical and discriminative analysis). The MaZda package is widely used by participants of COST B11 and successive B21 projects, by other collaborating scientists and students in numerous research areas. Further sections describe program functionality along with examples of selected applications.

2 Image Analysis Pathways in MaZda

There are several pathways of image analysis that can be handled by the MaZda package (Fig. 1). Starting with input data, there is a choice between the analysis of 2D grayscale, 2D color or 3D grayscale images. MaZda implements procedures for loading of most popular standards in MRI. Also it loads Windows Bitmaps, selected Dicom formats or unformatted grey-scale image files with pixels intensity encoded with 8 or 16

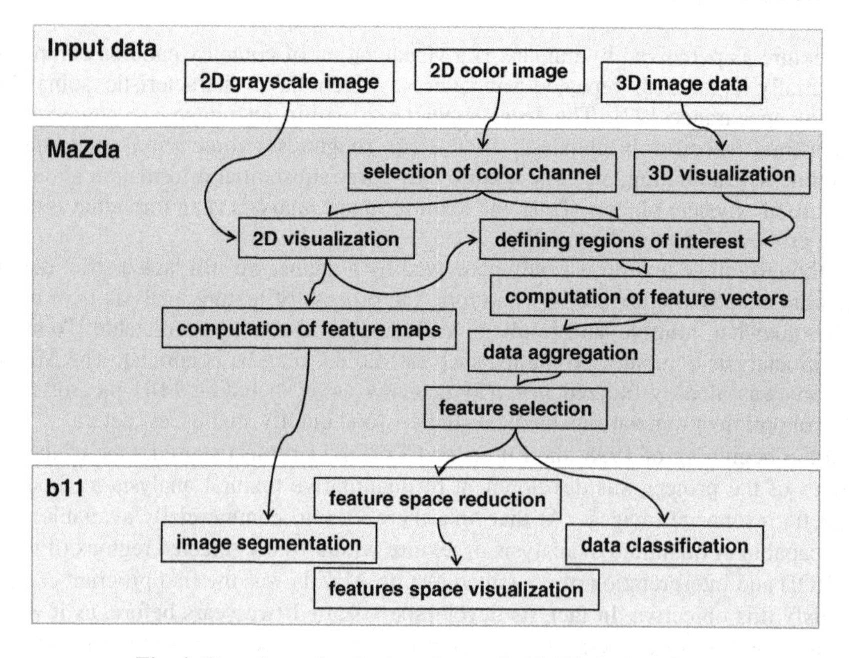

Fig. 1. Flowchart of analysis pathways in MaZda/b11 package

bits. Then, user is given a choice between analyzing the image as a whole or analyzing image within freely defined regions of interest (The region has to be shaped by means of MaZda's 2D or 3D region editors.) Depending on the choice made, the results of the image texture analysis are feature distributions within the image (feature maps), or text lists of features computed within regions of interest (feature vectors). Feature maps can be useful for image segmentation, as the feature vectors for classification of image content.

Feature vectors computed by MaZda may include up to several hundred features per individual region of interest. Such a number of features, creating several-hundred-dimensional spaces, are not easy to handle by statistical analysis or by classifiers implemented in b11. Thus, MaZda employs techniques for reduction of feature vector dimensionality by selecting the most discriminative features for further analysis. There are several methods for feature selection, which use various selection criteria, which can be chosen by the MaZda user.

Finally, there are three main pathways of analysis offered by b11 module. The data (feature vectors) can be statistically analyzed and visualized to find out relations between features and classes of textures. Moreover, there are methods implemented for supervised and unsupervised classification. The b11 may be used for formulating guidelines for texture classification or designing an artificial neural network classifier. Finally, feature maps can be used by b11 for image segmentation.

3 Textural Features

There are three major issues in texture analysis that MaZda may assist with. These are: feature extraction, texture discrimination and texture classification. Feature extraction is a computation of image characteristics able to numerically describe the image texture properties. Texture discrimination is to partition a textured image into regions, each corresponding to a perceptually homogeneous texture, which leads to image segmentation. Texture classification determines to which of a finite number of physically defined classes a homogeneous texture region belongs. Feature extraction is usually the first stage of image texture analysis. Results obtained from this stage are used for texture discrimination, classification or segmentation.

There are three categories of feature extraction approaches that MaZda includes: statistical, model-based and image transform. Statistical approaches represent the texture indirectly by the non-deterministic properties that govern the distributions and relationships between the grey levels of an image. Model based texture analysis [27], using fractal or stochastic models, attempt to interpret an image texture by use of generative image models and stochastic models respectively. Transform methods of texture analysis, such as Fourier, Gabor or wavelet transforms [28] represent an image in a space whose co-ordinate system has an interpretation that is related to the characteristics of a texture.

The user of MaZda package, by means of Options window controls, may select which group of features to generate. At choice are histogram, gradient, co-ocurrence matrix, run-length matrix, autoregressive model [27] and Haar wavelet [25] groups of features.

The most common, statistical method for image features extraction is based on image first-order histogram. The histogram is computed from pixels' intensity, without taking into consideration any spatial relations between the pixels within the image. Features are simply statistical parameters of the histogram distribution such as: mean brightness, variance, skewnes, kurtosis and percentiles. Another statistical method derives features from the image gradient's magnitude map. In similar way to the image histogram features, the histogram of the image gradient is computed and statistical parameters of such a histogram distribution are determined.

The gray-level co-occurrence matrix (COM or GLCM) is a second-order histogram, computed from intensities of pairs of pixels, where the spatial relationship of the two pixels in a pair is defined. The COM based features are derived from the matrix, and they demonstrate statistics, such as angular second moment, contrast, correlation, sum of squares, and various averages, variances, inverse moments and entropies [30].

The run-length matrix (RLM) holds counts of pixel runs, having the specified gray-scale level and length. In MaZda, there are four various run-length matrices computed, for four directions of pixel runs: horizontal, vertical, at 45° and at 135°. There are five run-length matrix based features computed for each of the matrices: short run emphasis inverse moment, long run emphasis moment, grey level nonuniformity, run length nonuniformity and fraction of image in runs [30].

There are also model-based textural features computed by the software, which are based on autoregressive model of image. The model assumes that pixel intensity, in reference to the mean value of image intensity, can be predicted as a weighted sum of four neighboring pixel intensities. These neighboring pixels are left, top, top-left and top-right adjacent. Therefore, the model has four parameters, which are weights associated to these pixels, plus the fifth parameter which is a variance of a minimized prediction error.

The transform method of texture analysis, implemented in MaZda, is based on discrete Haar wavelet. With the wavelet image is scaled up to five times, both in horizontal and vertical direction, resulting in transforming an image into twenty frequency channels. Energies computed within the channels provide data on texture frequency components. Thus, these energies are used as texture characterizing features.

To make sure the features characterize image texture exclusively and do not depend on some global image characteristics like overall brightness or image contrast, caused e.g. by varied illumination or some other biasing, the normalization procedure has been implemented. The normalization removes dependency of higher order parameters on first order grey-level distribution. There are two image histogram normalization options available. One of them remaps an image histogram in a range with mean luminance in the middle and span of 3 standard deviations, onto a white-to-black gray-scale range. The other remaps an image histogram in a range between the first and ninety ninth percentile onto white-to-black range. The image normalization step is performed prior to textural features computation.

The other image transformation that precedes features computation, and influences the way features are computed, involves altering the number of bits used to encode the image intensity. The number of bits can be set up between 4 and 12. This set-up substantially changes lengths of pixels in runs and size of the co-occurrence matrix, which in result affect the time and results of computation based on RLM and COM matrices, respectively.

Summarizing, the Mazda software allows for computation of 9 histogram-based textural features, 11 co-occurrence-matrix-based, derived from 20 co-occurrence matrices produced for 4 directions and 5 inter pixel distances, 5 run-length-matrix-based features at 4 different directions each, 5 gradient-map-based, 5 based on auto-regressive model and up to 20 based on Haar wavelet transform. Altogether 279 numbers, which can characterize a grey-scale image texture. All the features can be computed within the image of original histogram or within the image with normalized histogram, at various setups of bit per pixel option.

Methods for textural features computation implemented in MaZda require a gray-scale image as an input. On the other hand, it is evident that often color in color images carries essential information required for image differentiation or image recognition. In MaZda, it may be chosen to analyze selected color component (or channel) of the image, not only the image brightness. Therefore, there are several options for color to gray-scale transformation available, including conversions to Y, R, G, B, U, V, color saturation or hue channels. It is possible to combine features computed within different channels of the same image to get comprehensive characterization of color texture.

4 Regions of Interest

Regions of interest are sets of pixels in 2D images or voxels in 3D images selected to be processed. Defining specific region of interest (ROI) concentrates computation effort on image fragment that is relevant to a goal of computation and thus helps avoid processing of unnecessary image fragments. ROIs are of great interest in biomedical image processing applications. As illustration, tomography images of human body may present various kinds of organs or tissue. To analyze image properties in some selected organ and not in a surrounding tissue, the image fragment corresponding to the organ must be defined as a ROI for the analysis.

Any ROI in MaZda can be of arbitrary shape. The software allows for definition of up to 16 ROIs within a single image. These regions may overlap if required. If there are more then 16 regions in an image required for the analysis, they have to be analyzed successively, 16 at a time.

ROIs may be loaded from a disk file or defined with MaZda ROI editors. To edit 2D ROIs (Fig. 2 a), drawing tools such as pencil, draw line (with various line thickness), draw square, rectangle, circle, ellipsis are used. Also tools based on image grey level thresholding and flood-filling are available. In addition, to process a region shape, tools based on morphological transformations can be used, such as regions erosion (removes a layer of pixels), dilation (adds a layer of pixels), closing (smoothes boundaries, fills-in small holes) or opening (smoothes boundaries, removes small groups of pixels).

Volumetric ROIs within 3D (Fig. 2 b) images, e.g. images from magnetic resonance or computer tomography scanners, can be defined with other set of tools. The simplest way is to assemble ROI from predefined blocks, such as sphere, tube, cube and tetrahedron. Blocks can be placed within 3D image space at chosen location. The orientation, size and proportions of blocks can be adjusted freely. Other ways to create 3D ROI are to perform image segmentation with image grey-level thresholding

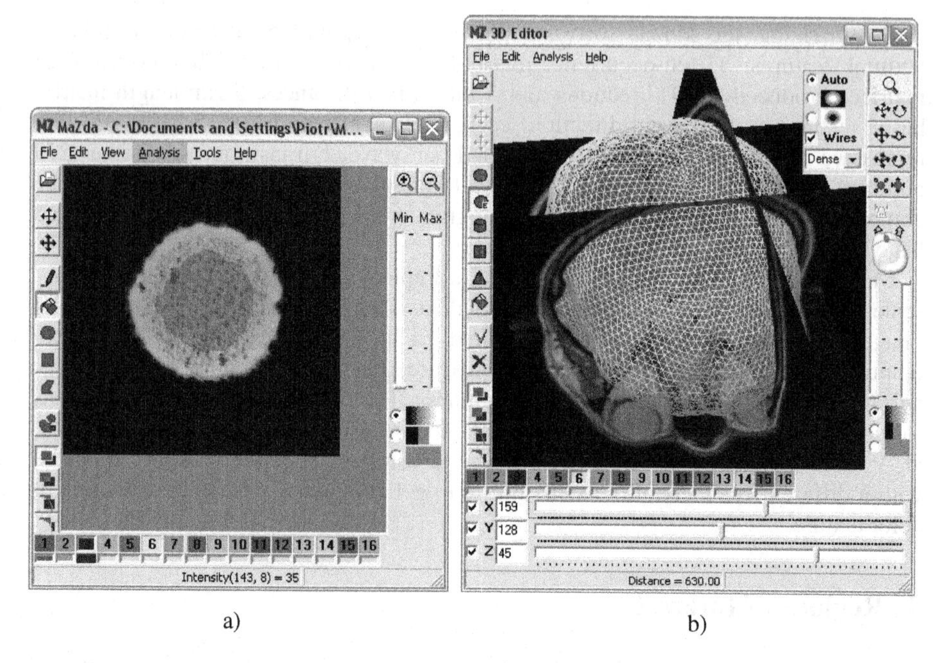

a) b)

Fig. 2. Region of interest editors: a) 2D ROI editor with a cheese image example and b) 3D ROI editor with human head volumetric data (deformable surface net detecting brain boundaries presented)

and flood-filling, or to edit regions cross-section with the 2D ROI editing tools. The most advanced tool for 3D region editing implemented in MaZda is deformable surface [26]. It is a mathematical model of enclosed surface that starts from ellipsoidal shape and deforms upon local image characteristics. The deformation process aims at fitting the surface at locations of high image gradient or locations having a gray-level close to selected threshold value. The final shape of the model strongly depends on initial shape and location of the surface, image contrast and some other parameters. Therefore, the deformable surface is implemented as an interactive tool allowing the user to adjust these parameters, to get the most satisfying shape.

5 Geometric Parameters

Two-dimensional regions of interest, which were primarily planned as masks for textural analysis, may be also viewed as images themselves. They represent silhouettes of two-dimensional objects that hey cover and they may carry key information for classification of such objects. Therefore, another approach for feature extraction [28] is to measure characteristics of these regions, such as location, orientation, size, geometric and topology descriptors, etc. The software computes parameters such as areas, perimeters, various diameters and radix, including Feret's and Martin's, as well as parameters of inscribed circle, circumscribed circle, ellipsis, rectangle and various ratios of these parameters. Most of such ratios are size invariant as elongation, compactness or roundness. Other parameters implemented in the software that are size invariant are first and second order binary moments.

Other group of parameters are based on transformations into a profile (wholes are removed from region), into a convex region (concavities are filled in) and skeletonization. Skeletonization is implemented through a thinning algorithm that removes outer pixels of a region to find a medial axis of the region. A result, called a skeleton, preserves information on region's topology. The skeletal descriptors computed by MaZda are: length of a skeleton, number of branches, branching points and loops, as well as minimal and maximal thickness of a region body surrounding the skeleton.

6 Feature Selection and Reduction

Using MaZda, one can produce a substantial set of features potentially carrying sufficient information for image texture characterization or region classification. On the other hand, the possible number of features computed by MaZda is enormous, may reach a few thousands per region of color image, and is difficult to handle. The several-hundred features turns into the problem of analysis of a several-hundred-dimensional space. This would be time consuming, inefficient or even not feasible.

Usually only a limited number of features carry relevant information needed for texture discrimination. MaZda allows for selection of these most effective ones and rejection of the others. There are four methods for feature selection implemented. These are supervised methods i.e. they require a-priori knowledge on which feature vector, or sample, belongs to which predefined class. Given the information, these methods select a subset of features according to a given mathematical criterion. There are four criteria used in MaZda: Fisher coefficient, classification error combined with correlation coefficient, mutual information and selection of optimal feature subsets with minimal classification error of 1-nearest neighbor classifier.

If the number of selected features is still unacceptably large, it is possible to perform their further reduction by transformation of the original features to a new space with lower dimensionality. This approach is called feature reduction or projection. Procedures implemented in the b11 module comprise principal component analysis (PCA), linear discriminant analysis (LDA) and nonlinear discriminant analysis (NDA) [5].

The two described steps, feature selection and feature reduction, lead to decrease of feature space dimensionality. This is usually a necessary step before further data analysis, like classification. None of the implemented methods for feature selection or reduction can be viewed as superior to the others. The choice should be made as a consequence of actual sample distributions and classification method to be used. Therefore, the purpose of developing the software is to allow for experimenting, verification and choosing the best solution to a problem being considered.

7 Texture Classification

The b11 allows visualization for viewing sample distributions within a feature space, statistical analysis of these distributions and classification of feature vectors. It displays clouds of samples presented in one-, two- or three-dimensional space of arbitrary selected features or within the transformed feature space (Fig. 3 a). Samples of different classes are represented with distinctive symbols. The user may conclude about feasibility of classification by determining whether clouds of samples group in separate clusters.

The b11 implements two procedures for nonlinear supervised classification: 1-nearest neighbors (1-NN) classifier and artificial neural network (ANN). The 1-NN incorporates a simple learning algorithm, in which generalization is done after collecting all the training data. During the training phase feature vectors and class labels of the training samples are simply stored. In the classification phase, distances from the new sample to all stored feature vectors are computed, k closest samples are selected and the new sample is assigned to the most numerous class within the k-samples set. The ANN implemented in b11 is a feed-forward network with two hidden layers of neurons. The neuron's nonlinearity is modeled with sigmoid function. The number of neurons in the hidden layers is adjustable. The user should prepare two sets of samples, one for training the other for validation. The training procedure fine-tunes neurons for best discrimination of the subsets of the training set. After the training, the resulting net should be validated with another, testing set of samples. The resulting net configuration and result of training may be stored to a disk file for further use.

Other methods implemented in b11 are useful for unsupervised data classification and cluster analysis [29]. These are the agglomerative hierarchical clustering (AHC), the similarity-based clustering method (SCM) and k-means algorithm. The AHC represent a bottom-up strategy of cluster analysis. The individual samples at first are viewed as separate clusters. The clustering algorithm computes distances between pairs of clusters in feature space. The distance between the two clusters characterizes their dissimilarity. Then, the clusters of the lowest dissimilarity are joined together. The process is repeated until the single cluster of samples forms.

The development of AHC may be visualized with a dendrogram (Fig. 3 b), which is a hierarchical tree. The tree leaves represent individual samples, branches represent links between samples or clusters, and a level at which branches join represent

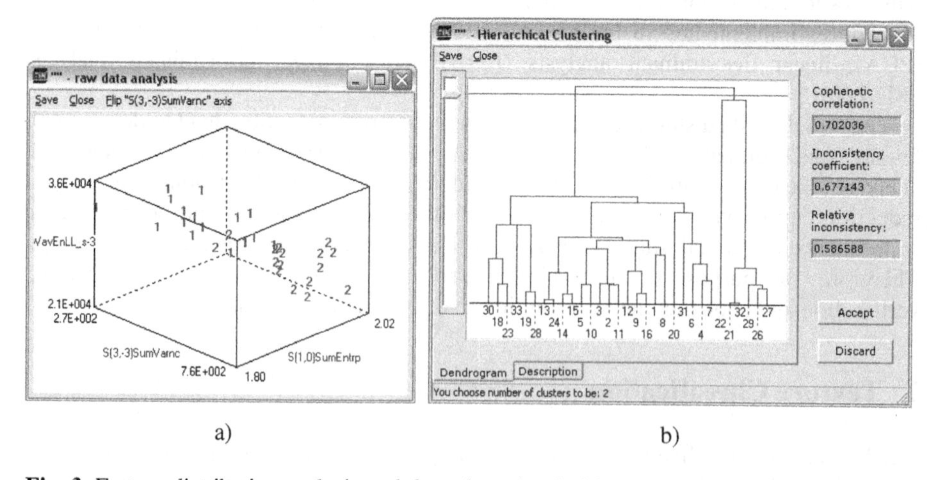

a) b)

Fig. 3. Feature distribution analysis and data clustering in b11: a) sample distributions and b) dendrogram of agglomerative hierarchical clustering

dissimilarity between the joined clusters. The user may adjust the clustering result in two ways: by selecting one of four available dissimilarity measures and by defining the dissimilarity level at which the dendrogram is split into clusters (sub-trees).

The SCM defines a continuous, parameterized similarity function, which corresponds to a density of samples within the feature space. The number of the function maxima determines the number of clusters. Each individual sample is iteratively relocated within the feature space by the function's gradient. Eventually, samples reach locations of certain maxima of the function, which in turns determine their membership to the corresponding cluster. The user can control the result of clustering by adjusting the parameter of the similarity function, which is responsible for the function's smoothness and the number of maxima.

The third clustering method implemented in b11 utilizes a k-means algorithm. The algorithm separates samples into a predefined number of k clusters by minimizing the total sum of distances between samples and centers of clusters they are assigned. To verify the result of clustering with the k-means algorithm, the user may examine silhouette plots or a silhouette value. There are as many plots as clusters. Plots that resemble a rectangle indicate accurate clustering.

8 Feature Maps and Image Segmentation

As already mentioned MaZda computes also feature distributions within the image (feature maps). The map is a grey-scale image, in which a gray level represents a particular textural feature value. The feature at a given image location is computed within a rectangular region (a mask) centered at this location. During the analysis process, mask slides over the image surface by a given vertical and horizontal step in order to fill the whole output image with computed feature values. User may select features for which maps should be computed, height and width of the mask and the horizontal and vertical steps.

Segmentation is an image processing task to partition an image into separate regions, which are in some way homogeneous. The most common segmentation routine is performed through image gray level thresholding. In this method, image pixels of intensity higher then the threshold level fall into one segmentation region, others fall into the other segmentation region. Unfortunately, if the goal is to segment texture, the image gray level thresholding alone usually fails. However, the thresholding may still be effective if preceded by a feature map computation. If the feature is found that discriminates two different textures, and then the feature map is computed on image containing such textures, the result would be an image showing one texture as a dark area and the other one as a bright area. Therefore, the thresholding of the feature map would separate the two textures visible in the input image.A visual inspection of maps produced by MaZda may lead to conclusions on which feature maps should be used for texture segmentation.

To study a feasibility of image texture segmentation based on multiple feature maps, the unsupervised method of k-means clustering was implemented in b11 module. The MaZda user can load a number of arbitrary selected feature maps, then to enter a number of segments or texture classes present in the image and run the segmentation algorithm. The result is an image that represents individual texture regions with unique colors.

9 Applications

Patterns or texture areas appear in almost every visual image and thus images can be investigated with textural analysis tools, such as MaZda. The MaZda software was already utilized in many domains including MRI measurement protocol optimization, various medical studies, food quality studies and others.

Within COST B11 and B21 projects several studies on MRI scanning are carried out. To assure a quality and provide means for MRI scanner calibration, test objects [19] (phantoms), which imitate characteristics of living tissues are used. Such phantoms are visualized with different MRI scanners to produce test images. The images serve for quality control of scanners, for testing and standardization of protocols. The phantoms' images obtained in various medical centers through several years were evaluated and compared with the MaZda program. These studies conclude on phantoms usefulness for scanner quality testing and on the phantoms invariability in time as to be used for scanner calibration.

Texture analysis was also performed to identify and discriminate biomedical image areas, which have different textural characteristics. In medical applications textural image analysis has been used for the characterization and discrimination of image areas that represent healthy and pathological tissues. The researches involved: detection of amygdale activation in rat brains [22], to detect and quantify hipocampal sclerosis, to distinguish between brain tumors [1], discrimination of healthy and cirrhotic livers, textural analysis of trabecular bone images targeted at osteoporosis detection [13, 23], monitoring of atrophy and regeneration of muscles [15], monitoring of teeth implants [12], analysis of myocardium tissue in ultrasound images [17], assessment of cellular necrosis in epithelial cell [18] and evaluation of anti-vascular therapy of mammary carcinomas in mice [2].

The textural analysis is useful not only in medicine. The other fruitful application of such analysis is in agriculture and food processing industry. The MaZda tools turned out to be useful in discrimination between potato varieties, cooked and raw potatoes, analysis of the influence of apple ripening process on storage [20], and assessment of soft cheeses quality [3]. More examples related to MaZda applications can be also found in [19].

The MaZda package is an efficient and reliable set of tools for analysis of image textures. Its efficiency was also confirmed by the COST projects participants and other researchers, who applied this software for many different texture analysis tasks. Compared to other texture analysis software, like Keyres [8] or LS2W [9], it provides complete analysis path of textures images, including feature estimation, statistical analysis of feature vectors, classification and image segmentation. Additional information on MaZda package and its executable code can be found on the web page [7] of the Institute of Electronics, Technical University of Łódź.

Acknowledgments

The development of MaZda package was in part done within the COST B11 and B21 European projects.

References

[1] Bonilha, L., Kobayashi, E., Castellano, G., Coelho, G., Tinois, E., Cendes, F., Li, L.M.: Texture Analysis of Hippocampal Sclerosis. Epilepsia 44(12), 1546–1550 (2003)

[2] Chen, G., Jespersen, S., Pedersen, M., Pang, Q., Horsman, M., Stødkilde-Jørgensen, H.: Evaluation of anti-vascular therapy with texture analysis. Anticancer Res. 25(5), 3399–3405 (2005)

[3] Collewet, G., Strzelecki, M., Mariette, F.: Influence of MRI acquisition protocols and image intensity normalization methods on texture classification. Magnetic Resonance Imaging 22, 81–91 (2004)

[4] Duda, R., Hart, P.: Pattern Classification and Scene Analysis. Wiley, Chichester (1973)

[5] Fukunaga, K.: Introduction to Statistical Pattern Recognition. Academic Press, New York (1991)

[6] Hecht-Nielsen, R.: Neurocomputing. Addison-Wesley, Reading (1989)

[7] http://www.eletel.p.lodz.pl/cost (visited: September 2007)

[8] http://www.keyres-technologies.com (visited: September 2007)

[9] http://www.maths.bris.ac.uk/~wavethresh/LS2W (visited: September 2007)

[10] Jain, A., Dubes, R.: Algorithms for Clustering Data. Prentice Hall, Englewood Cliffs (1998)

[11] Jirák, D., Dezortová, M., Taimr, P., Hájek, M.: Texture analysis of human liver. Journal of Magnetic Resonance Imaging 15(1), 68–74 (2002)

[12] Kozakiewicz, M., Stefanczyk, M., Materka, A., Arkuszewski, P.: Selected Characteristic Features of Radiotexture of Bone of the Dental Alveolus in the Human Maxilla and Mandible. Magazyn Stomatologiczny 3(181), 40–43 (2007) (in Polish)

[13] Lerouxel, E., Libouban, H., Moreau, M.F., Baslé, M.F., Audran, M., Chappard, D.: Mandibular bone loss in an animal model of male osteoporosis (orchidectomized rat): a radiographic and densitometric study. Journal Osteoporosis International 15(10), 814–819 (2004)

[14] Letal, J., Jirak, D., Suderlova, L., Hajek, M.: MRI 'texture' analysis of MR images of apples during ripening and storage. Lebensmittel-Wissenschaft und -Technologie 36(7), 719–727 (2003)

[15] Mahmoud-Ghoneim, D., Cherel, Y., Lemaire, L., de Certaines, J.D., Manier, A.: Texture analysis of magnetic resonance images of rat muscles during atrophy and regeneration. Magnetic Resonance Imaging 24(2), 167–171 (2006)

[16] Mao, J., Jain, A.: Artificial Neural Networks for Feature Extraction and Multivariate Data Projection. IEEE Trans. Neural Networks 6, 296–316 (1995)

[17] Punys, V., Puniene, J., Jurkevicius, R., Punys, J.: Myocardium Tissue Analysis Based on Textures in Ultrasound Images. Studies in Health Technology and Informatics 116, 435–440 (2005)

[18] Santos, A., Ramiro, C., Desco, M., Malpica, N., Tejedor, A., Torres, A., Ledesma-Carbayo, M.J., Castilla, M., García-Barreno, P.: Automatic detection of cellular necrosis in epithelial cell cultures. In: Sonka, M., Hanson, K.M. (eds.) Proceedings of SPIE, Medical Imaging 2001, vol. 4322, pp. 1836–1844 (2001)

[19] Hajek, M., Dezortova, M., Materka, A., Lerski, R. (eds.): Texture Analysis for Magnetic Resonance Imaging. Med4 Publishing, Prague (2006)

[20] Thybo, A.K., Szczypinski, P.M., Karlsson, A.H., Donstrup, S., Stodkilde-Jorgensen, H., Andersen, H.J.: Prediction of sensory texture quality attributes of cooked potatoes by NMR-imaging (MRI) of raw potatoes in combination with different image analysis methods. Journal of Food Engineering, 91–100 (2004)

[21] Yang, M., Wu, K.: A Similarity-Based Robust Clustering Method. IEEE Trans. on Pattern Analysis and Machine Intelligence 24(4), 434–448 (2004)

[22] Yu, O., Parizel, N., Pain, L., Guignard, B., Eclancher, B., Mauss, Y., Grucker, D.: Texture analysis of brain MRI evidences the amygdala activation by nociceptive stimuli under deep anesthesia in the propofol–formalin rat model. Magnetic Resonance Imaging 25(1), 144–146 (2007)

[23] Herlidou, S., Grebe, R., Grados, F., Leuyer, N., Fardellone, P., Meyer, M.-E.: Influence of age and osteoporosis on calcaneus trabecular bone structure: a preliminary in vivo MRI study by quantitative texture analysis. Magnetic resonance Imaging 22(2), 237–243 (2004)

[24] Szczypiński, P., Kociołek, M., Materka, A., Strzelecki, M.: Computer Program for Image Texture Analysis in PhD Students Laboratory. In: International Conference on Signals and Electronic Systems, Łódź-Poland, pp. 255–262 (2001)

[25] Kociołek, M., Materka, A., Strzelecki, M., Szczypiński, P.: Descrete Wavelet Transform-Derived Features for Digital Image Texture Analysis. In: International Conference on Signals and Electronic Systems, Łódź-Poland, pp. 99–104 (2001)

[26] Szczypinski, P.M.: Center Point Model of Deformable Surface Computer Vision and Graphics. In: International Conference, ICCVG 2004, Warsaw, Poland, September 2004, pp. 343–348 (2004)

[27] Materka, A., Strzelecki, M.: Texture Analysis Methods – A Review, Technical University of Lodz, Institute of Electronics, COST B11 report, Brussels (1998), `http://www.eletel.p.lodz.pl/cost/pdf_1.pdf`

[28] Kindratenko, V.: Development and Application of Image Analysis Techniques for Identification and Classification of Microscopic Particles. Ph.D. Thesis, University of Antwerp, Belgium (1997), `http://homepages.inf.ed.ac.uk/rbf/CVonline/LOCAL_COPIES/KINDRATENKO1/part2.pdf`

[29] Klepaczko, A.: Zastowanie algorytmów analizy skupień do selekcji cech dla zadań klasyfikacji wektorów danych. Ph.D. Thesis, University of Lodz, Poland (2006)

[30] Haralick, R.: Statistical and Structural Approaches to Texture. Proc. IEEE 67(5), 786–804 (1979)

Gilbert-Multiplier-Based Parallel 1-D and 2-D Analog FIR Filters for Medical Diagnostics

Rafał Długosz[1,2,3,*], Vincent Gaudet[2], and Ryszard Wojtyna[3,4]

[1] University of Neuchâtel, Institute of Microtechnology, Rue A.-L. Breguet 2, CH-2000, Neuchâtel, Switzerland
[2] University of Alberta, Department of Electrical and Computer Engineering 114 St – 89 Ave, Edmonton Alberta, T6G 2V4, Canada
[3] The College of Computer Science in Łódź, Poland, Department in Bydgoszcz, ul. Fordońska 246, 85-766, Bydgoszcz, Poland
[4] University of Technology and Life Sciences, Faculty of Telecommunication and Electrical Engineering, ul. Kaliskiego 7, 85-791 Bydgoszcz, Poland
rdlugosz@ualberta.ca, vgaudet@ece.ualberta.ca, woj@mail.utp.edu.pl

Abstract. A novel idea and CMOS implementation of power-efficient 1-D and 2-D finite-impulse-response (FIR) filters based on a current-mode Gilbert-vector-multiplier (GVM) have been proposed. MOS transistors included in the GVM multiplier work in a weak inversion resulting in an ultra low power consumption, with currents as low as several hundred nanoAmps to several microAmps. Due to the proposed multiplier, all output samples of the FIR filters can be calculated in parallel, making the filtration operation very fast. Moreover, the GVM enables a simple normalization of the output samples. As a consequence, not current values but current ratio values are significant here. As an example, a time-domain 1-D 3rd order filter has been presented which dissipates 8-μW of power enabling a 2-MHz sampling frequency (f_S). Another example is a 2-D filter with the frame resolution of 6x1 pixels that dissipates 7-μW at the data rate of 1 Mframe/s.

Keywords: FIR filters, Gilbert vector multipliers, parallel data processing.

1 Introduction

Modern medical devices often require high speed and ultra-low power integrated circuits (IC), which allow for increasing a system reliability and for device miniaturization. One of examples of diagnostic systems where the mentioned features are essential is so called camera endoscopic capsule that can be used in gastroscopy. This autonomous device can be swallowed by a patient, enabling an observation of the alimentary canal by means of a built-in low-power vision system with a micro-camera. The collected data are transmitted to an external computer using an embedded RF transceiver. In this paper, we propose ultra-low power analog filters suitable

[*] Fellow of the EU Marie Curie International Outgoing Fellowship.

E. Kącki, M. Rudnicki, J. Stempczyńska (Eds.): Computers in Medical Activity, AISC 65, pp. 85–99.
springerlink.com

for low-energy signal preprocessing inside the device. In this way, we can reduce the amount of data that must be sent via the RF and save the consumed energy.

In typical vision systems with charge coupled devices (CCD's), matrix analog data registered by a camera are directly converted into digital signals, using analog-to-digital converters (ADC's), and next processed by means of digital signal processors (DSP's) or field programmable gate arrays (FPGA's). This is sufficient in applications, where power dissipation is of secondary importance and a relatively low data rate is acceptable. Serial data processing in microprocessors is a bottleneck especially visible in processing high resolution images. For example, when an input image would have the resolution of 1000x1000 pixels, then to realize a simple (3x3) image filtering, a DSP would have to perform even 10 million operations per each image frame. This means that even a very fast DSP is able to calculate not more than several dozen of frames in a real time. The other problem are I/O circuitries in a DSP system, which contains relatively slow ADC's. For example, to calculate images with a resolution of 1000x1000 pixels with a data rate of 100 frames per second and an 8-bits color depth, the ADC must enable data rate that is equal to about 1 Gbit/s. Converters designed for such data rates dissipate at least several to several dozen mW of power [1]. In the other approach, a matrix of low-power and low-rate ADC's operating in parallel may be used [2], but the problem with a large amount of data is the same. The described constrains draw trade-offs that are between the data rate, the image resolution and the power dissipation.

One also observes various efforts to implement analog image processing. Such analog processors are very often realized using Cellular Neural Networks (CNN) [3]. An example circuit of this type has been described in [3]. This circuit designed in CMOS 0.5μm process enables a parallel data processing, calculating images with a 64x64 resolution for data rate of 1 MSamples/s and dissipating power of 1.5 W from the 3.3 V supply.

In this paper, anther approach to build data processing systems is proposed. Our circuits incorporate ultra low power analog circuitry, such as current mode Gilbert vector multipliers, which use transistors working in a weak inversion region. The Gilbert multipliers have been used in various applications for many years. FIR filtering is one of possible applications but so far only scalar Gilbert multiplication cells (SGM's) have been used in an implementation of FIR filter coefficients [4-6], mostly in adaptive equalization systems, where a high selectivity is not required. On the other hand, current-mode Gilbert vector multipliers (GVM's) working in a weak inversion have recently been successfully used to implement ultra low power analog decoders [7]. Here, we propose a novel application of these circuits – the current-mode FIR filters, which enable a parallel data processing with a mach better efficiency.

Our filters have been implemented in two versions, i.e. for filtering 1-D and 2-D signals. In both cases the core circuit is the Gilbert multiplier. The difference is in the domain of input data. In the first case, the GVM circuit receives samples of only one signal sampled in time domain. In this case a delay line is needed. In the second case, all inputs are independent data streams coming, for example, from particular pixels in a CCD matrix. In this case the image coordinates form the signal domain. Both cases are closely related and are discussed in this paper.

The proposed circuits enable initial low-power data preprocessing at the analog side. After that, some amount of data can usually be dropped off. As a result, the ADC that is used in the system as a next block can be simplified. One of examples is a decimation process, which allows for significant reduction of data amount in case, when a signal temporarily does not contain important information at high frequencies. When a decimation preceded by an antialiasing filtering is performed at the analog side, which can be easily performed using the proposed filters, this technique allows for a significant reduction of the power dissipation in the following ADC.

The text is organized as follows. In the next section, a short necessary information about 1-D and 2-D FIR filters is provided. The idea of using GVM circuits in implementation of parallel FIR filters has been presented in the following section. Then, in two sections we present implementation of both the 1-D and 2-D filters. Application of the proposed filters to realization of multirate systems is shown in the successive section. Finally, conclusions are drawn in the last section.

2 Basics of 1-D and 2-D FIR Filtration

As FIR filters are widely described in the literature, here we only present key aspects, which are important to explain some analogies between FIR filters and the GVM circuits. A general structure for a 1-D N^{th} order FIR filter is shown in Fig. 1. When an input signal, $X=\{x_0, x_1,\ldots, x_N\}$, is passing through a filter, particular samples, x_i, are stored in delay elements T. After multiplication by coefficients h_i , they are summed at the output. Thus, the output filter samples, y_i , are calculated using the following equation:

$$y_n = \sum_{i=0}^{N} h_i x_i \tag{1}$$

Various implementation techniques of FIR filters, both digital and analog, have been widely described in the literature. In existing implementations, usually only one output sample is calculated after each new sample enters the filter. In this paper, we propose a different approach where several output samples are calculated in parallel after receiving a certain input data block.

In 2-D filtering, an image frame is a 2-D signal, where pixels are samples of this signal in (x, y) image coordinates. In case of 2-D FIR filtering, particular input pixels (brightness) are multiplied by filter coefficients given by a 2-D mask and summed to produce output image samples. The principle mentioned is illustrated in Fig. 2 for an example (3x3) filter mask H. In this case, pixels of the output image, B, are calculated on the basis of the input image, A, using the following equation:

$$B(x, y) = \sum_{n=1}^{3}\sum_{m=1}^{3} A(x+n-2, y+m-2)h(n,m) \tag{2}$$

The lowpass filter mask, H, is often used in multirate systems to realize anti-aliasing or anti-imaging filtering. A highpass filtering, that is useful for example in detection of edges, requires a mechanism that enables realizing negative coefficients.

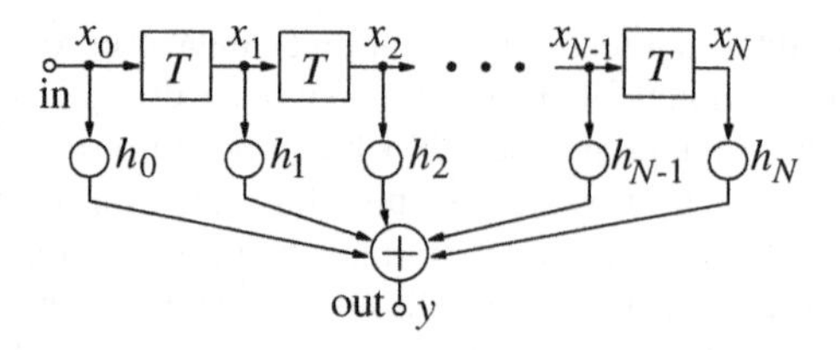

Fig. 1. Block diagram of a finite impulse response (FIR) filter

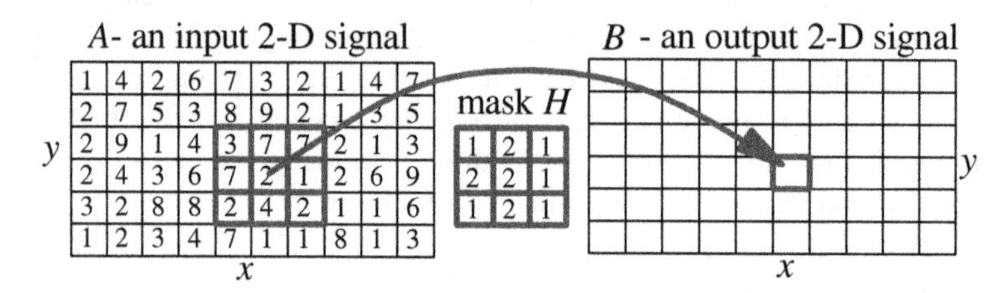

Fig. 2. Block Two-dimensional FIR image filtration [9]

3 Implementation of FIR Filters Using Gilbert Vector Multipliers

To realize the multiplication operations required in the filtration process, we propose to utilize so called Gilbert multiplier adapted to multiply two vectors [7]. Scheme of the adapted vector-by-vector Gilbert multiplier, denoted by GVM, is shown in Fig. 3 (a). One of the multiplied vectors (denoted by *X*) includes the currents I_{xi} while the other (denoted by *H)* the currents I_{hi}. In Fig. 3 (b) we have the Gilbert multiplier adapted for multiplying the vector *H* by the scalar I_x.

The vector-by-vector GVM block calculates components of a matrix denoted by *P*, which presents I_p currents resulting from multiplication of *X* and H^T, according to (3):

$$P = \frac{XH^{\mathrm{T}}}{\sum_{i=0}^{N} h_i} = X|H|^{\mathrm{T}} \quad \text{or} \quad P = \begin{bmatrix} x_0|h_0| & x_0|h_1| & x_0|h_2| & \cdots & x_0|h_N| \\ x_1|h_0| & x_1|h_1| & x_1|h_2| & \cdots & x_1|h_N| \\ x_2|h_0| & x_2|h_1| & x_2|h_2| & \cdots & x_2|h_N| \\ \vdots & \vdots & \vdots & \ddots & \vdots \\ x_M|h_0| & x_M|h_1| & x_M|h_2| & \cdots & x_M|h_N| \end{bmatrix} \tag{3}$$

It is worth noting that particular elements of the *P* matrix are divided by the sum of all components of the vector *H*, which enables an automatic normalization of *H*. The normalized vector *H* in (3) is denoted as |*H*|. Comparing equations 1 and 3 we see that all elements of the *P* matrix needed in equation 1 are situated along the matrix diagonal (provided that *X* represents input signals and *H* coefficients of the filter). The *H* normalization possibility is a very important superiority of our FIR filter realization over the ones reported earlier, based on scalar multipliers. This is because in our approach not absolute values but ratios of the currents forming the *H* vector are important, which simplifies the filter controlling significantly.

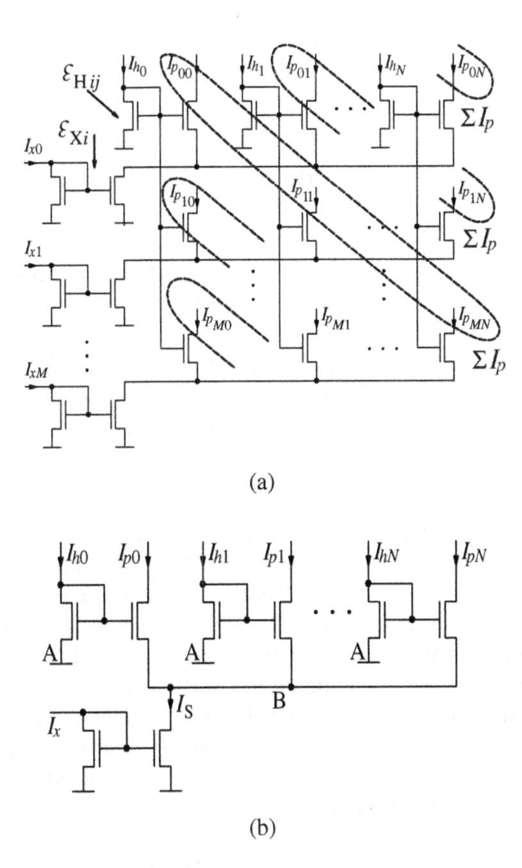

Fig. 3. Gilbert multipliers: (a) vector-by-vector multiplier (GVM) and (b) scalar-by-vector multiplier (GSVM)

One of the GVM multiplier features is that it also calculates other elements, which in the P matrix are placed off the diagonal. In a typical implementation of FIR filters, these currents would be treated as parasitic currents, which only increase the filter power consumption and are never used in calculations of the output samples. Assuming that both vectors, X and H, include the same number of components, i.e. $M = N$, a number of these off-diagonal currents is equal to $N{\cdot}(N\text{-}1)$. Then, the filter efficiency decreases hyperbolically with the filter order N. As the number of parasitic currents increases with a square of the filter order, N, the number of the currents equals about $1/N$.

Originality of our approach is that the P-matrix off-diagonal elements have been utilized in parallel calculations of other than the diagonal output samples, y, in order to increase the filtration speed and reduce a power consumption associated with one sample (improve power per sample efficiency). To explain the principle of our method, consider an example GVM block where N=4 and M=4. In a given k^{th} cycle, where the cycle starts with introducing a new set of M input samples, the GVM block calculates $N{\cdot}M$ of new elements $p_{n,m}$. These elements are used in calculations of the following signals:

$$
\begin{aligned}
y_{0,1}(k) &= x_0h_0+x_1h_1+x_2h_2+x_3h_3 \mid y_{0,2}(k)=0 \\
y_{1,1}(k) &= x_0h_1+x_1h_2+x_2h_3 \mid y_{1,2}(k)=x_3h_0 \\
y_{2,1}(k) &= x_0h_2+x_1h_3 \mid y_{2,2}(k)= x_2h_0+x_3h_1 \\
y_{3,1}(k) &= x_0h_3 \mid y_{3,2}(k)=x_1h_0+x_2h_1+x_3h_2
\end{aligned} \tag{4}
$$

Note, that the first sum, $y_{0,1}(k)$, is a complete output sample from equation 1. The GVM block calculates also partial sums $y_{m,1}(k)$, which will be used in calculations of other output samples in the next $(k + 1)$ cycle. The block calculates also partial sums $y_{m,2}(k)$, which in a kth cycle supplement the partial sums $y_{m,1}(k - 1)$ calculated in the previous cycle, creating in the same time next complete output samples. In general, in a kth cycle, the following samples are generated concurrently:

$$y_m(k)= y_{m,1}(k-1)+ y_{m,2}(k),\ m = 0, .. , M \tag{5}$$

In our approach, all elements from the P matrix are utilized in the calculations, i.e. there are no parasitic currents which are useless. It is worth noting that the case when $N>M$ makes no sense from the practical point of view because the number of samples must be not lower than the number of filter coefficients. The main advantage of our technique is that in one cycle, which lasts M / f_S [s], we calculate M signal samples concurrently. As a result, the GVM block has sufficient time (M times more than the sampling period duration) for calculating the new P matrix. As a result, the GVM block can work with significantly smaller currents, which means power saving. Another question is, how to solve in practice the problem of introducing the parallel data in a cyclical pattern. This problem is discussed in the following sections.

3.1 Implementation Issues of the Proposed 1-D Filter

In the previous section, a conception of cyclic delivering parallel data has been outlined. In practical implementations, however, some problems occur. The most important of them is storing partial sums created in the previous cycle. Using intermediate analog memory cells to store partial sums is not a proper solution. This is because values of particular sums may differ significantly when particular sums contain a different number of the P-matrix elements.

Nonlinear properties of analog memories cause the final output samples to have different DC levels. In addition, the DC levels depend on temperature, which makes an easy level correction impossible. We have decided to solve this problem in a different way. Instead of using an N x M dimension GVM multiplier block, a block with an N x $2M$ resolution was applied. The proposed circuit is shown in Fig. 4 together with the required clock phases. In this solution, the number of sample-and-hold (S&H) elements is doubled, but all output samples are calculated under equal conditions and their DC levels are the same for each output sample. As a consequence, there are two groups of outputs that are read-out alternately.

The filter has been implemented in a TSMC CMOS 180-nm technology and verified using HSPICE post-layout simulations. Transfer properties of the filter can be controlled by means of currents collected in the H vector and different transfer functions can be realized depending on the current values. Results of simulations in time

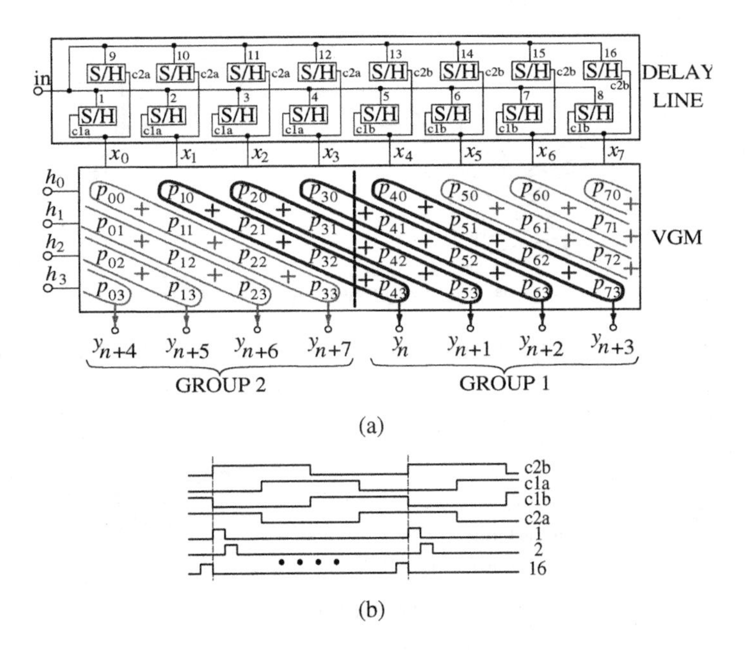

Fig. 4. Example of a 8x4 1-D GVM FIR filter: (a) general structure (b) clock generator

domain, concerning passband and stopband of an example filter, are shown in Fig. 5. Frequency-domain amplitude-characteristics of the filter are shown in Fig. 6 for two cases, i.e. for H={1/4, 1/4, 1/4, 1/4} (currents: 200, 200, 200, 200 nA) and H={1/8, 3/8, 3/8 1/8} (currents: 200, 600, 600, 200 nA).

As can be seen from Fig. 6, for some frequencies the simulated attenuation is about 55 dB. This value, however, is achievable provided that transistors used to build the current mirrorshave equal dimensions. In real applications, various mismatch components affect the filter performance. Variations in the transistor threshold voltage, V_{TH}, are usually regarded as the main reason for the mismatch problem. As a result, relation between input and output currents in the mirror is given by [7]:

$$I_{\mathrm{out}} = I_{in}(1+\varepsilon) \tag{6}$$

where: ε is a zero-mean Gaussian random variable that results from the threshold voltage mismatch [7]. Taking (6) into account, particular elements in the P-matrix can be described as:

$$p_{ij} = \frac{x_i(1+\varepsilon_{\mathrm{X}i})\cdot h_j(1+\varepsilon_{\mathrm{H}ij})}{\sum_{k=0}^{N} h_k(1+\varepsilon_{\mathrm{H}ik})} \tag{7}$$

For a properly designed layout, with sufficiently large transistor dimensions, the mirror gain variation is kept below 2 % [8]. To perform analysis for the worst case scenario, values of particular ε variables in equation 7 have been selected to be equal to

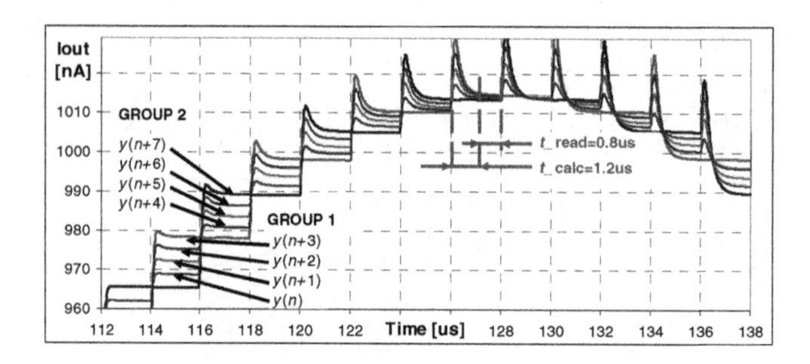

Fig. 5. Filter's output signal in the passband for f_S=2 MHz, and input data frequency 10 kHz

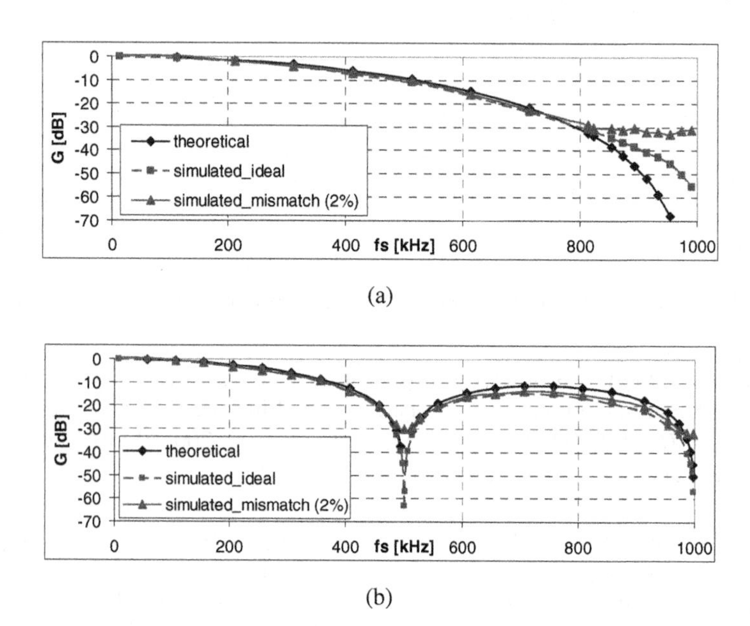

Fig. 6. Simulated and theoretical filter transmittances: (a) H=[1/4 1/4 1/4 1/4] (b) H=[1/8 3/8 3/8 1/8]

+/- 2%. As sum of all filter coefficients is equal to one, the maximum (worst case) error level introduced by the mismatch is not greater than approximately (MAX(ε))·2, i.e. not greater than about 4% in our case. This has been verified for several transfer functions and for different distributions of mismatch components in the P matrix. In most of the tested cases (roughly 70%), the attenuation was larger than 30-dB, which in case of color picture filtering means a possible color depth of 4-5 bits. Such a value is sufficient in many diagnostic tasks and other applications of the filters [10]. This is worth noting that values of ε parameters are for a given chip constant, resulting in systematic errors that load particular p components, which can be corrected at the digital side, after device calibration.

4 Implementation of 2-D Programmable Image Filter

General idea as well as initial results concerning an image filter considered in this section have been presented in [9]. In some respects, the filter is similar to the 1-D FIR one described in the previous sections. Its basic block, like in the 1-D filter, is a GSVM circuit shown in Fig. 3, for which the following expression holds:

$$P_{xy} = \frac{I_{xy} H^{\mathrm{T}}}{\sum_{i=0}^{N} h_i} = I_{xy} |H|^{\mathrm{T}} \tag{8}$$

Each input signal (pixel) in a vision system is associated with one GSVM circuit, which calculates currents, I_p, that are products of a given input sample, $A(x, y)$, at the I_{xy} input, and a H vector. Length of the output vector, P_{xy}, is determined by the number of coefficients, whose values are unique. For example, for the lowpass filter mask shown in Fig. 2, length of the P_{xy} vector equals 2 only, as this mask contains only two distinguished coefficients, namely 1 and 2. To simplify the filter analysis, it is convenient to present particular vectors, P_{xy}, as if they were columns of a 3-D P-matrix with p_{xyz} elements, which is shown in Fig. 7. In such a case, the x and y coordinates indicate a given input pixel, $A(x,y)$, while the z coordinate indicates a given product of this pixel and a given filter coefficient. To calculate the output image, B, particular elements of the P matrix must be summed in a proper way.

If the mask size is N x M, in calculations of $N \cdot M$ output samples, $B(x, y)$, elements of each P_{xy} vector are used. In our image programmable filter, to enable a realization of different filter masks, each p_{xyz} product is copied into $N \cdot M$ independent output branches, using PMOS current mirrors. This is shown in Fig. 8. The block presented in Fig.8 is associated with each input signal. As a result, the I_{xy} signal is multiplied by the I_h coefficients, using the GSVM circuit. There are two types of the circuit outputs denoted in Fig. 8 by (-) and (+). Currents in the (-) branches are used to create negative coefficients by means of the "b" circuit of Fig. 8. In this circuit, all products representing the samples to be multiplied by negative coefficients are summed in one node and then are subtracted from the sum of the products representing samples multiplied by positive coefficients. A problem may occur when the first sum becomes larger than the second one. Then, an additional biasing I_{DC} current is added to the output signal. Our approach is a very simple solution to this problem as only one additional NMOS current mirror per each output pixel has to be applied. The required map of connections is programmed using a 4-dimensional matrix D. The first two dimensions (x and y) in D indicate a given output pixel, while the 3rd one indicates the p element to be used in calculating a given sample $B(x, y)$. The 4th dimension of D indicates, whether the product must be added of subtracted at the output. Note that only particular elements, d, of this matrix control given switches in each circuit of Fig. 8. This means that to program a 2-D image filter with any resolution, only one D matrix is necessary.

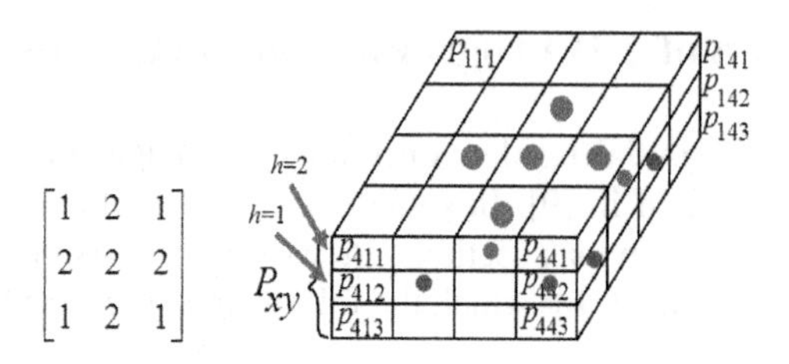

Fig. 7. Simulated and theoretical filter transmittances: (a) H=[1/4 1/4 1/4 1/4] (b) H=[1/8 3/8 3/8 1/8]

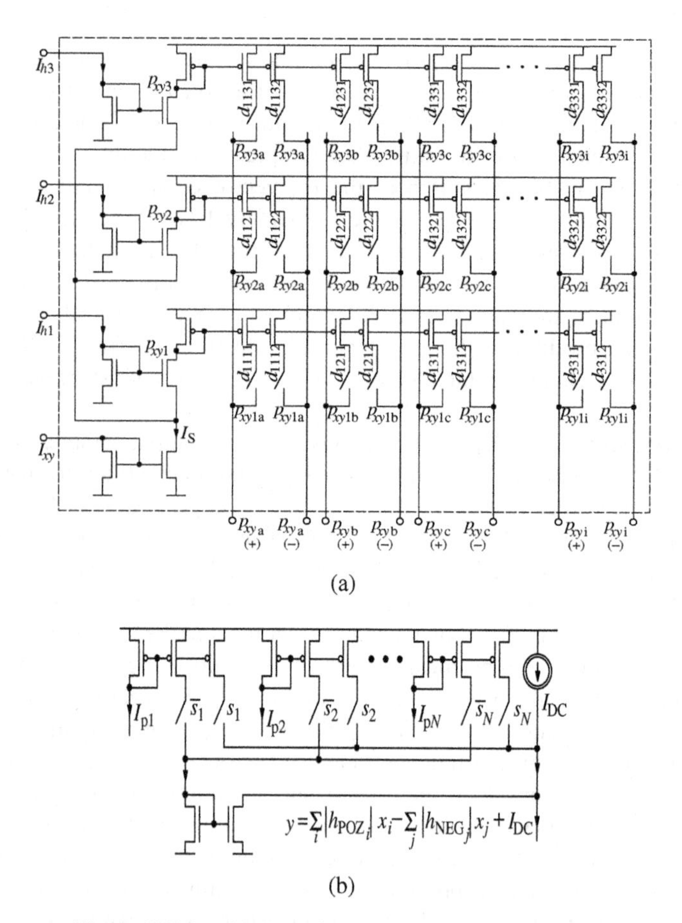

Fig. 8. GVM multiplier suited for parallel image filtration

The connection map is constructed in a way that enables fully parallel data processing, where all output pixels are calculated in the same time. This means an increase in the data processing rate (important advantage). Furthermore, the D matrix is setting up only ones (at the beginning). Then, the filter works asynchronously without the clock generator (another advantage).

Table 1. Input and output signals in the designed image filter for small input currents

In and out No.	A1/B1	A2/B2	A3/B3	A4/B4	A5/B5	A6/B6
Input [nA]	200	200	200/250	200/270	200/300	200
Theoretical out [nA]	400	650	720	820	770	500
Post-layout simulations [nA]	***296***	354.2	365.9	382	373.4	***312***
Normalized output [nA]	***285***	649	722	822	768	***385***
Error [%]	***28.87***	0.20	-0.21	-0.22	0.23	***23.05***

Table 2. Input and output signals in the designed image filter for larger input currents

In and out No.	A1/B1	A2/B2	A3/B3	A4/B4	A5/B5	A6/B6
Input [nA]	2000	2000	2000/2500	2000/2700	2000/3000	2000
Theoretical out [nA]	4000	6500	7200	8200	7700	5000
Post-layout simulations [nA]	***2770***	3283	3372	3492	3426	***2893***
Normalized output [nA]	***2202***	6481	7224	8225	7674	***3228***
Error [%]	***44.95***	0.29	-0.33	-0.30	0.34	***35.44***

To experimentally test the proposed idea, a 2-D FIR image filter has been implemented in a 0.18 μm CMOS process. The image resolution in the designed filter was 6 x 1, while a resolution of the filter masks was 3 x 1, which is sufficient to verify the proposed filter concept. In this paper, post-layout simulation results are presented. In our simulations, presence of parasitic elements, such as unwanted node capacitances and signal path resistances, was taken into account. The obtained results confirm the observation made in [9] that the proposed circuit exhibits a low sensitivity to parasitic elements.

From our studies it follows that the filter operates correctly for a wide range of the input current values. Experimental results obtained for $H = [1, 1, 1]$ (filter mask) and for different average values of the input currents are presented in Tables 1 and 2. To enable investigating dynamic features of our filter, the input image, A, was varied in time. The A1, A2 and A6 input samples were constant during the whole test while the others (A3, A4 and A5) oscillated not exciding values 200 and 300 nA in the case of Table 1, and between 2000 and 3000 nA in the case of Table 2 (second row in both Tables). Theoretical values of the output pixels are gathered in the 3rd row while real values of them in the 4th one.

To make a comparison between the theoretical and experimental results to be more clear, the latter have been normalized in such a way to obtain comparable values of the theoretical and experimental currents (rows 5 in both tables). Differences (errors) between these signals are given in the last row of each table. Notice that average errors in the columns 2, 3, 4, and 5 and are much below 1%. This is a regularity observed for different input images and filter masks as well. On the other hand, errors concerning the B1 and B6 outputs (columns 1 and 6) are much larger than 1%, due to a border effect, which is associated with the fact that these samples are calculated using only two input signals.

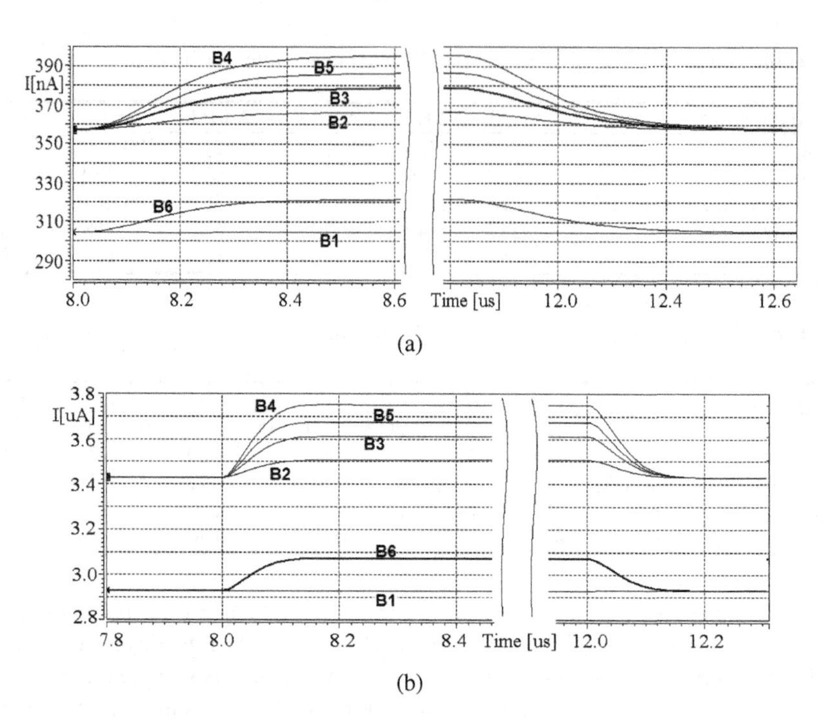

Fig. 9. Time domain post-layout simulations for input signals from (a) Table 1 and (b) Table 2

Dynamic parameters, like a maximum data rate, can be assessed on the basis of time-domain results shown in Fig. 9 (for currents given in Tables 1 and 2). All output samples are calculated in parallel. In the case of higher currents (bottom), time required to calculate the output image is about 7 times shorter than in the low-current case (upper). Power consumption equals to about 7μW in the first case and 70 μW in the second one. The power increase gives, fortunately, a shorter calculation time. Since our filter works in an asynchronous way, energy per one pixel is the right measure characterizing the power aspect. In both cases the energy per pixel is almost the same and equals approximately 1 pJ.

5 Multirate Systems Realized Using the GVM FIR Filters

The proposed GVM filters can be used in power-efficient multirate signal processing. The idea of decimation and interpolation systems has already been presented for a 1-D FIR filter case. Decimation consists in down-sampling in the input signal preceded by an antialiasing lowpass filtering. Our GVM filter calculates N+1 output samples in parallel. Decimation in this case is simply realized by selecting one or more output samples y. Superiority of such an approach over typical solutions is that samples at the filter output are available within a time period equal to $(M+1) / f_S$ [s], while in typical multirate systems within a time period equal to $1 / f_S$ [s] only. As a result, the subsequent block in the system, that gets the GVM filter output signal, does not need to be as fast as in typical solutions.

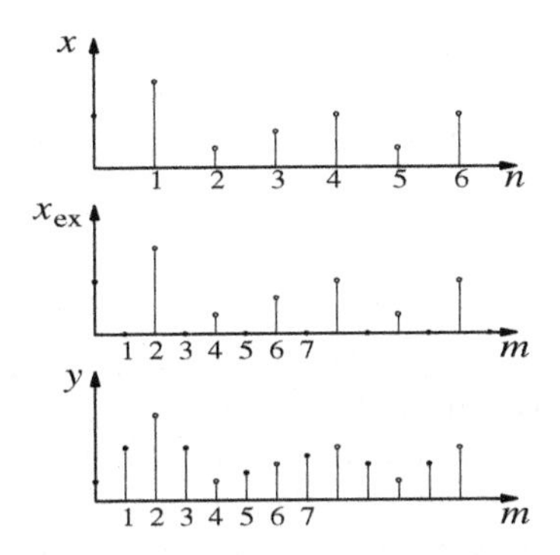

Fig. 10. Interpolation principle: x - input signal, x_{ex} - signal beyond expander, y - output signal

Interpolation by a non-fractional up-sampling factor, K, consists of two stages, as illustrated in Fig. 10. In the first stage, K-1 uniformly spaced zero-valued samples are placed between each pair of samples of the input signal x, shown in the upper diagram, producing the signal x_{ex} – the expander output – shown in the middle diagram. In the next stage, the anti-imaging lowpass filter is used to eliminate undesired spectrum components, which occur in the signal after the up-sampling operation, producing the signal, y, that is shown in the bottom diagram.

In a typical approach, the anti-imaging filter operates with the sampling frequency of the output signal, which is K-times higher than the input sampling frequency [11]. As the proposed GVM filter calculates the p products in parallel, the interpolation is simply realized by summing only selected products p. For example, consider the example 8x4 GVM filter shown in Fig. 4 and assume that anti-imaging filter has the coefficients $h = \{1,\ 2,\ 1\}$ and an up-sampling factor $K = 2$. The output signal (y) shown in Fig. 10 can be calculated using the expander output signal, x_{ex}, like in the equation 9(a) or using the expander input signal, x, like in equation 9(b), which can be simplified to the form 9(c).

$$\text{(a)}\quad \begin{aligned} y_1 &= x_{ex2}h_0 + 0\cdot h_1 + x_{ex0}h_2 \\ y_2 &= 0\cdot h_0 + x_{ex2}\cdot h_1 + 0\cdot h_2 \\ y_3 &= x_{ex4}h_0 + 0\cdot h_1 + x_{ex2}h_2 \\ y_4 &= 0\cdot h_0 + x_{ex4}\cdot h_1 + 0\cdot h_2 \\ &\dots \end{aligned} \qquad \text{(b)}\quad \begin{aligned} y_1 &= x_1h_0 + 0\cdot h_1 + x_0h_2 = x_1h_0 + x_0h_2 \\ y_2 &= 0\cdot h_0 + x_1\cdot h_1 + 0\cdot h_2 = x_1\cdot h_1 \\ y_3 &= x_2h_0 + 0\cdot h_1 + x_1h_2 = x_2h_0 + x_1h_2 \\ y_4 &= 0\cdot h_0 + x_2\cdot h_1 + 0\cdot h_2 = x_2\cdot h_1 \\ &\dots \end{aligned}$$

$$\text{(c)}\quad \begin{aligned} y_1 &= x_1h_0 + x_0h_2 \\ y_2 &= x_1\cdot h_1 \\ y_3 &= x_2h_0 + x_1h_2 \\ y_4 &= x_2\cdot h_1 \\ &\dots \end{aligned} \qquad (9)$$

P matrix of the GVM shown in Fig. 4 contains all necessary products required to calculate output samples, y, in parallel. In this case, at least eight samples can be calculated on the basis of this matrix. An advantage of this approach is that such an anti-imaging filter still works with the sampling frequency of the x input signal and not with the K-times higher sampling frequency of the expander, like in typical systems of this type. Thus, our solution is power efficient (important advantage).

6 Conclusions

New 1-D and 2-D analog current-mode FIR filters have been proposed in this paper. The main block in our filters is the Gilbert vector multiplier (GVM), which enables an automatic normalization of filter coefficients represented by vector of currents. The filter transfer function depends only on relationships between particular currents (current ratios) and not on the current values. Normalization performed in the GVM block allows for keeping the filter gain stable and equal to one. This is of prime importance in the filtration tasks. Our filers are characterized by concurrent data processing and lead to power economic implementations of multirate systems.

To verify the proposed idea, two filters have been design in a CMOS 0.18 μm technology The first circuit is a 1-D 3rd-order filter. Operating with a sampling frequency of 2 MHz it dissipates power of 8 μW. Attenuation observed in post-layout HSICE simulations reaches the level of about 55 dB. Theoretical analysis concerning an influence of the transistor-threshold-voltage mismatch on the filter properties shows that even in the worst case scenario, attenuation higher than 30-dB can be achieved. This makes the 1-D filter to be attractive in many low-precision applications.

The second circuit presented in this paper is an asynchronous image processor. The processor calculates all output pixels in a parallel way and requires no clock generator. This is an important advantage because clock generators are a typical source of feedthrough noises. An image resolution in this experimental circuit is 6 x 1, while a filter mask has resolution of 3 x 1. An effective data rate depends on values of input signals. For example, for a power dissipation of 7 μW and an average level of input currents equal to about 300 nA, the possible data rate equals 1 Mframes/s, while for a power dissipation of 70 μW, the data rate is 7 Mframes/s. Energy consumption per a single pixel is as low as 1 pJ. Another significant advantage of the processor is that the number of frames per a given time unit does not depend on the image resolution. This feature allows for implementing very large and low power image processors operating with a very high data rate. It is possibly, for instance, to build a circuit with the resolution of 100x100 pixels (10000 pixels in parallel every 1 μs), which will dissipate a power of about 10-20 mW only. The effective data rate in this case will be equal to about 60-70 Gbit/s. The filter is easily programmable by means of only several bits and several DC currents. Both lowpass and high-pass filters can be realized using our approach.

References

1. Długosz, R., Iniewski, K.: Flexible Architecture of Ultra-Low-Power Current-Mode Interleaved Successive Approximation Analog-To-Digital Converter for Wireless Sensor Networks. Hindavi VLSI design (2007)

2. Tanner, S., Heubi, A., Ansorge, M., Pellandini, F.: An 8-bit low-power ADC array for CMOS image sensors. In: 1998 IEEE International Conference on Electronics, Circuits and Systems, September 1998, vol. 1, pp. 147–150 (1998)
3. Linan, G., Foldesy, P., Espejo, S., Dominguez-Castro, R., Rodriguez-Vazquez, A.: A 0.5 μm CMOS 106 transistors analog programmable array processor for real–time image processing. In: 25th European Solid-State Circuits Conference (ESSCIRC), pp. 358–361 (1999)
4. Alini, R., et al.: A 200-MSample/S Trellis-Coded PRML Read/Write Channel With Analog Adaptive Equalizer and Digital Servo. IEEE Journal of Solid-State Circuits 32(11), 1824–1838 (1997)
5. Brown, J.E.C., Hurst, P.J., Rothenberg, B.C., Lewis, S.H.: A CMOS Adaptive Continuous-Time Forward Equalizer, LPF, and RAM-DFE for Magnetic Recording. IEEE Journal of Solid-State Circuits 34(2), 162–169 (1999)
6. Vahidfarl, M.B., Shoaei, O., Fardis, M.: A Low Power, Transverse Analog FIR Filter for Feed Forward Equalization of Gigabit Ethernet. In: IEEE International Symposium on Circuits and Systems (ISCAS), Kos Greece (2006)
7. Winstead, C.: Analog Iterative Error Control Decoders, Ph.D dissertation. University of Alberta, ECE Department, Edmonton, Alberta (2004)
8. Croon, J.A., Rosmeulen, M., Decoutere, S., Sansen, W., Maes, H.E.: An easy-to-use mismatch model for the MOS transistor. IEEE Journal of Solid-State Circuits 37(8), 1056–1064 (2002)
9. Długosz, R.: Analog, Continuous Time, Fully Parallel, Programmable Image Processor Based in Vector Gilbert Multiplier. Paper submitted to International Conference Mixed Design of Integrated Circuits and Systems (MIXDES), Poland (June 2007)
10. Hoffmann, H.: Perception through visuomotor anticipation in a mobile robot. Neural Networks 20(1), 22–33 (2007)
11. Vaidyanathan, P.P.: Multirate systems and filter banks. Prentice Hall, Englewood Cliffs (1993)

Biomedical Image Segmentation Based on Aggregated Morphological Spectra

Juliusz L. Kulikowski[1], Małgorzata Przytulska[2], and Diana Wierzbicka[3]

[1,2,3] Institute of Biocybernetics and Biomedical Engineering, Polish Academy of Sciences, 4 Ks. Trojdena Str, 02-109 Warsaw, Poland
jlkulik@ibib.waw.pl, gosia@ibib.waw.pl, diana@ibib.waw.pl

Abstract. It is described a method of biomedical images segmentation by discrimination of textures based on their morphological spectra. Basic notions concerning morphological spectra are given. Their properties making possible to characterize basic morphological structures independently on spatial orientation or shifts of the analyzed specimens are described. It is shown that spectral components can be chosen and used in aggregated form so as to make discrimination of textures invariant with respect to scale changing and to basic geometrical image transformations. Analysis of two types of biomedical images: aorta tissue and pancreas tissue, based on comparison of histograms of selected spectral components values illustrate the methods presented in the paper.

1 Introduction

Image segmentation is one of preliminary steps to computer-aided biomedical image processing. It is aimed at a selection of a limited number of regions of interest (*ROI*) for a deeper analysis within a research or a medical diagnostic procedure. Effective image segmentation reduces the image area subjected to examination and, as a consequence, it reduces the total time consumption of image analysis. Two basic approaches to image segmentation can be mentioned. The first one concerns images with well-visible and easily contoured objects of interest (e.g. X-ray images with distinct bone structures). In such case standard (say, luminance-gradient based) object contouring methods to image segmentation can be used. Another approach is needed if ill-visible, smooth objects are of interest. In such case image segmentation on more sophisticated objects' contours detection methods should be based. The contours of segments then can be considered as lines separating adjacent image areas covered by different textures. However, this approach needs at least two problems to be explained: 1st what is a texture, and 2nd what is a distance measure between two different textures. Various answers to the above-given questions can be found in the literature [1,4]. In this paper texture is considered as a pattern, homogenous due to its morphological, spectral or statistical features, covering a compact image area and visualizing the surface properties of an examined object. The definition is intuitive rather than a formal one. Moreover, it suggests that a lot of methods of texture analysis, according to the formal models describing the patterns, can be used. In fact, various morphological, spectral, Markov chains or fields based, statistical, fractal and many other methods have been presented in literature [1,2,3,4]. According to [1], a great deal

E. Kącki, M. Rudnicki, J. Stempczyńska (Eds.): Computers in Medical Activity, AISC 65, pp. 101–112.
springerlink.com

(about 53%) of papers concerning texture analysis is devoted to statistical and about 11% to morphological methods. Despite the fact that most of them are universal, no strongly optimal texture analysis method can be distinguished. However, in any given application area or for any given class of textures some effective texture analysis methods can be recommended.

When choosing a suitable texture analysis method the following general texture properties should be taken into account:

1. Single- vs. multi-level structure of the type of pattern constituting the given texture;
2. Dependence vs. invariance of the texture with respect to:

   * Geometrical transformations:
     * Scale changing,
     * Parallel shifting (horizontal, vertical),
     * Rotation,
   * Photo-optical transformations:
     * Mean luminance changing,
     * Contrast changing,
     * Color changing;
3. Existence of any other characteristic texture features to be taken into account.

The below-presented texture analysis, on morphological spectra based method, among the morphological and partially statistical methods can be counted. Basic concepts of morphological spectra (*MS*) and of their hierarchical structure have been described in [5,6]. Invariance to geometrical transformations of morphological spectra based texture analysis are presented in [7]. This paper is an extended version of a presentation delivered to a Conference on Computers in Medical Activity in Lodz, 2007. It is focused on theoretical and practical aspects of using *MS* to discriminate textures for image segmentation. In the next Section basic notions concerning *MS* are shortly presented. Then a principle of uncertainty in discrimination of textures is formulated. The effects of textures discrimination by using combined components of morphological spectra are illustrated by several examples. In the last Section final conclusions are given.

2 Basic Notions of Morphological Spectra

Monochromatic images are here assumed to be given in the form of a rectangular bitmaps:

$$S^{(0)} = \begin{bmatrix} x_{11} & x_{12} & x_{13} & x_{14} & \ldots \\ x_{21} & x_{22} & x_{23} & x_{24} & \ldots \\ x_{31} & x_{32} & x_{33} & x_{34} & \ldots \\ x_{41} & x_{42} & x_{43} & x_{44} & \ldots \\ \ldots & \ldots & \ldots & \ldots & \ldots \end{bmatrix} \quad (1)$$

x_{ij} being integers denoting pixel values (brightness levels) within an interval $[0, 2^K-1]$, K being a fixed natural number. It is also assumed that the size of image frame is $I \times J$ where I and J denote, respectively, the number of rows and columns of the image. For the sake of simplicity it is also assumed that $I = 2^p$, $J = 2^q$ where p, q are some natural numbers. Formally, $S^{(0)}$ will be considered as a 0-th level (initial) *MS*.

Higher-level *MS* are defined as ordered collections of 2^{2n} numerical matrices of $2^{p-n} \times 2^{q-n}$ size called n-th level spectral components of the image. Therefore, it is assumed that for any fixed p, q an inequality $n \leq min(p,q)$ limiting the highest *MS* level holds. Each collection of the above-mentioned matrices is called a n-th level *MS* and it is denoted by $S^{(n)}$, $n = 0,1,2,\ldots, n_{max}$. Spectral components' notations are coded (and, if necessary, lexicographically ordered) using a 4-elements alphabet (Σ, H, V, X). This makes it possible to present the system of *MS* components in the form of a hierarchical tree as shown in Fig. 1.

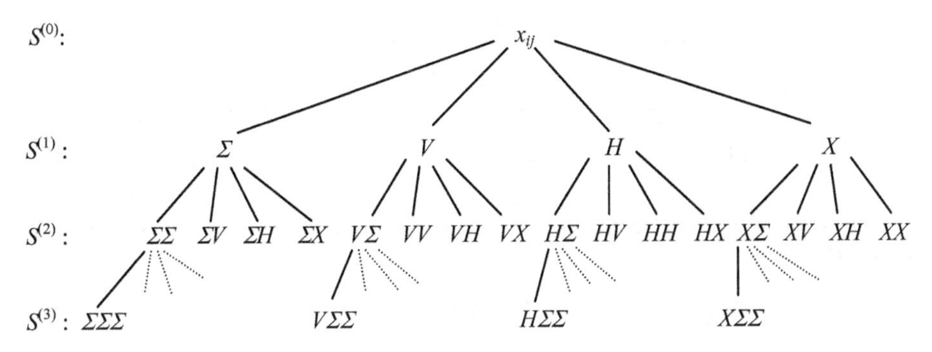

Fig. 1. Tree of morphological spectral components

For calculation of the elements of a given n-th level spectral component the original image $S^{(0)}$ is divided into 2^{p+q-2n} square windows of $2^n \times 2^n$ size called n-th level basic windows. The given spectral components' value is calculated as a linear algebraic function of values of pixels covered by the corresponding basic window. In the given image, textures are analyzed and recognized within testing areas being some compact subsets of pairwise adjacent basic windows of the n_{max} level. The image partition into basic windows of a fixed level and testing areas is illustrated in Fig. 2; the minimum (lowest level) squares correspond there to single pixels.

For the sake of simplicity it will be assumed below that testing areas are rectangular, consisting of $r \times s$ basic windows of the highest level $N = n_{max}$. Of course, it should be $r \cdot 2^N \leq I$, $s \cdot 2^N \leq J$. Such assumptions correspond to the case of image segmentation when testing areas can not fixed in advance.

Calculation of spectral components is simplified if so-called component masks are used. A component mask is a square matrix of the size corresponding to this of a basic window of the given level. The elements of component masks are +1 or –1; they are interpreted as weights assigned to the corresponding pixels in the basic window covered by the mask. Then the spectral component is calculated as a weighted sum of pixel values within the given basic window. In particular, the masks corresponding to the four spectral components of $S^{(1)}$ are numerical matrices of size 2×2 of the form graphically presented in Fig. 3. where □ stands for +1 and ν for –1.

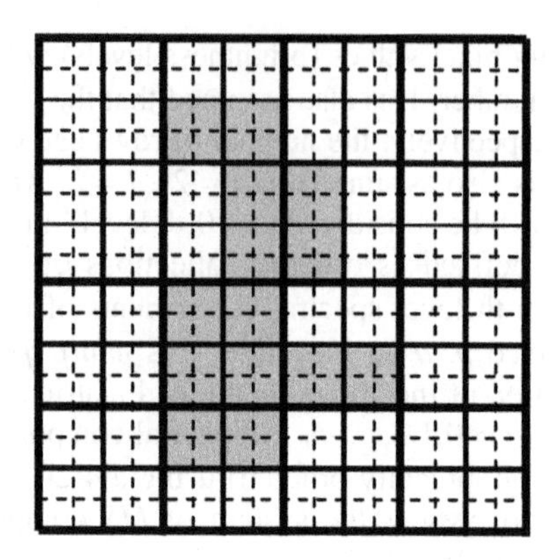

Fig. 2. Image partition into 2 × 2 basic windows and selection of a testing area (grey)

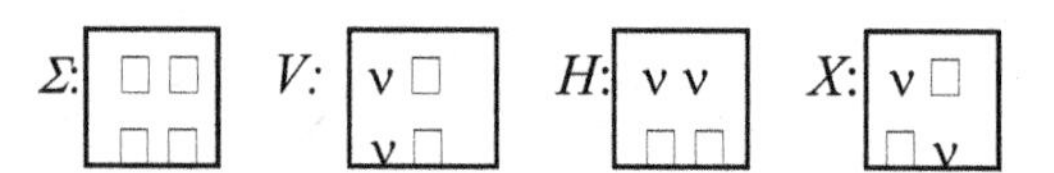

Fig. 3. Masks for calculation of the $S^{(1)}$ spectral components

The way of spectral components calculation using the above-given masks is illustrated below:

A bitmap:

5	8
6	4

Calculations:

$$s_\Sigma = 5 + 8 + 6 + 4 = 23,$$
$$s_V = -5 + 8 - 6 + 4 = 1,$$
$$s_H = -5 - 8 + 6 + 4 = -3,$$
$$s_X = -5 + 8 + 6 - 4 = 5.$$

MS:

23	1
–3	5

In certain applications the weights assigned to the *Σ*-component may be ¼ instead of 1; this leads to normalized *MS* avoiding dealing with large values of the *Σ, ΣΣ, ΣΣΣ*, etc. components. Full collections of masks for calculation of *MS* of the 2nd level have been given in [5], higher (up to 4th) level masks are available in the form of unpublished reports. It is convenient to present the higher-level *SM* in the form of hierarchically ordered matrices. For example, for $S^{(2)}$ it takes the form:

$$S^{(2)} = \begin{bmatrix} \begin{bmatrix} \Sigma\Sigma & \Sigma V \\ \Sigma H & \Sigma X \end{bmatrix} & \begin{bmatrix} V\Sigma & VV \\ VH & VX \end{bmatrix} \\ \begin{bmatrix} H\Sigma & HV \\ HH & HX \end{bmatrix} & \begin{bmatrix} X\Sigma & XV \\ XH & XX \end{bmatrix} \end{bmatrix} \qquad (2)$$

However, taking into account that similar matrices should be calculated for any basic window of a given testing area, for a better visualization of the effects of morphological transformation it is better to collect all values of any given *MS* component in a table corresponding to the testing area or to the total original image. In the last case, $S^{(0)}$ will be represented on the n-th level by a collection of 2^{2n} matrices representing spatial distribution of the *MS* components' values, the size of each matrix being 2^n times lower than the size of $S^{(0)}$. The elements of such matrices of the n-th level can take, in general, values within the interval $[-n(2^k-1), n(2^K-1)]$ (excepting the Σ^n-type components that can take only non-negative values). In order to visualize the spatial distribution of the *MS* components' values it is thus necessary to transform the matrices so that the transformed values are represented by non-negative integers between 0 and 2^K-1. The corresponding transformation is thus given by the formula:

$$s' = C[\frac{s + 2^K - 1}{2n}] \quad (3)$$

where s denotes the spectral component value before transformation, s' – the corresponding value after transformation, and $C[x]$ denotes an integer part of x. The matrices of so transformed values s' will be called morphological maps of the given image.

As an illustration, two types of microscopic biomedical images: 1/ human aorta tissue, and b/ human pancreas tissue with selected morphological maps are presented in Fig, 4.

In the first row (the a/, b/ and c/ images) the sensitivity of the $V\Sigma$ and $H\Sigma$ morphological components to isotropic image orientation is visible. In the second row, corresponding to an anisotropic pancreas image, it can be observed that the $X\Sigma$ component

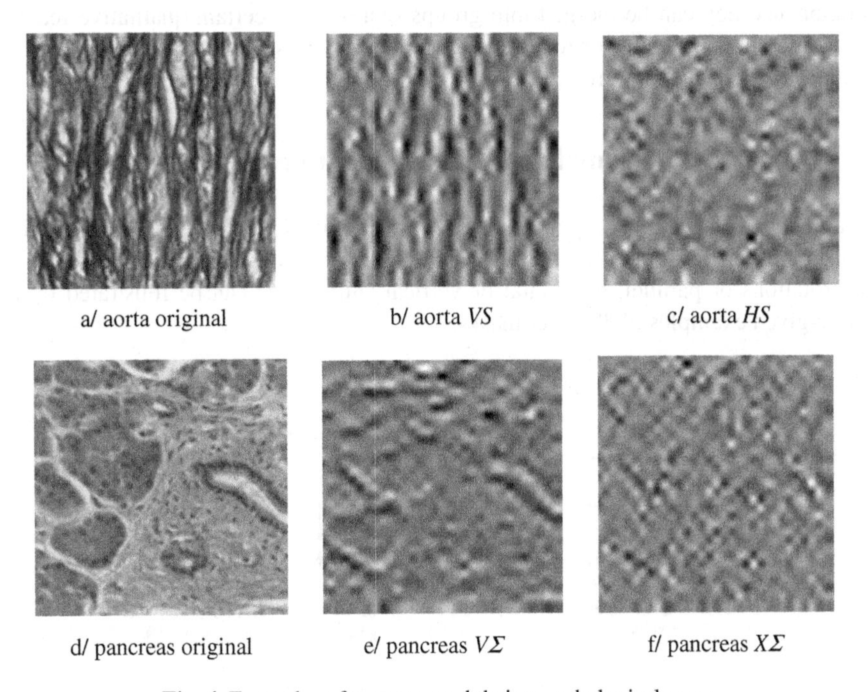

a/ aorta original b/ aorta *VS* c/ aorta *HS*

d/ pancreas original e/ pancreas $V\Sigma$ f/ pancreas $X\Sigma$

Fig. 4. Examples of textures an d their morphological maps

shows (better than the $V\Sigma$ one) the spatial distribution of lower-level image granularity, independently of the luminance level.

Any-level *MS* of an image makes it possible to reconstruct the original image. However, the effectiveness of the method of texture analysis based on *MS* depends on choosing:

* *MS*-level adequate to the mean size (granularity) of typical morphological structures constituting the texture under consideration,
* the most characteristic *MS* components of the texture,
* functional combinations of the selected components supporting effectiveness of texture discrimination.

Selection of *MS* components means that the primary information contained in $S^{(0)}$ is irreversibly compressed by rejection of some spectral components. Taking into account that the *n*-th level *MS*, $n = 1,2,3,\ldots,$ contains, in general, 4^n types of spectral components characterizing the contents of a basic window of 2^n x 2^n size, the *compression rate* η of a *MS*-based approach to the analysis of a given class of texture can be roughly defined as

$$\eta = 1 - 4^{-n}m \tag{4}$$

where m, $1 \leq m \leq 4^n$, denotes the number of spectral components (or based on them secondary parameters) that should be used in order to characterize the textures with a satisfying quality. It will be shown below that instead of neglecting some spectral components they can be merged into groups representing certain qualitative features substantial and sufficient for textures discrimination. by several examples. In the last Section final conclusions are given.

3 Invariance to Geometrical Transformations

Examination of spectral components' masks of any given *MS*-level show that some of them represent the same morphological structures within the groups of scale changing, rotations or parallel, horizontal or vertical shifts. This can be illustrated by the below-given examples of 3rd-level masks.

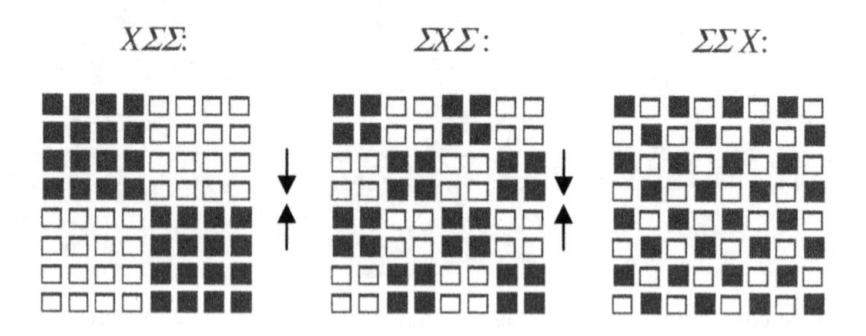

Fig. 5. Illustration of scale changing effects

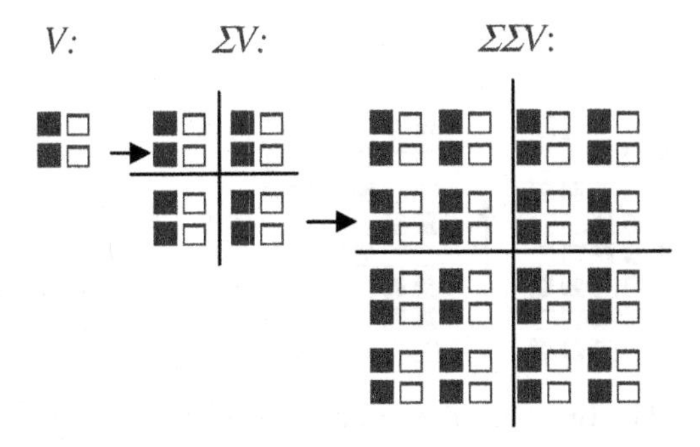

Fig. 6. Illustration of lower-level structures multiplication effect

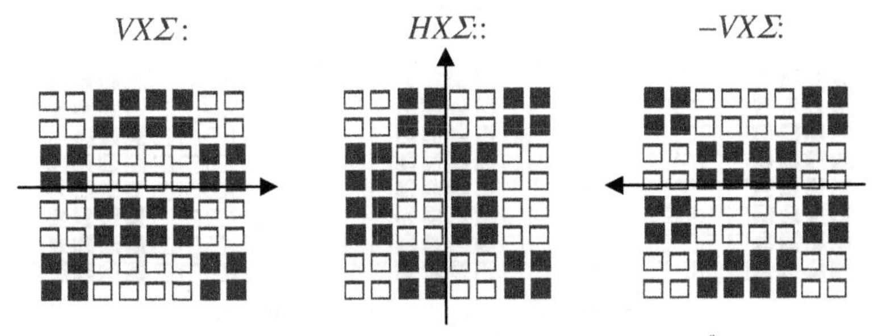

Fig. 7. Illustration of the effect of rotations by -90^0

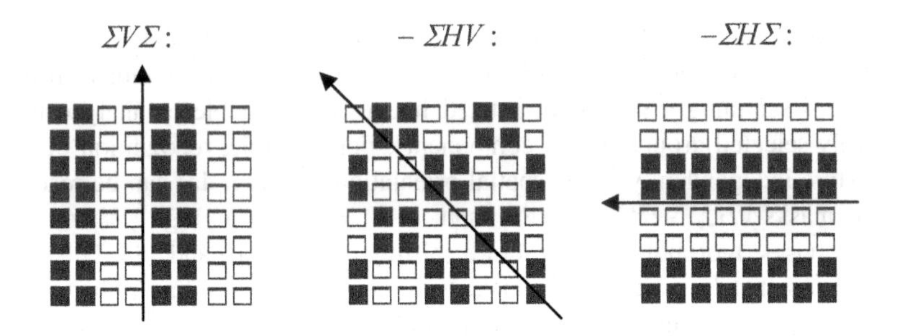

Fig. 8. Illustration of the effect of rotations by -45^0

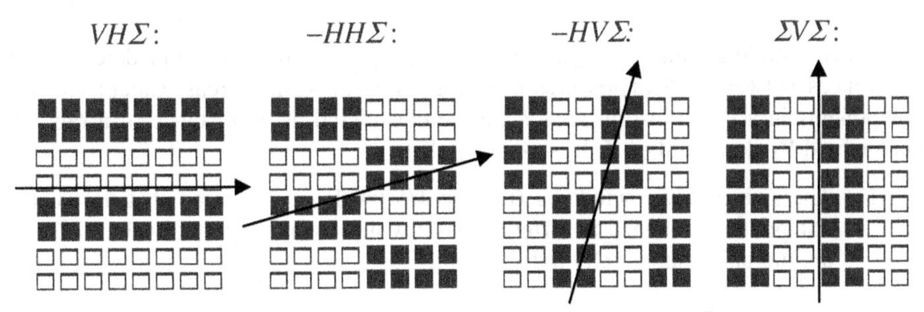

Fig. 9. Illustration of the effect of rotations by -30^0

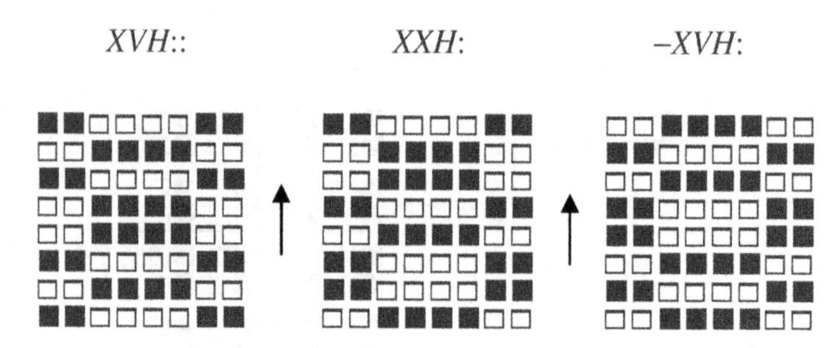

Fig. 10. Effects of vertical structure shifts by 2 pixels

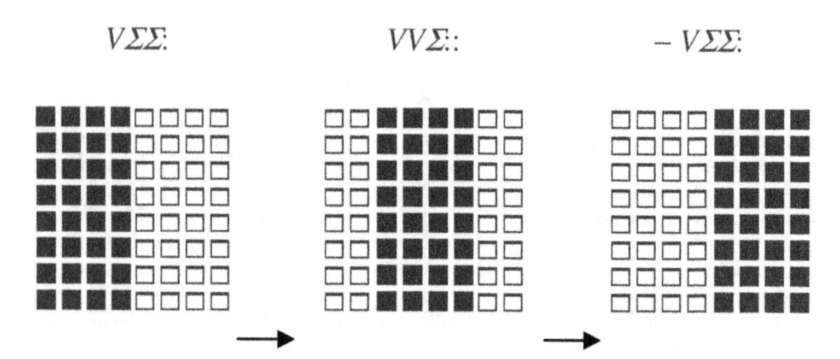

Fig. 11. Effects of horizontal structure shifts by 2 pixels

The above-presented *MS* properties give us an opportunity of making texture recognition invariant to certain types of image geometrical transformations. Instead of several times scanning a shifted or rotated image it is possible to analyze it using respectively selected groups of *MS* components. For example, recognition of an isotropic texture independently on its spatial orientation (see Fig. 4a) can be reached by using the masks $VH\Sigma$, $-HH\Sigma$, $-HV\Sigma$, and $\Sigma V\Sigma$, as shown in Fig. 9. Using a negative mask causes morphological structure shifting (see Fig. 10 and 11). This leads to the conclusion that for shifts-invariant texture recognition absolute rather than real values of *MS* components should be taken into consideration.

4 Image Segmentation Based on *MS* Discrimination

Generally speaking, image segmentation is based on comparison and detection of differences between *MS* of textures covering adjacent testing areas. Calculated *MS* components in a given testing area *T* can be considered as an instance of a random vector field $\mathbf{V}_T$ described on *T*. It is assumed that:

1) The size of basic windows (i.e. the *MS*-level) is chosen so that the vector components assigned to different basic windows (i.e. the local values of $\mathbf{V}_T$) are mutually statistically independent;

2) The size of T is such that the set of the MS components' values taken from the basic windows belonging to T form a statistically representative sample of V_T.

Under such assumptions discrimination of textures can be based on statistical analysis of histograms of MS components' values taken from the testing areas. Generally speaking, if T' and T'' are two different testing areas then the problem consists in verifying a non-parametric statistical hypothesis:

I. Statistical samples drawn from T' and T'' represent the same statistical population,

versus:

II. Statistical samples drawn from T' and T'' represent different statistical populations.

The testing areas T' and T'' can be merged within a common segment $T' \cup T''$ if hypothesis I is valid on a sufficient credibility level [7]. There is a lot of non-parametric statistical tests leading to the solution of the above-formulated problem [8]. In the simplest case a comparison of basic statistical parameters calculated on the basis of compared histograms can be used. This can be observed on the below shown histograms of two MS components ($X\Sigma$ and $V\Sigma$) of *aorta* tissue presented in comparable scales: a concentration of $X\Sigma$ component values around 0 is caused by the fact that their spatial variations within the given (32×32 pixels) testing area are random in nature and represent low-level image granularity. On the other hand, large values of the $V\Sigma$ components indicate a substantial role of this MS being played by this component in the fibrous texture representation. However, in this case the sign (+ or –) of the component value is unimportant as being dependent on a horizontal shift of the mask with respect to the analyzed image. Therefore, instead of real, absolute values of

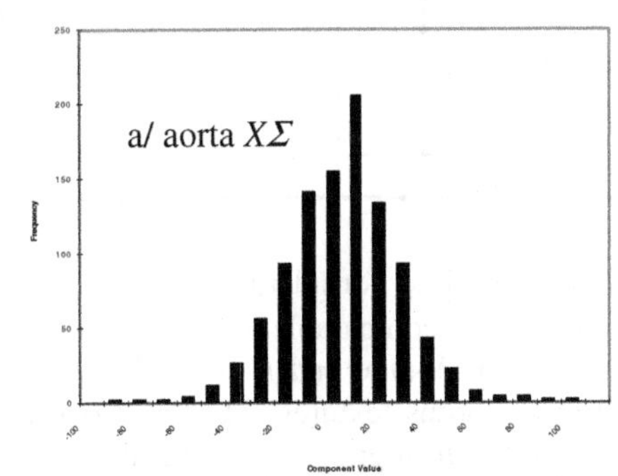

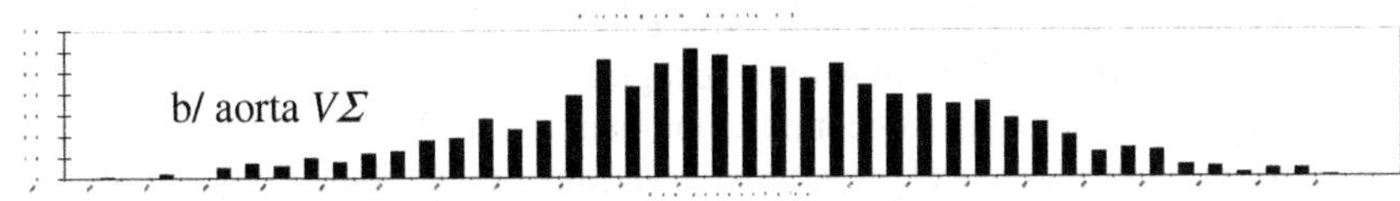

Fig. 12. A comparison of histograms of two selected MS components

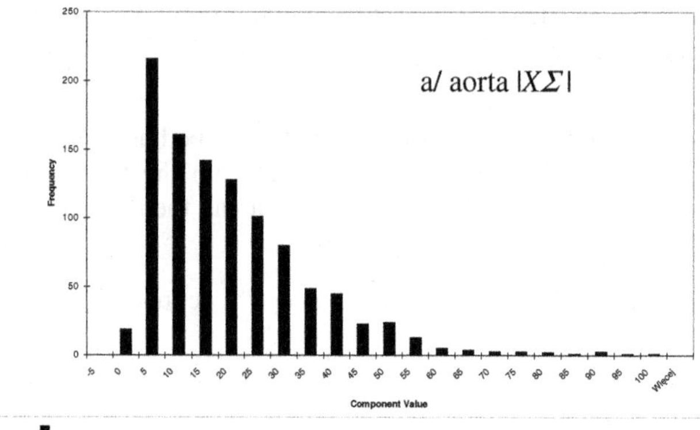

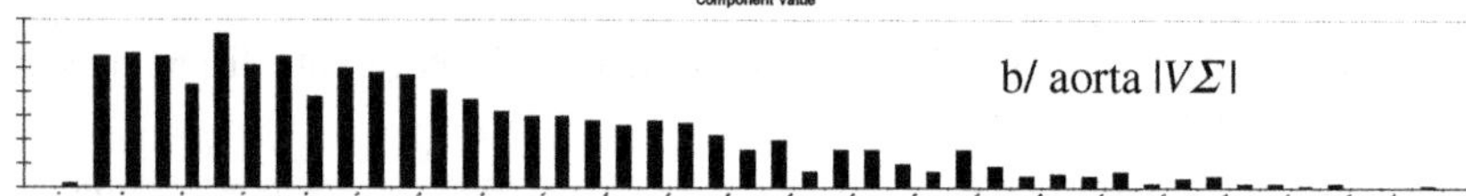

Fig. 13. Histograms of the *aorta MS* components $|X\Sigma|$ and $|V\Sigma|$ in comparable scales

Table 1. Basic statistical parameters of histograms of selected MS components

Type of *MS* component		*MS* component's parameter			
		u_{min}	u_{max}	U_{mean}	$U_{st.dev.}$
Aorta texture	$X\Sigma$	–95	95	–0.1035	23.58
	$V\Sigma$	–431	408	2.238	143.6
	$H\Sigma$	–285	239	0.6660	58.98
	$\|X\Sigma\|$	0	96	17.99	15.23
	$\|V\Sigma\|$	0	431	118.2	304.8
	$\|H\Sigma\|$	0	285	44.38	38.82
Pancreas texture	$X\Sigma$	–79	71	–0.05762	18.23
	$V\Sigma$	–193	245	1.024	61.62
	$H\Sigma$	–303	317	2.304	78.23
	$\|X\Sigma\|$	0	79	13.84	11.86
	$\|V\Sigma\|$	0	246	45.96	41.03
	$\|H\Sigma\|$	0	317	58.62	51.83

MS components should be taken into consideration. In Fig. 13 a,b the histograms of $|X\Sigma|$ and $|V\Sigma|$ for the aorta tissue in comparable scales are presented.

The histograms show that the *V*-type and *H*-type *MS* components suite well for discrimination of anisotropic fibrous textures. This is also visible in Table 1 where basic statistical parameters of histograms of several other *MS* components of anisotropic (*aorta*) and isotropic (*pancreas*) textures are presented.

In the case if a fibrous texture is to be recognized independently to its spatial orientation it is reasonable to use algebraic combinations of *MS* components sensible to linear (fibrous) morphological structures of various orientations. For example, it follows from the masks shown in Fig. 8 and Fig. 9 that the following combination of 3rd level *MS* components:

$$S' = |\Sigma V \Sigma| + |\Sigma H \Sigma| + |\Sigma HV| + |VH\Sigma| + |HV\Sigma| + |HH\Sigma| \quad (5)$$

as well as its extension on the 4th level combination of *MS* components:

$$S'' = |\Sigma\Sigma V \Sigma| + |\Sigma\Sigma H \Sigma| + |\Sigma\Sigma HV| + |\Sigma VH\Sigma| + |\Sigma HV\Sigma| + |\Sigma HH\Sigma|, \quad (6)$$

etc. can be used to a detection or discrimination of fibrous textures of various spatial orientation.

The general concept of using *MS* components combinations to characterize textures is illustrated in Fig. 14 where histograms of two combinations of 1st and 2nd level *MS* components of *pancreas* texture are shown.

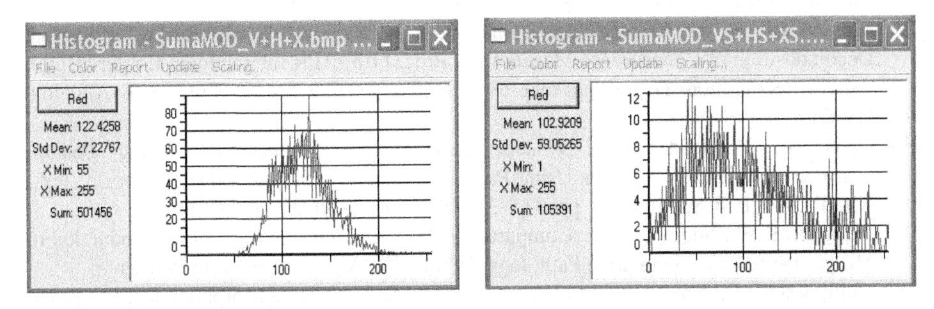

Fig. 14. Histograms of two combinations of *MS* components of a *pancreas* texture: a/ $|V| + |H| + |X|$, b/ $|V\Sigma| + |H\Sigma| + |X\Sigma|$

Like in the former cases, statistical parameters extracted from the histograms should be taken as a basis of discrimination of textures. For this purpose not only the two first-order (mean value and variance) but also higher-order moments can be taken into account. Let us also remark that texture discrimination can be based, in general, on comparison of several histograms corresponding to different *MS* components or combinations of different components.

5 Conclusions

Texture analysis plays a basic role in radiological images segmentation and analysis. Morphological spectra are a novel tool of textures recognition and/or discrimination. The method of texture analysis based on *MS* should be considered as a complementary one to other methods described in literature. Morphological spectra make it possible to analyze the properties of textures on various levels of morphological structures' organization.

They make also possible to discriminate anisotropic textures of various spatial orientation in two cases: 1st discriminating spatial orientation of the examined testing areas or 2nd neglecting it. In the last case algebraic combinations of *MS* components corresponding to different spatial orientations of the fragments of anisotropic texture can be taken into consideration. Final decision about statistical similarity or dissimilarity of two compared testing areas covered by textures should be based on analysis and comparison of histograms of adequately chosen *MS* components or of their algebraic combinations.

The paper shows that the above-presented approach to textures discrimination is, in general, possible; however, its effectiveness in practical biomedical applications on larger number of real cases should be proved.

References

[1] Bruno, A., Collorec, R., Bezy-Wendling, J., et al.: Texture Analysis in Medical Imaging. In: Roux, C., Coatrieux, J.-L. (eds.) Contemporary Perspectives in Three-Dimensional Biomedical Imaging, pp. 133–164. IOS Press, Amsterdam (1997)

[2] Haddon, J.F., Boyce, J.F.: Texture Segmentation and Region Classification by Orthogonal Decomposition of Cooccurence Matrices. In: Proc. 11th IAPR International Conference on Pattern Recognition, Hague, pp. 692–695. IEEE Computer Society Press, Los Alamitos (1992)

[3] Ojala, T., Pietikajnen, M.: Unsupervised Texture Segmentation Using Feature Distributions, Texture Analysis Using Pairwise Interaction Maps. In: Del Bimbo, A. (ed.) ICIAP 1997. LNCS, vol. 1310, pp. 311–318. Springer, Heidelberg (1997)

[4] Zielinski, K.W., Strzelecki, M.: Computer Analysis of Biomedical Images. Introduction to Morphometry and Quantitative Pathology. WN PWN, Warsaw (2002) (in Polish)

[5] Kulikowski, J.L., Przytulska, M., Wierzbicka, D.: Application of Morphological Spectra to Computer-Aided Analysis of Textures. In: Proc. of the XI Int. Conf. Medical Informatics & Technology, MIT 2006, Wisla, pp. 3–8 (2006)

[6] Kulikowski, J.L., Przytulska, M., Wierzbicka, D.: Recognition of Textures Based on Analysis of Multilevel Morphological Spectra. GESTS Int. Trans. on Computer Science and Eng. 38(1), 99–107 (2007)

[7] Kulikowski, J.L., Wierzbicka, D.: Texture Analysis Based on Application of Non-Parametric Serial Statistical Tests. Biocybernetics and Biomedical Engineering 24(2), 27–39 (2004)

[8] Kulikowski, J.L., Przytulska, M., Wierzbicka, D.: Morphological Spectra as Tools for Texture Analysis. In: Kurzynski, M., et al. (eds.) Computer Recognition Systems. Springer, Heidelberg (2007) (to be published)

[9] Runyon, R.P.: Nonparametric Statistics. A Contemporary Approach. Addison-Wesley Publishing Company, Reading (1977)

Application of Artificial Neural Network to Predict Survival Time for Patients with Bladder Cancer

Marta Kolasa[1], Ryszard Wojtyna[1,2], Rafał Długosz[2,3,4], and Wojciech Jóźwicki[5]

[1] University of Technology and Life Sciences, Faculty of Telecommunication & Electrical Engineering, ul. Kaliskiego 7, 85-796 Bydgoszcz, Poland
markol@utp.edu.pl

[2] The College of Computer Science, Dept. in Bydgoszcz, ul. Fordońska 246, 85766 Bydgoszcz, Poland
woj@utp.edu.pl

[3] University of Neuchâtel, Institute of Microtechnology, Rue A.-L. Breguet 2, CH-2000, Neuchâtel, Switzerland
rdlugosz@ualberta.ca

[4] University of Alberta, Department of Electrical and Computer Engineering 114 St – 89 Ave, Edmonton Alberta, T6G 2V4, Canada

[5] The Ludwik Rydygier Collegium Medicum in Bydgoszcz, Nicolaus Copernicus University in Toruń, Department of Pathology, The F. Lukaszczyk Oncology Center, Bydgoszcz, Poland
wojtekj@cm.umk.pl

Abstract. This paper presents an application of an artificial neural network to determine survival time of patients with a bladder cancer. Different learning methods have been investigated to find a solution, which is most optimal from a computational complexity point of view. In our study, a model of a multilayer perceptron with a training algorithm based on an error back-propagation method with a momentum component was applied. Data analysis was performed using the perceptron with one hidden layer and training methods with incremental and cumulative neuron weight updating. We have examined an influence of the order in the training data file on the final prediction results. The efficiency of the proposed methodology in the bladder urothelial cancer prediction after cystectomy is on the level of 90%, which is the best result ever reported. Best outcomes one achieves for 5 neurons in the hidden layer.

Keywords: artificial neural network, bladder cancer, prognosis, survival analysis.

1 Introduction

Development of applications that use artificial neural networks (ANNs) in biomedical signal analysis is gaining popularity over last years [1-4]. This is mostly due to the fact that biomedical signals like EKG, EMG, EEG are nonlinear and non-stationary and therefore are difficult to analyze using standard linear systems. An interesting comparison between statistical methods and ANN-based approaches has been presented by Wei [5]. For example, a genetic adaptive neural network (GANN) reaches

E. Kącki, M. Rudnicki, J. Stempczyńska (Eds.): Computers in Medical Activity, AISC 65, pp. 113–122.
springerlink.com

an accuracy of 85% in predicting a 12-month survival after surgery for nonsmall cell lung carcinoma, while accuracy of the logistic regression model is on the level of only 70 % [6].

Neural networks are widely used in urology as a diagnostic tool suitable to determine a patient state in prostate or bladder cancer cases [1, 2,5, 7-11]. One of examples of such an application has been reported in [5]. In the case of [5], the ANN has been used to predict a biochemical failure in patients undergoing radical prostatectomy and accuracy of 80 % has been reached in predicting highrisk patients that would develop early prostate-specific antigen (PSA) recurrence. An application of ANN has been also demonstrated in calculi regrowth estimation following shock wave lithotripsy. In this case, ANN utilizing previous calculi events, metabolic abnormalities, medical therapies, infections and caliectasis was able to predict outcomes with an accuracy of 91 %[11].

In this paper, the perceptron ANN has been used for another task, namely to predict a survival time of patients with a bladder urothelial cancer. So far, this task was addressed to statistical methods, which have limitations due to requirements of linear relationships between particular variables. Hence, they often fail when used in clinical urologic practice due to biomedical data which exhibit significant nonlinear intervariable relationships. This is a specific of biomedical data [9,10].

In practice, traditional statistical methods can only be used to deliver a comparative analysis for some population, but due to their limitations have no power as a prediction tool in individual prognosis [1]. As a result, the survival prognosis in bladder cancer is still uncertain in number of clinical cases. For example, in solution presented by Shariat et al. [12], more than 20 % of patients had unpredictable prognosis, which means that efficiency of this method was below 80%.

The other problem is insufficient amount of the prognostic markers, which does not allow for high efficiency of the statistical methods. The commonly used prognostic variables, such as a tumor stage (T), a histological grade (G) and a lymphnode status (PLN), are not sufficient to predict a survival time in case of patients with the bladder cancer [13,14].

This creates a high demand for a new analysis methodology as well as new systems that will be able to overcome limitations of linear systems. Such new methods are required, for example, in effective therapy planning.

In this paper, we propose a new analytical methodology of investigation based on information taken from histopatologically evaluated bladders with a cancer and information about age and sex. In our approach, a training vector contains universally accepted prognostic markers as input data. By means of the applied ANN, authors developed a new tool to predict survival time of patients with bladder urothelial cancer. Several training methods were examined to find the one leading to the most accurate prediction (smallest prediction error). Prediction efficiency as high as 94 % has been reached.

2 Problem Overview

Existing biological models of the bladder cancer try to find relationships between survival time and factors influencing tumor growth and histological pattern. Complexity of a biological model depends on different types of variables which may be grouped as follows: (1) The environmental carcinogen hazards such as smoking, medicines, industrial chemicals, (2) biological disposition of the organism like age, sex, psychophysical condition during the diagnosis, (3) a real progression stage of the bladder cancer, which includes grading, staging and lymphnode status, (4) morphological features of the process described from the macro- and microscopic point of view: size, histological type, and the way of infiltration [12,15].

A factor that is also required for proper prognosis is time that passed since the beginning of an optimal treatment to appearing recurrence symptoms as well as body reaction to the applied treatment [16].

In existing biological models, one observes a tendency to enlarge the number of model parameters (variables) for better planning individual treatment [7]. A large number of variables described in the literature [12,15] as well as nonlinear relationships describing biological models are the main reason for difficulties in survival predictions when using classical statistical methods.

3 Applied Methodology and the Input Training Data

This paper presents a software model for predicting the postoperative survival in patients treated by cystectomy because of bladder urothelial cancer and examined histopathologically in the Department of Urology of the Dr. Biziel Hospital in Bydgoszcz. The applied pre-classification includes 133 patients fulfilling the condition for bladder urothelial cancer in the T1-4 progression. In the next qualification stages, excluded were patients:

a) Who died owing to reasons not related to the bladder cancer,
b) With a high risk of death owing to such reasons,
c) In case when values of variables qualified to the input training vector does not Differ significantly from others patients to avoid data redundancy.

For these reasons, the preliminary data set has been reduced by 4, 16 and 7 patients, respectively, eliminating 27 persons. After that, the obtained training file contained data of 106 patients, which have been divided into four subsets, i.e. training, validating and two testing sets relating to 52, 14, 11 and 29 patients, respectively. The number of training vectors in particular subsets has been determined on the basis of the following assumptions: (1) the training subset should by as large as possible, (2) particular types of data should be evenly distributed over each subset. The second assumption has been verified using a t-Student distribution. This methodology allowed for determining sizes of the training, the validating and the first testing set. The second testing set contained patients who were still alive during experiments.

All bladders have been evaluated histopathologically, considering standard survival predictors such as: T and N, histological differentiation grade (G), positive lymphnode number (PLN), the number of removed lymphnodes (LN) but additionally also the patient's age and sex.

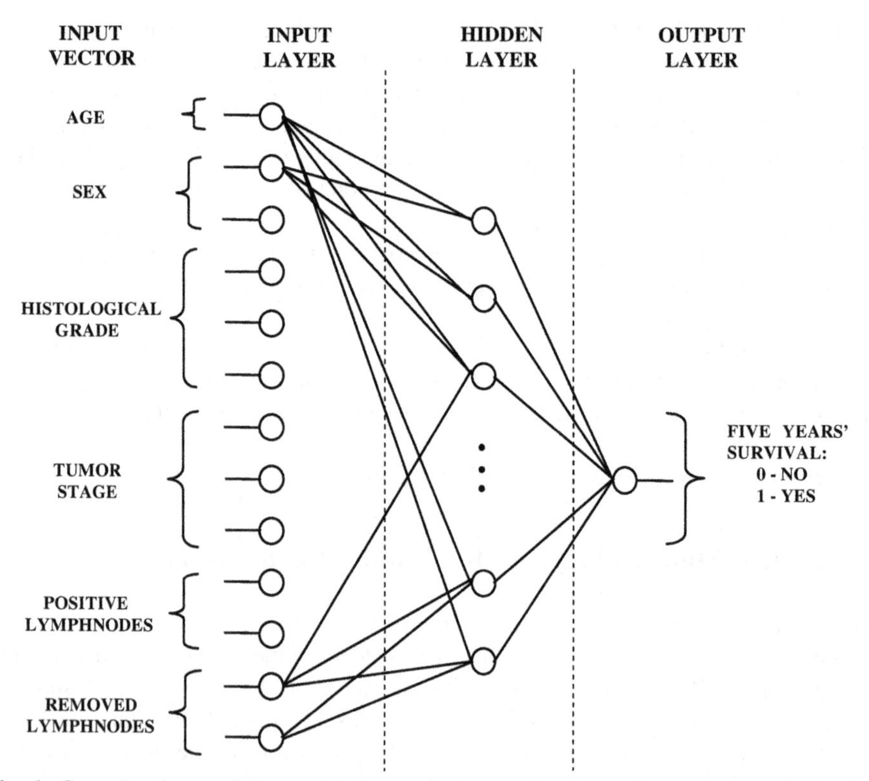

Fig. 1. General scheme of the model for predicting survival time for patients with bladder cancer

Analysis of data described above has been performed using Matlab model of the considered neural network. We have used a multilayer perceptron network, which is widely applied for prediction tasks [1, 2, 17, 18]. Model of our network is shown in Figure 1. In this model, neurons possess sigmoidal activation functions. A classic error back-propagation algorithm with a momentum factor has been applied [3, 19] as a training method. We examined a network with one hidden layer and different number of neurons in this layer. The number of neurons at the network input has been selected to be equal to 13, because this covers the entire training vector described in Table 1. Output layer of the network of Figure 1 contains only one neuron.

Values of the applied training vectors are expressed in a digital form using binary variables as shown in the fourth column of Table 1. At the network output we obtain a binary information about the patient survival for particular cases, i.e. whether the patient will survive the period of 5 years or not.

The learning rate, η, and the momentum coefficient in the training process have been selected to be equal to 0.01 and 0.9, respectively. Both values have been determined experimentally to achieve the final prediction error to be minimal. During the learning process, these values were kept constant. Such an approach is often used in tasks similar to ours [19].

Table 1. Input training signals and their features

Input data groups	Notation of all categories included in a given group	Group category description	Binary coded categories of given input data group	Required number of network inputs needed to indicate each category for a given input data group
Sex	1	Woman	0	1
	2	Man	1	
Age	1	<50	00	2
	2	<50;60)	01	
	3	<60;70>	10	
	4	>70	11	
G	1	Low	000	3
	2	Low/High	001	
	3	Low-High	010	
	4	High/Low	011	
	5	High	100	
T	1	Lamina propria invasion	000	3
	2	Muscularis propria invasion (up to half of thickness)	001	
	3	Muscularis propria invasion (over half of thickness)	010	
	4	Subserous tissue invasion microscopically	011	
	5	Subserous tissue invasion macroscopically	100	
	6	Prostate invasion	101	
	7	Other tissue and organs invasion	110	
PLN	1	0	00	2
	2	{1;2}	01	
	3	{3;4}	10	
	4	>4	11	
LN	1	<0;5>	00	2
	2	<6;10>	01	
	3	<11;15>	10	
	4	>15	11	

Three different training algorithms have been applied and tested:

- The method with cumulative updating network weights (CUNW),
- The method with incremental updating network weights without changes in the order of imputing training patterns (IUNWa),
- The method with incremental updating network weights with changes in the order of imputing training patterns (IUNWb).

In cases of the IUNW methods (the second and third method), weights of the network neurons were updated immediately after using each training vector. In both cases, the prediction efficiency was estimated using a mean-square error measure described by:

$$E_j(W) = \frac{1}{2}\sum_{k=1}^{N}(y_{jk}^{(j)} - d_{jk}^{(j)})^2 , \tag{1}$$

In the CUNW method (the first one), neuron's weights were updated after presenting the network all training vectors. In this case, the prediction error was evaluated using the expression given by [20]:

$$E(W) = \frac{1}{2}\sum_{j=1}^{p}\sum_{k=1}^{N}(y_k^{(j)} - d_k^{(j)})^2 , \tag{2}$$

Particular symbols used in both equations have the following meaning:

p – number of the training pattern,
N – number of the output layer neuron,
X – training vector defined as: $X = [x_1,\dots\dots, x_M]$,
Y – output vector defined as: $Y = [y_1,\dots\dots, y_N]$,
D – expected answer vector defined as: $D = [d_1,\dots\dots, d_N]$,
W – weight vector of a given neuron $W = [w_1,\dots\dots, w_R]$.

Notice that in our network the output vector, Y, contains only one element, i.e. N=1.

4 Experimental Results

For each of the training methods, our network was optimized in terms of the number of neurons in the hidden layer. When designing the network architecture, one should determine an optimum number of these neurons, according to a given biological model. This is important as the effective training process strongly depends on the number of neurons in the hidden layer. The following numbers of neurons in this layer have been used during the experiments: 3, 4, 5, 6, 7, 8, 10, 13, 15, 20, 25 and 30. In each experiment, 10 learning cycles were performed, where the number of iterations in each cycle varied between 80 and 1200. Initial values of the neuron's weights were selected randomly in the range from -1 to 1 [18].

The training process was stopped when the mean-square error, described by (1) or (2), reached a minimum for a given validation data set [21]. Then, a percentage of false predictions of our network (prediction error) was calculated for the training, validation and testing subsets. The prediction error is defined as a ratio of the number of wrong responses to the total number of the network responses.

Table 2. Mean percentage of false predictions for 10 cycles in three training algorithms versus the number of neurons in the hidden layer for the training (Tr) and validation (V) subsets

Training algoritm		CUNW		IUNWa		IUNWb	
Set		Tr	V	Tr	V	Tr	V
Neuron number in a hidden layer	3	5,77	6,43	6,73	7,14	6,34	6,43
	4	5,38	5,71	6,34	6,43	5,58	6,43
	5	4,61	5,71	6,92	7,14	5,96	7,14
	6	4,61	6,43	5,77	6,43	5,00	6,43
	7	5,00	5,71	5,38	6,43	4,61	6,43
	8	5,77	7,14	6,54	7,14	6,54	7,14
	10	5,96	6,43	5,77	6,43	5,38	6,43
	13	5,38	7,14	6,34	7,14	5,77	7,14
	15	6,70	7,14	7,69	7,14	6,92	7,14
	20	7,88	7,14	7,69	7,14	6,92	7,14
	25	9,04	7,14	8,08	7,14	7,12	7,14
	30	10,58	7,14	9,43	7,14	8,08	7,14

After finishing the training, a mean percentage of the false predictions was calculated for each training method and 10 training cycles applied for each method. The obtained results are presented in Table 2. In case of the testing subset, the percentage error was zero for all training cycles and, for this reason, the testing-subset results are not included in the table.

Results gathered in Table 2 are illustrated in Figure 2. The curves show the prediction error versus the number of neurons included in the hidden layer for the applied three training methods (CUNW, IUNWa and IUNWb) when using the training subset (Tr). Notice that all curves exhibit a minimum when the neuron number lies in the range between 5 and 7. This means that increasing the number of the hidden-layer neurons not necessarily is the best solution. The optimal number of neurons, for which the prediction error reaches the minimum, depends on the type of the used learning methods but always equals 5, 6 or 7. We expect that the difference in the error minimum value and the optimum neuron number, obtained for different learning methods, may be greater when applying a larger number of learning vectors. This problem is a subject of further investigations.

From Figure 2 it also follows that an efficiency of the survival-time predictions (ratio of correct predictions to the total number of predictions), obtained for the optimal or close to optimal value of the hidden-layer neuron number, is approximately 94%. For the neuron number less than 30, the efficiency is above 90%. This is a better result than that obtained when using statistical prediction methods published in the literature.

In our another experiment, particular subsets have been enlarged by adding data for those patients that have been excluded from testing in the previous experiment, due to the reasons listed in Section 3. The network has been examined applying the

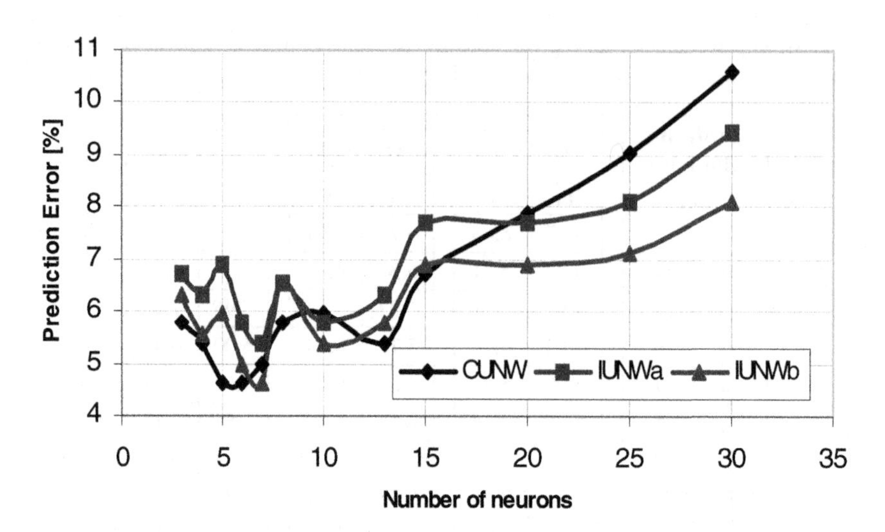

Fig. 2. Prediction error as a function of the number of neurons in the hidden layer for three tested learning methods when using the training set (Tr)

second testing subset containing data of 29 patients that were observed too short. Our network predicted the survival-time being longer than 5 years in case of 9 patients, which equals 31% of the whole patient group in the second testing subset. As compared to the 27% representation of the predictions achieved when using the training set, the 31% representation of the 5-year survival-time predictions amongst the alive patients with a too short observation time period (the subset 2 test) may show oncological representation of this group of patients in the future.

5 Conclusions

The paper presents effectiveness of applying an Artificial Neuron Network (ANN) to predict survival time of patients with a bladder cancer. This is the first reported attempt of using a neural network for the problem, which so far was treated only by means of statistical methods. Unfortunately, the statistical methods exhibit a low efficiency in solving prediction tasks, i.e. not more than 80% of all predictions are correct. In our application, the efficiency obtained for optimal network parameters is larger than 94 %, which is the best outcome ever reported.

The paper is one of stages of a larger project we deal with and, therefore, the presented studies should be considered as preliminary. The results obtained so far will have to be verified using a greater amount of data concerning a bigger group of patients. The presented methodology will be further optimized by including other variables to the training vector, i.e. taking into account other factors influencing the survival problem.

In this paper, three different training methods have been verified and optimized for the specific task considered. The presented results show that the applied two IUNW methods are more efficient than the CUNW one, although the difference between them is not very large. This is probably due to a relatively small amount of the training data taken into consideration.

Worsening the generalizing abilities of the network, observed when increasing the neuron number, occurred definitely faster in case of the method with cumulative updating of the network weights compared to the method with incremental updating. In our researches, the error of survival-time predictions for the training set was considerably lower when changing the sequence of training patterns introduced during the incremental training of the neural network (Fig. 2). Introducing the training patterns in a variable sequence during the process of the network training has a positive influence on the final result of the prediction.

An important task undertaken in this paper was to optimize the number of the network-hidden-layer neurons. In our study, the optimal number of the neurons depends on the applied training methods and takes values in the range from 5 to 7. This shows that a relatively small network is able to solve complex diagnostic problems. The number of the neurons should be optimized for each set of the training data.

References

1. Abbod, M.F., Catto, J.W.F., Linkens, D.A., Wild, P.J., Herr, A., Wissmann, C., Pilarsky, C., Hartmann, A., Hamdy, F.C.: Artificial Intelligence Technique for Gene Expression Profiling of Urinary Bladder Cancer. In: 3rd International IEEE Conference Intelligent Systems, pp. 646–651 (2006)
2. Catto, J.W.F., Linkens, D.A., Abbod, M.F., Chen, M., Burton, J.L., Feeley, K.M., Hamdy, F.C.: Artificial Intelligence in Predicting Bladder Cancer Outcome: A Comparison of Neuro-Fuzzy Modeling and Artificial Neural Networks. Clinical Cancer Research 9, 4172–4177 (2003)
3. Naguib, R.N.G., Qureshi, K.N., Hamdy, F.C., Neal, D.E.: Neural Network analysis of Prognostic Markers in Bladder Cancer. In: 19th International Conference IEEE/EMBS, Chicago, vol. 3, pp. 646–651 (1997)
4. Tkacz, E.J., Kostka, P., Jonderko, K., Mika, B.: Supervised and Unsupervised Learning Systems as a Part of Hybrid Structures Applied in EGG Signals Classifiers. In: IEEE Annual Conference Engineering in Medicine and Biology, Shanghai, China (2005)
5. Wei, J.T., Tewari, A.: Artificial Neural Networks in Urology: Pro. Urology 54, 945–948 (1999)
6. Jefferson, M.F., Pendleton, N., Lucas, S.B., et al.: Comparison of a Genetic Algorithm Neural Network with Logistic Regression for Predicting Outcome after Surgery for Patients with Nonsmall Cell Lung Carcinoma. Cancer 79, 1338–1342 (1997)
7. Habuchi, T., Marberger, M., Droller, M.J., et al.: Prognostic markers for bladder cancer: International Consensus Panel on Bladder Tumor Markers. Urology 66, 64–74 (2005)
8. Tewari, A., Narayan, P.: Novel staging tool for localized prostate cancer: a pilot study using genetic adaptive neural networks. J. Urol. 160, 430–438 (1998)
9. Snow, P.B., Rodvold, D.M., Brandt, J.M.: Artificial Neural Networks in Clinical Urology. Urology 54, 787–790 (1999)
10. Snow, P.B., Smith, D.S., Catalona, W.J.: Artificial neural networks in the diagnosis and prognosis of prostate cancer: a pilot study. J. Urol. 152, 1923–1926 (1994)
11. Michaels, E.K., Niederberger, C.S., Golden, R.M., et al.: Use of a Neural Network to Predict Stone Growth After Shock Wave Lithotripsy. Urology 51, 335–338 (1998)

12. Shariat, S.F., Karakiewicz, P.I., Palapattu, G.S., Amiel, G.E., Lotan, Y., Rogers, C.G., Vazina, A., Bastian, P.J., Gupta, A., Salagowsky, A.I., Schoenberg, M., Lerner, S.P.: Nomograms Provide Improved Accuracy for Predicting Survival after Radical Cystectomy. Clin. Cancer Res. 12(22), 6663–6676 (2006)
13. Shariat, S.F., Karakiewicz, P.I., Palapattu, G.S., Amiel, G.E., Lotan, Y., Rogers, C.G., Vazina, A., Bastian, P.J., Gupta, A., Salagowsky, A.I., Schoenberg, M., Lerner, S.P.: Nomograms Provide Improved Accuracy for Predicting Survival after Radical Cystectomy. Clin. Cancer Res. 12(22), 6663–6676 (2006)
14. Colquhoun, A.J., Jones, G.D., Moneef, M.A., et al.: Improving and predicting radiosensitivity in muscle invasive bladder cancer. J. Urol. 169, 1983–1992 (2003)
15. Lopez-Beltran, A., Sauter, G., Gasser, T., et al.: Infiltrating urothelial carcinoma. In: Eble, J.N., et al. (eds.) WHO classification of tumours. Pathology and genetics. Tumours of the urinary system and male genital organs, Lyon, France, pp. 97–104. IARC Press (2004)
16. Karakiewicz, P.I., Shariat, S.F., Palapattu, G.S., Gilad, A.E., Lotan, Y., Rogers, C.G., Vazina, A., Gupta, A., Bastian, P.J., Perrotte, P., Sagalowsky, A.I., Schoenberg, M., Lerner, S.P.: Nomogram for predicting disease recurrence after radical cystectomy for Transitional Cell Carcinoma of the Bladder. J. Urol. 176, 1354–1362 (2006)
17. Osowski, S.: Neural Networks. Depicted Algorythmically, Wydawnictwo Naukowe. PWN, Warsaw (1996) (in Polish)
18. Tadeusiewicz, R.: Neural Networks. Akademicka Oficyna Wydaw. RM, Warsaw (1993) (in Polish)
19. Khashman, A., Dimililer, K.: Neural Network Arbitration for Optimum DCT Image Compression. In: Eurocon 2007, Warsaw (2007)
20. Żurada, J.: Introduction to Artificial Neural Networks. West Publishing Company (1992) (in Polish)
21. Electronic Statistics Textbook PL StatSoft, Krakow (2006) (in Polish), `http://www.statsoft.pl/textbook/stathome.html`
22. Magnotta, V.A., Heckel, D., Andreasen, N.C., Cizadlo, T., Corson, P.W., Ehrhardt, J.C., Yuh, W.T.: Measurement of brain structures with artificial neural networks: Two- and three-dimensional applications. Radiology 211(3) (1999)

Artificial Inteligence Methods in the Problems of Drug Side-Effects

Joanna Stempczyńska[1,2] and Edward Kącki[2]

[1] Medical University, Paderewskiegostr. 4, 93-548 Łódź, Poland
joasia53@poczta.onet.pl
[2] College of Computer Science, Rzgowskastr. 17A, 93-008 Łódź, Poland
ekacki@neostrada.pl

Abstract. The paper has been devoted to the problems of prognosis of drag side-effects of chemotherapy application and it shows the possibility of effective use of artificial neural networks to this perpose. Based on meny years obsevations of chemotherapy patients have been gathered and elaborated the suitable training sets and testing sets for the neural networks. In the paper following cases has been taken into considerations: a) five kinds of chemotherapy programmes (schedules): fluorouracyl + leukovorin, with the application of platinum derivative, with the taxan application, with the irynotecan application and with the antracyclin application); b) 45 kinds of side–effects symptoms with proper types of scales.; c) five features describing a patient condition. The paper ends with conclussions describing practical uses of the created neural networks.

Keywords: drug side-effect, neural networks, prognosis.

1 Introduction

In many cases, the site-effects occur as a result of drug administrations and they are usually very burdensome and require suitable intervention and special medical care. Prognosis of undesirable drug effects and their great intensity makes it possible to prevent their occurrence, prepare the patient, and his suffering. The aim of the authors' work is to investigate the conditions of drug side-effects occurrence considering all the possible parameters characterising the conditions of the application of the therapeutic schedule, as well as those characterising the state of the patient.

As a result, the procedure oughts to result in creation of easy access and simple tools used to forecast side effects of drugs and their escalation. Authors decide to use for this purpose a three-layer artificial neural network training with the metod of backpropagation error.

For formalization and uniformity of the patient's state description and undesirable drug-effect intensities, estimation scales of patient states and forecasted intensities have been introduced. As a result the notion of general coeficient side effect state allowing to crieate formulations for their classifications has been introduced.

E. Kącki, M. Rudnicki, J. Stempczyńska (Eds.): Computers in Medical Activity, AISC 65, pp. 123–127.
springerlink.com

2 Material from Observation and Clinical Activity

The suitable preparation of teaching sets had essential meaning for right action of the network. The questionnaire forms based on the observation from the clinical practice and on sets of the patients' illnesses stories have been filled, lasted for many years. The obtained materials served to creature the teaching sets prepared for five following kinds of the cancer chemotherapy schedules: fluorouracyl + leukoworyn, with the application of platinum derivative, with the taxan application, with the irynotekan application and with the antracyclin application. At the same time, one of the following five classes has been assigned to every patient: corpulence (obese, normal, emaciated), age (15-30, 30-50, 50-70, 70-90), lifestyle (busy, normal, resting), general state health (very bad, bad, normal, good), level of stress (0, 1, 2, 3).

In the questionnaire examinations 45 kinds of side effect symptoms of intensity $y_k \in \{0, 1, 2, 3\}$ for k= 1, 2,..., 45 have been favoured. To every symptom a number $u_k = A_k\, y_k$ has been ascribe, where k is the number of symptoms and A_k is the weight. Following list contains all kinds of symptoms taken into considerations in the questionnaire.

1. difficulty in doing tiring works, $A_1 = 1$
2. getting tired of a long walk, $A_2 = 1$
3. getting tired of a short walk, $A_{32} = 2$
4. the need of lying down (resting), $A_4 = 2$
5. help needed while doing simple activities e.g. eating or dressing, $A_5 = 3$
6. feeling the a dysponeas, $A_6 = 3$
7. difficulty with the dream, $A_7 = 1$
8. the absence of appetite, $A_8 = 2$
9. tediousness, $A_9 = 2$
10. vomiting, $A_{10} = 3$
11. constipation, $A_{11} = 1$
12. diarrhoeas, $A_{12} = 2$
13. blood on/in stool, $A_{13} = 3$
14. difficulty with concentration, $A_{14} = 1$
15. psychological tension, $A_{15} = 1$
16. fear/worry, $A_{16} = 2$
17. pain interfering with normal activities, $A_{17} = 3$
18. irritation, $A_{18} = 2$
19. depression, $A_{19} = 2$
20. problems with memory, $A_{20} = 2$
21. disturbed family life, $A_{21} = 2$
22. disturbed social life, $A_{22} = 1$
23. fever, $A_{23} = 3$
24. infections, $A_{24} = 3$
25. bruises and disturbances in the blood coagulability, $A_{25} = 3$
26. muscle weakness, $A_{26} = 3$
27. cramp of muscles, $A_{27} = 3$
28. trance, $A_{28} = 3$
29. numbness of limbs, $A_{29} = 3$
30. disturbances in giving urine, $A_{30} = 3$
31. blood in urine, $A_{31} = 3$
32. pain of the heart, $A_{32} = 3$
33. irregular heartbeat, $A_{33} = 3$
34. hearing deterioration, $A_{34} = 2$
35. vision deterioration, $A_{35} = 2$
36. stomach upset, $A_{36} = 2$
37. problems with swallowing, $A_{37} = 3$
38. pain in the mouth, $A_{38} = 3$
39. cough, $A_{39} = 2$
40. oversensitivity to the light, $A_{40} = 2$

41. headache, $A_{41} = 2$
42. stomach-ache, $A_{42} = 2$
43. skin changes, $A_{43} = 2$
44. hair loss , $A_{44} = 1$
45. weight change, $A_{45} = 2$

For each of the above mentioned symptoms one of four following numbers {0, 1, 2, 3} describing the rank of the symptom escalation has been assigned. In the questionnaire form they also took into consideration general patient's condition on a scale of 1 - 10, both before therapy, as well as after applying of the chemotherapy schedule.

Preliminary examinations of using the artificial neural network allowed to formulate a several conclusions concerned with its practical usefulness and the way of supplementing and modyfication.

As a result of a detailed analysis of the material obtained from the described questionnaire, a total coefficient and limited coefficient of the chemotherapy schedule arduousness has been suggested to introduce in the work, and next a possibility of applying this material has been shown to forecast the effectiveness of the giventherapy program on a scale of 0 - 10 and improvements in the quality of the life of the patient also on a of scale 0 - 10.

After a discussion with a group of oncologists the authors have proposed a side effect coefficient U as a measure of suffering intensity.

$$U = 45^{-1} (A_1 y_1 + A_2 y_2 + \ldots + A_{45} y_{45})$$

3 Artificial Neural Networks

In this work five neural networks composed of two layers of artificial neurons have been used. In literature such nets are often called a three-layer nets with the so-called input layer being in fact, a fictitious layer.

Accordingly, we can say that the considered two-layer net consists of the first layer with 15 neurons (the neuron number has been established in an experimental way) and of the second (output) layer with 45 neurons adequate to the number of side-effect kinds mentioned above. The neural network has been taught by the method of backpropagation error method.

Every neuron in the first layer possesses five inputs, because the vector $\bar{s}$ of input signal has five components s_1, s_2, s_3, s_4, s_5 describing the patient's condition before the treatment.

$$\bar{s} = \{ s_1, s_2, s_3, s_4, s_5 \}$$

where: s_1 - obesity (obese, normal, emaciated),

s_2 - age (15-30, 30-50, 50-70, 70-90),
s_3 - lifestyle (busy, normal, resting).
s_4 – general state health (very bad, bad, normal, good)'
s_5 - level of stress (0, 1, 2, 3).

For every kind of the chemotherapy schedule a separate neural network of the type described above has been created.

4 Experimental Study and Its Results

For the following five kinds of the cancer chemotherapy schedules: fluorouracyl + leukoworyn, with the participation of platinum derivatives, with taxan participation, with irynotecan participation and with antracyclin participation there have been gathered five sets of pairs { $\bar{s}$, $\bar{y}$}, where $\bar{s}$ - the vector of patient's condition before the treatment, $\bar{y}$ – the vector of symptom intesity. Every set included 350 elements and it has been divided onto two parts (320 elements in the teaching subset and 30 elements in the testing subset).

For each kind of chemotherapy shedule the network has been taught by randomly chosen initial value of the weight vector. The table shows mean square errors obtained by teaching and by testing for each neural network.

No	Chemotherapy schedules	Teaching	Testing
1	fluorouracyl + leukovorin	0,004215	0,004523
2	platinum derivatives	0,004834	0,005122
3	Taxan	0,003958	0,003204
4	Irynotecan	0,004509	0,004237
5	Antracyclin	0,003877	0,003711

The period of teaching of the created neural networks was very long and it lasted about sixty hours.

5 Ending Remarks and Conclusions

The preliminary examinations of using the artificial neural network have confirmed its practical usefulness. The applications (30 instances) of the created and taught neural networks confirmed that 80% of the obtained results gave sufficient well informations on the forecasted intensity of side effects of the adopted therapy. Therefore, the patients were able to cope with the arduosness caused by the coming therapy side-effects more easily.

As a result of a detailed analysis of the material obtained from the described questionnaire and experimental study and from the preliminary neural networks applications the authors have confimed to mark a total coefficient as U (measure of suffering intensity) of the chemotherapy schedule arduousness by four coefficients U_1, U_2, U_3, U_4 crresponding to the subsets of adequately selected all kinds of symptoms taken into considrations in the questionnaire. The application of the mentioned procedure can result in the decrease the the number of neural network inputs (only four neurons in an input layer) and next in shortening of the teaching time of the neural networks without losing any information being important for clinical practice.

References

1. Kącki, E., Stempczyńska, J.: Neural Network in Communication with Medical Computer System. Journal of Medical Systems 25(2), 109–118 (2001)
2. Kącki, E., Zakrzewska, D., Stempczyńska, J.: Computer Assistance in Oncology Education. In: Proceed. of Intern. Conf. on System-Modelling-Control, Zakopane, pp. 27–28 (1990)

3. Kącki, E., Małolepszy, A.: Comparison Efficiency of the Artificial Intelligence Methods for the Diagnosis of Acid – Base and Anion Gap Disorders. Connecting Medical Informatics and Bio-Informatics. Technology and Informatics 116, 235–240 (2005)
4. Krzakowski, M.: Clinical oncology. WM Borgis, Warszawa (2001) (in polish)
5. Nałęcz, M. (ed.): Biocybernetyka, vol. 6, 7. Publ. AOW EXIT, Waszawa (2002) (in polish)
6. Stempczyńska, J., Kącki, E.: Information Technology Problems in Medical Expert Systems. Inform. Systems Architecture and Technology, Wrocław, 217–224 (1994)
7. Stempczyńska, J.: Problems of Oncology Computerization. Medical Journal 5(6), 10–12 (1994)
8. Stempczyńska, J., Kącki, E.: Multimedia Applications in Medical Systems. In: Proceed. of Intern. Conf. on System-Modelling-Control, vol. 2, pp. 265–268 (1995)
9. Stempczyńska, J., Kącki, E.: STUD2 System for Computer Assistence in Oncology Education. In: Proceed. of MedInfo 1995 Congress, Vancouver, vol. 2, pp. 1233–1237 (1995)
10. Tadeusiewicz, R.: Neural networks. AOW RM, Warszawa (1993) (in polish)

1. [illegible] Comparison Study of the Artificial Intelligence Methods for the Diagnosis of [illegible] Connecting Medical Informatics and Bio-Informatics [illegible] 779–784 (2005)
2. [illegible]
3. [illegible]
4. [illegible] Information [illegible] Problems in Medical [illegible] Systems [illegible] (1995)
5. [illegible]
6. [illegible]
7. [illegible]
8. [illegible]

Programming Symbian Smartphones for the Blind and Visually Impaired

Pawel Strumillo, Piotr Skulimowski, and Maciej Polanczyk

Institute of Electronics, Technical University of Lodz, 211/215 Wolczanska, 90-924 Lodz, Poland
pawel.strumillo@p.lodz.pl, piotr.skulimowski@p.lodz.pl, maciej@polanczyk.eu

Abstract. A set of software procedures for the Symbian OS mobile smartphone making the device more easily usable for a blind user is described in the paper. The application was written in the Carbide C++ environment, tested both on the S60 series phone emulator and the phone platform itself. The main task was to create a dedicated speech enabled menu, rather than a simple screen reader. Along with ordinary phone functions (calls, SMSs) the programmed phone can be used as a speech recorder, a web browser (RSS feeds are used), and a colour recognizer in images captured by the phone's camera. Added functionality makes the smartphone a very useful personal assistance tool for the blind who tested the developed application.

Keywords: visually impaired, smartphone, Symbian, speech synthezis.

1 Introduction

Current generations of cellular phones are much more than portable phones, they are in fact mobile microcomputers. Moreover, they are being frequently equipped with digital cameras, colour displays of increasing resolutions and are capable of performing functions of voice recorders, MP3 players, radios or even GPS receivers. Thus, these devices slowly take over the role of personal digital assistants (PDAs) with a growing number of capabilities. This view is particularly appropriate for the smartphones running under operating systems (OS) like Symbian, Mobile Linux or Windows CE.

Our aim is to develop a dedicated software package for the Symbian mobile platform that would meet the two following objectives:

– Make the device more friendly for the blind or visually impaired users,
– Equip the device with novel functions that would make it a useful tool in aiding everyday live activities of the visually handicapped.

Nuance TALKS [1] is an example of software that makes use of a speech synthesizer to read text displayed on a phone's screen. However, the drawback of such an aid is that the blind users still have to use the phone menu that was designed explicitly for persons with normal sight. The software solution proposed in our work adopts a different approach that is specially suited for the blind user and is more than just a screen reader.

E. Kącki, M. Rudnicki, J. Stempczyńska (Eds.): Computers in Medical Activity, AISC 65, pp. 129–136.
springerlink.com

2 Symbian Operating System (OS) for the Mobile Platforms

Symbian is a proprietary operating system designed for running on mobile platforms featuring limited resources. The operating system is owned mainly by Nokia and shared with other world's biggest mobile phone manufacturers. Symbian OS comes with associated libraries, user interface (UI) frameworks and software services (base, application, OS and kernel services) [2, 3]. The current market share of Symbian based smart mobile devices exceeds 70% with 18 mln shipments yearly [4].

The main advantage of the Symbian OS is its universality (many smartphone models are supported) and the flexible environment that is made available for implementing user applications. Also, the availability of a free developers' platform, i.e. the Series 60 Platform has focused programmers' interest in writing new software applications for this system. Table 1 lists advantages of this OS over other simpler operating systems dedicated to specific models of mobile devices.

Symbian OS features advanced software techniques for keeping low demand for memory and disk space. Event-driven concept of system operation enables swithing the CPU on and off to reduce power consumption. Symbian has its roots in the EPOC system that was designed for Psion palmtops in 1990th. Recently, version 9.5 of the Symbian OS has been released.

Table 1. Comparison of the Symbian OS vs. other dedicated systems

	Operating system	
Functionality	**Symbian**	**Other**
Access to files	Yes	No or limited
Data transmission via interfaces	Yes	Limited
Running user programs	Yes	No
Programs run in background	Yes	No

3 Programming for the Symbian Platforms

Although, the Symbian OS is not open source software, the Application Programming Interfaces (API) are made available for the users. Starting from version 9.1 (released in 2005) Symbian applications accessing GSM payable services (e.g. data transfers) need to be verified by electronic signature certified by Symbian Ltd.

Software projects developed for the Symbian OS are recommended to feature the following properties:

- Minimum number of tasks allocated for the system kernel,
- All resources shared between users, services and applications,
- All applications (except services) feature graphical user interface,
- Event driven application model,
- Libraries shared between applications.

Compilers offered for the Symbian OS are Java, OPL, and Python, nevertheless, C++ is recognized as the native compiler for this platform.

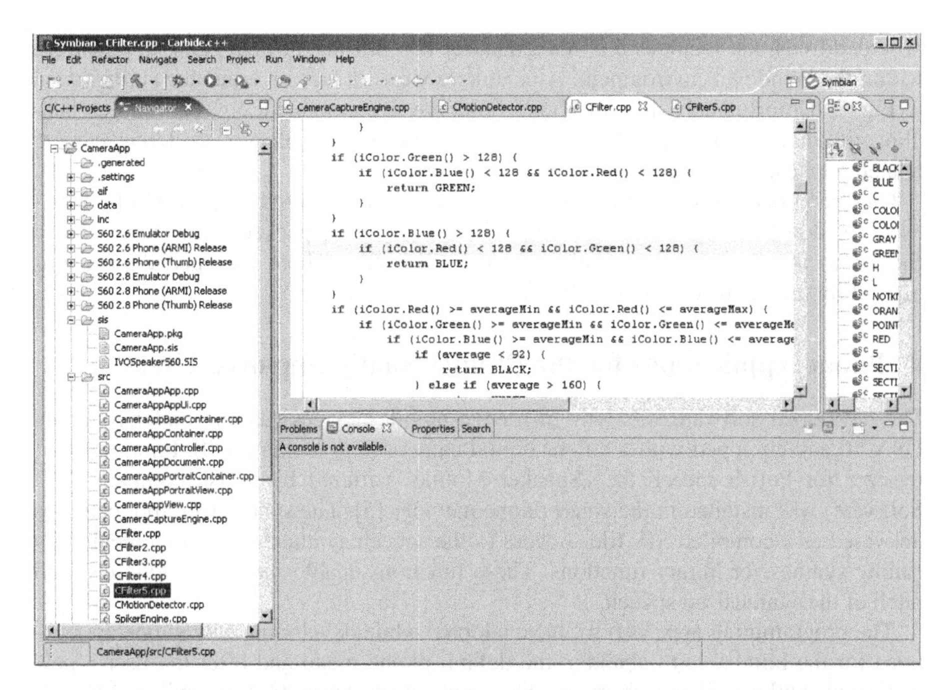

Fig. 1. An integrated programming environment of the Carbide C++ Express v. 1.1

C++ compilers developed for the Symbian OS differ from standard C++ compilers, e.g. the STL (Standard Template Library) is not supported. On the other hand, they support specific software technologies that are not available in other compilers. Active objects and active scheduler technologies enable parallel processing of a number of predefined applications. The active scheduler runs in a separate thread and its role is to link asynchronous events with the associated active objects.

Other important technology used specifically in Symbian OS compilers is the so called descriptor. Such objects are used for storing 8 and 16 bit data strings. They contain a header specifying the string length. The methods they implement are: data search, store and compare. Descriptors can be subdivided into the three following classes: Pointer (store pointers seemingly as for standard C++), Buffer (data stack e.g. for storing file names) and Heap (for storing large data volumes).

There are a number of Windows OS C++ compilers available for developing projects on the Symbian platform. A popular compiler, the Code Warrior, was succeeded in 2006 by the Carbide C++ development tool for Symbian OS S60 and S80 platforms (see Fig. 1). Other available C++ compilers are: Visul Basic, VB.NET, C#, and Bornald C++ Mobile Edition. Also, there are compilers available for Linux and Macintosh systems.

For non-commercial applications, the only freely available Windows OS development tool supported by Nokia is the Carbide C++ Express [6]. See Fig. 1 illustrating the Eclipse-based style of the integrated environment of this development tool that is available on Nokia's website: http://forum.nokia.com/. In order to compile and run projects developed in C++ a Software Development Kit (SDK) is required. The SDK provided by Nokia includes a phone emulator that allows for debugging applications within the Windows environment. An example view of such an emulator is illustrated in Fig. 2. Unfortunately, not all phone functions are emulated, e.g. procedures handling the digital camera are not included, forcing the developers to debug camera related applications directly on the phone platform.

C++ compiled application for the Symbian platform is stored in „*.app" file. However, for downloading it onto the smartphone it must be packed (with other related files) into the Symbian Installation Source (SIS) file. There are special programs offered for automatic creation of the SIS files.

4 Phone Applications for the Blind/Visually Impaired Users

The developed software was written for the mobile devices running under Symbian OS v7.0 and equipped with a colour digital camera (e.g. Nokia 6600). First, the synthesizer for Polish speech the „Speaker Mobile" (offered by Polish company IVO Software) was installed in the smart phone memory [5]. The synthesizer application is delivered as a compiled SIS file. Access to the speech synthesizer is implemented by calling synthesizer library functions. These functions enable settings of loudness and pitch of the synthesized speech.

The programming approach we have adopted while developing new phone applications for the blind was to abandon the default phone menu and offer the user a new dedicated synthesized speech menu. This application (termed "Asystent", see Fig. 2) is activated immediately after switching the phone on. It remains continuously active and its termination by typical use of the phone keyboard is blocked. Within the "Asystent" environment only a simple menu, specially designed for the blind user, is accessible. While browsing the menu (or submenus) each entry is read by the synthesizer, informing the user about the currently selected phone function and the possible actions. This style of the user interface is similar to creators that are extensively used on the PC platforms to aid the user in performing complicated program installations or actions. Such solution makes the phone more user friendly for the blind, visually impaired or even the elderly with normal sight who find difficulty in efficient use of new, complicated phone models.

The following functional capabilities (all speech enabled) are offered within the "Asystent" application:

- phone functions,
- writing and reading SMS,
- calculator,
- access to list of contacts and calendar functions,
- voice recording,
- time and date available from a keyboard shortcut,
- capture of images and recognition of the major scene colour,
- access to web pages,
- interfacing to other devices by using Symbian Bluetooth API (e.g. file exchange with a personal computer).

Further, the use of standard phone functions, access to the internet by using the RSS channels and basic image applications using the phone's camera are described.

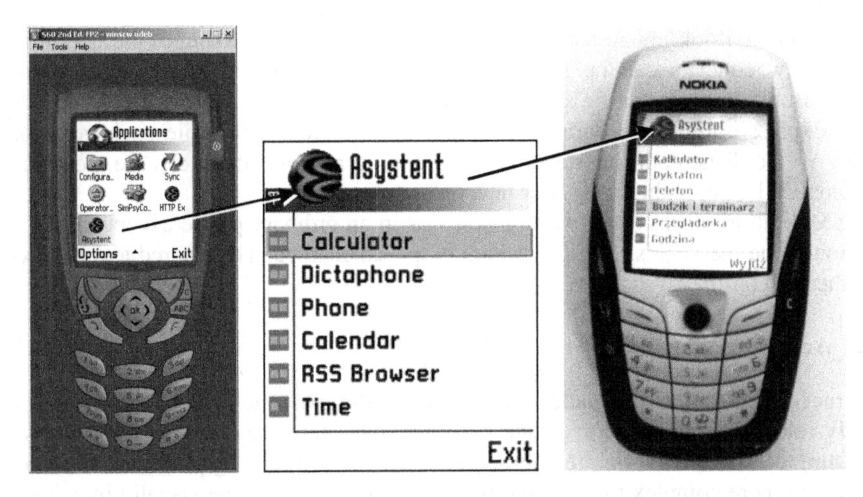

Fig. 2. Views of the Nokia series 60 emulator (left), menu entries of the developed software (centre), and a view of Nokia 6600 phone with the menu displayed on the screen

4.1 Phone Functions

'Phone' is the speech enabled application that allows for use of typical phone functions. The main menu of this application contains the following commands: 'Call', 'Text messages', 'PhoneBook', 'SMS editor', 'Help' and 'Exit'. Example views of the menu 'Phone' are shown in Fig. 3.

The 'Call' menu entry enables making phonecalls to recipients by entering the phone number from the speech enabled phone keyboard or by selecting a recipient's name from the 'PhoneBook' (also speech enabled). Once the call is terminated the phone automatically returns to the 'Phone' menu.

By selecting the 'Text messages' menu entry the user gets access to the list (sorted by dates) of senders and dates of the received short messages. The message is automatically speech synthesized if the phone user chooses to do so by entering the predefined shortcut key.

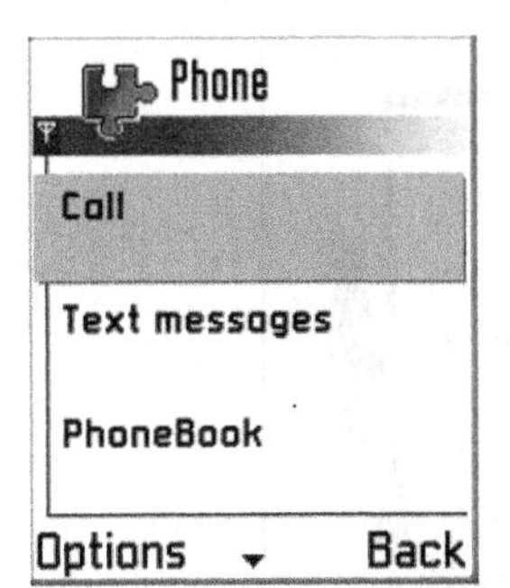

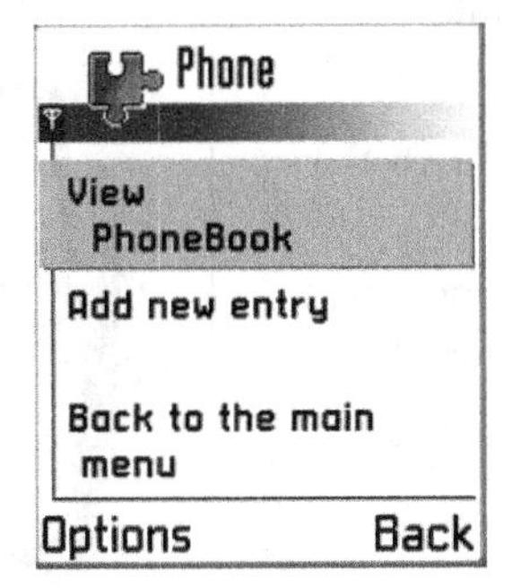

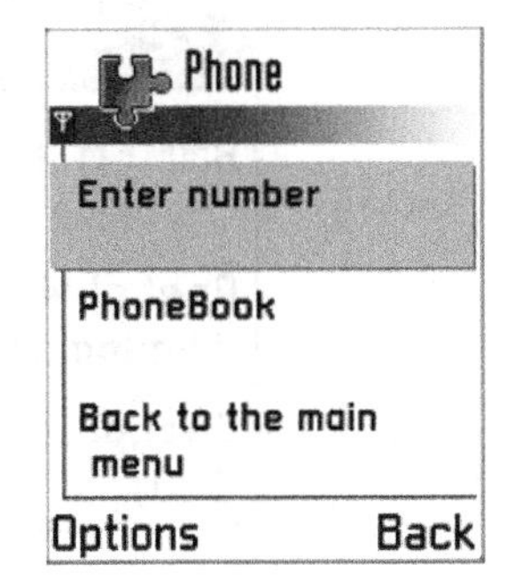

Fig. 3. Views of sample screen captures of the menu 'Phone' displayed in the phone emulator environment

The 'PhoneBook' menu entry can be used for auditory browsing of the list of contacts. New contacts can be added and stored in the 'PhoneBook'. Also, current 'PhoneBook' content can be synchronized with the PC Microsoft Outlook and Outlook Express e-mailing programs by using the free Nokia PC Suite package. Moreover, if the Bluetooth interface is used this synchronization can be performed automatically, i.e. without any user intervention.

'SMS editor' works in the same manner as in an ordinary phone except for the selection of the message's recipient, which is speech enabled. The entered text is speech synthesized on-the-fly.

4.2 Accessing Web Sites

Internet sites become overloaded with graphics and dynamic content that are not directly related to web page's default message. This tendency complicates access to meaningful information on the internet. Also, the screen reading programs need to be more and more complex to make the web pages accessible to the visually impaired or the blind (except for the web pages addressed to the visually impaired community, see e.g. www.pfron.org.pl). This situation also complicates thematic search within very many web sites performed by normally sighted users.

In order to resolve these problems, a growing number of web sites offer the so called RSS (Rich Site Summary) feeds. RSS is a format for distributing messages derived from web contents in the XML (Extensible Markup Language). This structured format is excellently suited for "filtering out information" from web pages. By using RSS feeds, summarized messaging of the web contents to blind users is considerably simplified. In order to gain access to the RSS feeds a special application (the so called RSS reader) is required.

The RSS feeds were used for providing access to the web pages from the Symbian OS smartphone. The 'RSS reader' application was developed to be run on the phone platform. Once the 'RSS reader' is called it connects to the predefined web server and fetches the list of message titles, i.e. the text tagged by <title>... </title> from the RSS list available on the server. This list of messages is continuously updated by the

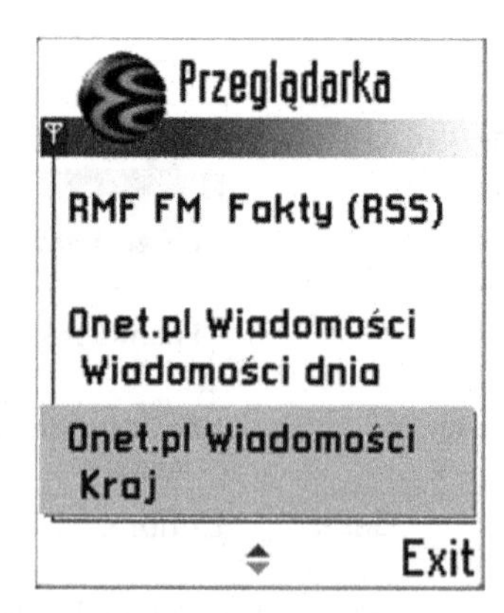

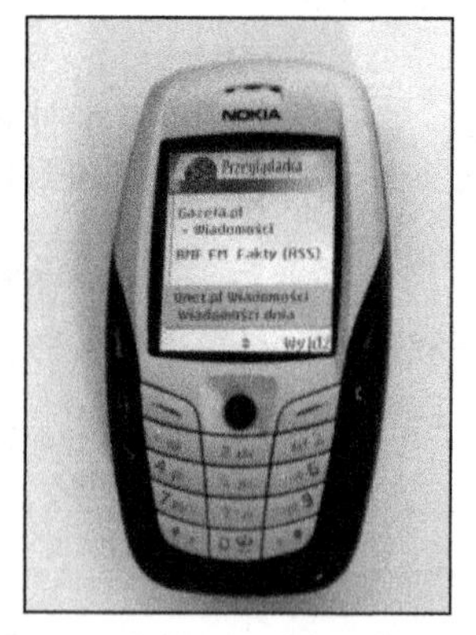

Fig. 4. List of RSS feeds viewed in the emulated „RSS reader' (left) and the corresponding list displayed on the Nokia 6600 phone screen (right)

web page provider offering such a service. For the testing purposes access to the RSS channels available on news portals such as www.gazeta.pl, www.interia.pl and www.onet.pl was implemented by the phone 'RSS reader' application. After the message titles are loaded onto the phone, their list can be browsed by the phone user (each message title is speech synthesized). If the particular message is selected its content that is linked to the selected title is loaded from the web server and read by the speech synthesizer. Only the plain text of the message is fetched to minimize loading time and the cost of the GPRS transmission. In Fig. 4 the list of RSS generated feeds viewed in the emulated 'RSS reader' are shown along with its version displayed on the phone platform.

4.3 Image Processing Applications

Currently an application is under development that is aimed at using the phone's on-board digital camera for processing and analysis of captured images. The processed images are the RGB colour images of size 640x480 pixels.

Tests were carried out that have revealed that special programming techniques need to be applied to minimize computing time of procedures for handling digital images [7]. Convolution lowpass and highpass filters for mask sizes of 3x3, 5x5 and 7x7 pixels were implemented. For masks with integer coefficients, the achieved computing times varied from below 1 sec to a few seconds for the Nokia 6600 phone. If no code optimization was used, image filtering took more than 1 min.

First successful results were also obtained for the task of recognizing colours in the captured images. However, due to the lack of access to the image RAW format, the phone camera user has to rely only on the automatic white balance settings. No custom settings are made available as it possible in typical digital photo cameras. First, the RGB color model format was converted into the HSI (Hue Saturation Intensity) colour sestem. For colour recognition purposes only the Hue component was analysed. Tests under different lighting conditions (color temperature of the light source), i.e. for both natural (direct sunlight, overcast sky) and artificial lighting conditions (fluorescent, incandescent) were performed. Light intensity for these light sources measured by Sekonic FLASHMATE L–308 S varied from 7 to 14 EV (Exposure Values). Reliable recognition of colours was obtained for the Hue component that was partitioned into six subregions: red, orange, yellow, green, blue and the extra region for unrecognized colours. The recognition result is communicated to the phone user by voiced speech.

5 Conclusions

The mobile Symbian OS smartphone equipped with the special purpose software is intended to serve as a personal assistant for the blind or visually impaired user. It was shown that this computing platform can be efficiently programmed to make it more friendly for such users by implementing a dedicated menu and an on board speech synthesizer. By using voiced commands the user is navigated within this specialized environment. Ordinary phone functions were speech synthesized and new software procedures written: like an internet browser (via RSS feeds), a voice recorder, and colour recognition in images captured by the on-board digital camera. The first version of the software package was tested by blind users. Enthusiastic reviews were given to the offered speech enabled phone functions. There were also suggestions for improving the phone's functionality, e.g. control over the speed of the synthesized speech was indicated as an important missing feature. These improvements are planned when new, more customizable synthesizers are made available for the phone platforms.

Acknowledgements. This work has been supported by the Ministry of Education and Science of Poland grant no. R02 013 03 in years 2007–2010.

References

1. Nuance website, `http://www.nuance.com/talks`
2. Symbian website,
   `http://www.symbian.com/about/fastfacts/fastfacts.html`
3. Edwards, L., Barker, R.: Developing Series 60 Applications. A guide for Symbian OS C++ Developers. Nokia Mobile Development Series (2004)
4. Canalys website: Mobile device trends, `http://www.canalys.com`
5. IVO Software website, `http://www.ivo.pl`
6. Nokia website: Carbide Development Tools,
   `http://forum.nokia.com/main/resources/tools_and_sdks/carbide/`
7. Polanczyk, M.: Implementation of image processing and analysis algorithms on the Symbian mobile platforms. MSc Thesis, Technical University of Lodz (2007) (in Polish)

CARDIO$^{©}$ – Environment for Computer-Aided Learning and Testing of Interpretation of ECG Signals

Jacek Cichosz and Marek Kurzynski

Wroclaw University of Technology, Chair of Systems and Computer Networks,
Wyb. Wyspianskiego 27, 50-370 Wroclaw, Poland
jacek.cichosz@pwr.wroc.pl

Abstract. We present an environment for ECG signal visualization, learning of its analysis, diagnostic interpretation and ECG software testing. The functional description of the system is given with focus on analysis module based on energy measure of fuzziness and the interpretation eveluation unit. In the latter, some evaluation criteria have been proposed. We also describe a proposal of testing ECG interpretation algorithm by means of artificial generation of ECG parameters. Some design ideas ensuring flexibility and reusability of our system are also suggested.

Keywords: Computerized ECG interpretation, ECG analysis.

1 Introduction

The regular work of a cardiologist includes reading of electrocardiograms (ECGs) because electrocardiography is a non-invasive investigative method that provides information for the detection, diagnosis and therapy of cardiac conditions [1]. In the last period the reader has often computer generated diagnostic suggestions, which can considerably speed up the process of physician decision making and help prevent errors in the ECG interpretation [3, 4, 5].

Usually, computer programs for ECG diagnosis have in its structure two modules: module for the ECG analysis and ECG interpretation. Analysis of an ECG signal includes an automatic detection of the signal characteristic points, amplitudes and durations (P wave, PQ segment, QRS complex, ST segment, T wave, QT interval). Interpretation however, on the base of the ECG characteristic measurement points, provides diagnostic information.

In order to ensure high quality of computerized ECG interpretation, manufacturer should perform empirical investigations of his software performance on the biological ECG signals. Such tests can help to evaluate analysis and interpretation accuracy of computer system before it will be recommended to clinical practice.

Unfortunately, existing ECG signal data bases are solely assigned for testing of ECG analysis (measurements) procedures. As an example we can refer to Common Standards of Electrocardiography (CSE) database [2], which is a well annotated reference database for ECG measurement. The golden standard has been derived here by an international group of cardiologists (referees), who have visually determined the onset and offset points of P, QRS and T waves. Another testing tool,

E. Kącki, M. Rudnicki, J. Stempczyńska (Eds.): Computers in Medical Activity, AISC 65, pp. 137–145.
springerlink.com

developed during the Conformance Testing Services for Computerized Electrocardiography (CTS-ECG) project [6] are extremely valuable for evaluating the accuracy of ECG signal analysis in computerized ECG systems. They are documented graphically and numerically in the CTS-ECG Test Atlas and available in the electronic version [7].

Today there is still a lack of diagnostic ECG signal databases, which can help of manufacturer of ECG interpretation software to evaluate his product.

This paper presents a multifunctional software system that, among other possibilities, can be used for testing and performance evaluation of software components designed for diagnostic interpretation of ECG signals. It can also play an educational role in teaching medical students and verifying their knowledge.

The structure of the paper is as follows. Section 2 addresses the functions that can be performed by the system in the form of a flowchart. Possible use cases depend on the available initial knowledge and the features offered by a computer system to be verified. In particular, software test routines are presented including analysis and the module artificially generating of analysis output, essential in the CARDIO system.

Section 3 addresses system's architecture and its computer implementation. Example user sessions are described in section 4. Section 5 concludes the paper.

2 Functions of the System

CARDIO system, is assigned to testing and quality evaluating of computer software for diagnostic interpretation of ECG signals. Its structure is depicted in Fig. 1. CARDIO states the computer environment, which makes possible evaluate the software for different cases presented in Table 1.

Table 1. Concepts of CARDIO system activity for different cases of available information

Available signal		Is in the tested software analysis module?	Testing/evaluating procedure
ECG with annotations	1	Yes	ECG signal is processed by analysis and interpretation modules of the tested software and next results are compared with interpretative annotations
	2	No	Procedure as in 1, but ECG signal is processed by CARDIO analysis module instead of analysis module of the tested software
ECG without annotations	3	Yes	Procedure as in 1, but interpretative annotations are added by user
	4	No	Procedure as in 2, but interpretative annotations are added by user
None	5	Yes/No	User defines the demanded pathological type of ECG signal, generator of analysis results generates parameters of ECG (artificial results of analysis) which are processed by interpretation module. Results are compared with interpretative annotations created by user

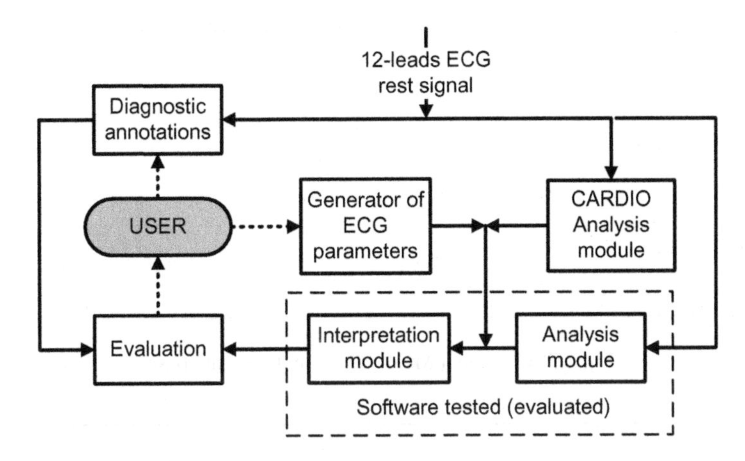

Fig. 1. Structure of the CARDIO system

2.1 Analysis Module of CARDIO System

The most important stage of ECG analysis consists in detection of fiducial points (onset and offset of P, QRS and T waves), because its quality has significant influence on the quality of the whole system. Usually, the detection of QRS complexes and P and T waves is composed of two-stages [4, 5]. First the so-called detection function is constructed, which has a smooth shape with local maxima for each QRS complex and P and T wave. Next, the location of QRS complexes and P and T waves on the time axis is estimated, applying some rules concerning the detection function.

In the analysis module of CARDIO system to the construction of detection function the energy measure of fuzziness method was applied, which has been reported as a powerful tool for ECG signal processing [16]. The energy measure of fuzziness is a method for quantitative assessment of fuzzy uncertainty in signals, which fulfils two postulates [17, 18]:

- For the constant signal containing no fuzzy uncertainty, the energy measure of fuzziness is equal to zero, which means that the information conveyed by such a signal is maximal.
- Higher dynamics of the changes of the original signal denotes the higher value of energy measure of fuzziness. It means that the amount of information is smaller for the variable signal than for the constant one.

As an example, an ECG signal MO1_004 (II lead) from data-base CSE is shown in Fig. 2. However Fig. 3 illustrates a course of energy measure of fuzziness for this signal. Since the course corresponds to a single peak of QRS complexes and furthermore, P and Q waves are represented by peaks with small amplitude, the presented course of energy measure of fuzziness may be used as a detection function.

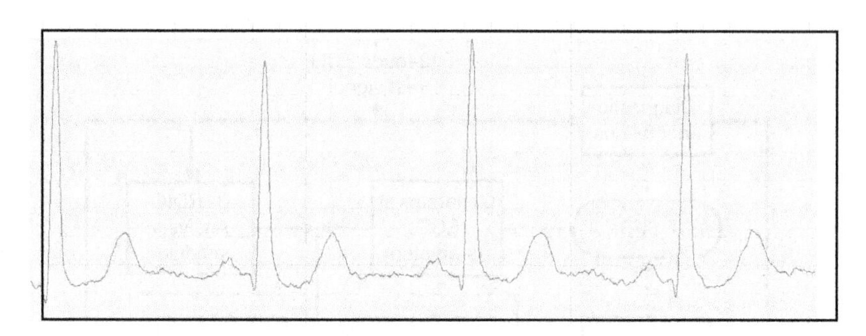

Fig. 2. ECG signal MO1_004 from CSE data base

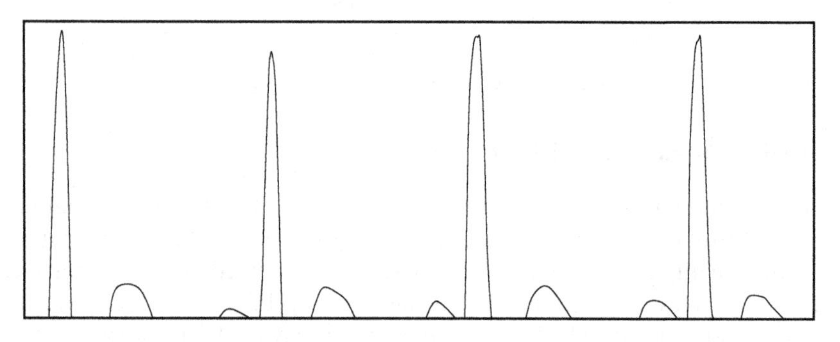

Fig. 3. Energy measure of fuzziness for signal from Fig. 2

2.2 Generator of ECG Parameters (GEP)

The generating module of ECG parameters plays the crucial role in the case, when ECG signals are not available. In such a situation, the concept of testing procedure consists in replacement of biological ECG signal with defined kind of pathology by the set of parameters into which this pathology manifests itself. Next, this set of parameters (or in other words the result of analysis of ECG signal) is supplied to the interpretation module as the basis of its activity.

The set of ECG disorders supported by the GEP module is presented in the Table 2. As an result of the performance of GEP module, we receive the following ECG parameters:

- Amplitudes of P, Q, R, S, T waves, amplitude and slope of ST interval (for each lead),
- Duration of Q, R, S waves (for each lead), duration of P wave, PQ segment, QT interval and QRS complex (absolute values),
- Number of P waves, localization of PM spikes (if any), flags for F/f waves detection

For a given kind of ECG disorder, parameters are generated according to the rules containing the universally applied clinical criteria [10, 11, 12, 13, 14] and Einthoven

Table 2. The available ECG disorders (according to AHA systematics [8] and Novacode classification system [9])

NORMAL TRACING: Normal ECG TECHNICAL PROBLEMS: Leads misplaced, Artifacts SINUS NODE RHYTHMS AND ARRHYTHMIAS: Sinus rhythm, Sinus tachycardia (>100 beats per minute), Sinus bradycardia (<50 beats per minute), Sinus arrhythmia, Sinus arrest or pause, Sino-atrial exit block OTHER SUPRAVENTRICULAR RHYTHMS: Atrial premature complexes, Ectopic atrial rhythm, Ectopic atrial tachycardia, Atrial fibrillation, Atrial flutter, Junctional premature complexes, Junctional escape complexes or rhythm, Accelerated junctional rhythm, Junctional tachycardia, Supraventricular tachycardia VENTRICULAR ARRHYTHMIAS: Ventricular premature complexes, Ventricular escape complexes or rhythm, Accelerated idioventricular rhythm, Ventricular tachycardia, Ventricular fibrillation ATRIAL VENTRICULAR CONDUCTION: First-degree AV block, Mobitz Type 1 second-degree AV block (Wenckebach), Mobitz Type 2 second-degree AV block, AV block or conduction ratio, 2:1, AV block, varying conduction ratio, AV dissociation INTRAVENTRICULAR CONDUCTION: Left bundle branch block, Right bundle branch block (complete or incomplete), Left anterior fascicular block, Left posterior fascicular block, Wolff-Parkinson-White syndrome QRS AXIS AND VOLTAGE: Right axis deviation, Left axis deviation, Indeterminate axis, Low voltage (less than 0.5 mV total QRS amplitude in each extremity lead and less than 1.0 mV in each Precordial lead) CHAMBER HYPERTROPHY OR ENLARGEMENT: Left ventricular hypertrophy (with or without ST-T abnormality), Right ventricular hypertrophy (with or without secondary ST-T abnormality) MYOCARDIAL INFARCTIONS AND/OR ISCHEMIC ABNORMALITIES: Q wave MI, Isolated ischemic abnormalities, Isolated minor Q and ST-T abnormalities PACEMAKER: Atrial-paced rhythm, Ventricular-paced rhythm, Atrial-sensed ventricular-paced rhythm, Failure of appropriate capture, Failure of appropriate inhibition, Failure of appropriate inhibition, Failure of appropriate pacemaker firing

rule [10]. For example, procedures of generation of crucial ECG parameters for the left anterior fascicular block are as follows:

- QRS complex duration [ms] – uniformly distributed random number from [80, 120],
- Amplitudes of $R(II)$, $R(III)$ and $R(aVF)$ waves [mV]:

  $R(II)$ - uniformly distributed random number from [0.05, 0.1]

  $$R(III) = R(II) - c_1, \quad R(aVF) = R(II) - c_2$$

  where c_1, c_2 - uniformly distributed random numbers from [0.02, 0.03]
- Amplitudes of $S(II)$, $S(III)$ and $S(aVF)$ waves [mV]:

  $$S(II) = aR(II), \quad S(III) = aR(III), \quad S(aVF) = aR(aVF)$$

  where a - uniformly distributed random number from [4, 8],
- Amplitudes of $Q(I)$ and $Q(aVL)$ waves [mV] - uniformly distributed random numbers from [0, 0.1].

2.3 Module of Interpretation Evaluation

As a result of evaluation of ECG interpretation software, CARDIO system produces so called confusion matrix, containing the numbers of correctly and incorrectly

Kind of	Computer interpretation of ECG signal				
ECG signal	Normal	Disorder 1	Disorder 2	...	Disorder n
Normal	*TN*	*FP1*	*FP2*	...	*FPn*
Disorder 1	*FN1*	*TP1*	*D12*	...	*D1n*
Disorder 2	*FN2*	*D21*	*TP2*	...	*D2n*
...	...	...	...	...	...
Disorder n	*FNn*	*Dn1*	*Dn2*	...	*TPn*

Fig. 4. Confusion matrix of interpretation results

interpreted signals. Its rows and columns correspond to kinds of ECG pathologies and diagnoses made by interpretation module, respectively. *TN* (true negative) denotes the number of normal signals interpreted as normal, *FPi* (false positive) denotes the number of normal signals interpreted incorrectly as signals with *i*-th disorder, *FNi* (false negative) denotes the number of signals with *i*-th disorder interpreted incorrectly as normal, *TPi* (true positive) denotes the number of signals with *i*-th disorder correctly classified and *Dij* denotes the number of signals with *i*th disorder interpreted incorrectly as signal with *j*-th disorder.

In particular, the results from confusion matrix allow us to calculate for *i*-th disorder (i=1,2,...n) the following indices, which are required by the European Standard [15]:

Sensitivity:

$$Se_i = \frac{TPi}{TPi + FNi} \cdot 100\%$$

Specificity:

$$Sp_i = \frac{TN}{TN + FPi} \cdot 100\%$$

Positive predictive value:

$$Pp_i = \frac{TPi}{TPi + FPi} \cdot 100\% .$$

3 Architecture of the CARDIO System

The CARDIO system was designed as an extensible environment for ECG visualization, testing of software modules and educational purposes. To achieve those goals its software architecture was developed as a processing framework with exchangeable plug-ins connected to the main control unit MCU as dynamic linked libraries (DLLs) with carefully designed interfaces implementing communication protocols with the MCU (fig. 5) to exchange information necessary for ECG processing. The system offers its own functionality consisting of essential ECG processing modules, eg. filtering kit, ECG analysis procedures and interpretation module – all encapsulated behind

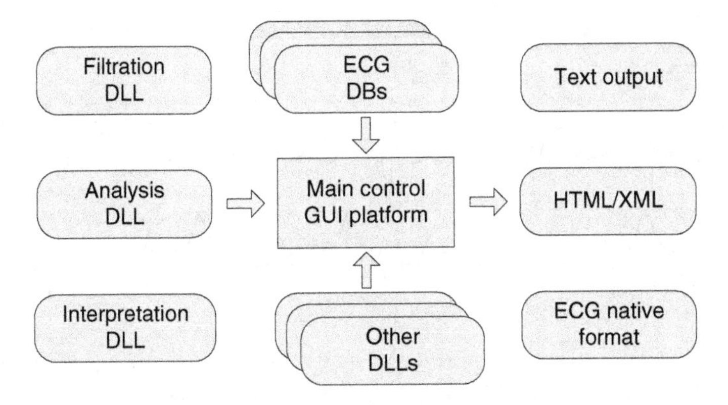

Fig. 5. CARDIO system architecture

the interfaces decoupling its technical and implementation details from the main processing framework configured in the MCU by a user.

The software piece to be tested must be wrapped up in a DLL (one or more), and provided with the appropriate interface in accordance with the specification in analogical way as the native CARDIO modules. Such an organization ensures easy exchangeability of functional modules implementing separate processing stages. The system is equipped with a knowledge base including ECG signals accompanied by expert annotations. Most frequently used ECG file formats import is provided, and the native XML-based storage format was elaborated, mainly for unified treatment of input data and possible future extensions. The MCU integrates all the software units and is responsible for communication with a user which interacts with the system through easy-to-use graphical user interface GUI. ECG processing framework is understood by a chain of sequential exchangeable operations implemented by DLL modules. Such a structure allows for easy configuration of a processing scheme by including/excluding/exchanging an operation from the chain. Implementing system enhancements as DLL modules allows for easy configuration without rebuilding of the whole. This feature is particularly useful for software testing.

4 Demonstration of Working Sessions

A typical working session begins with a configuration stage (ie. setting-up necessary parameters and user options determining the processing profile). The first step can be skipped in case of default processing scheme. ECG signal is then imported to the system together with the attached annotations, if there are any. The signal then appears in the left window (fig. 6) and the characteristic point markers visible as the green vertical lines corresponding to the input annotations. At the same time, in the right window, one can observe the exact values of ECG parameters of interest. The GUI of the MCU shown in fig. 6 offers also other features for taking measurements by means of the mouse cursor (not visible in the screenshot).

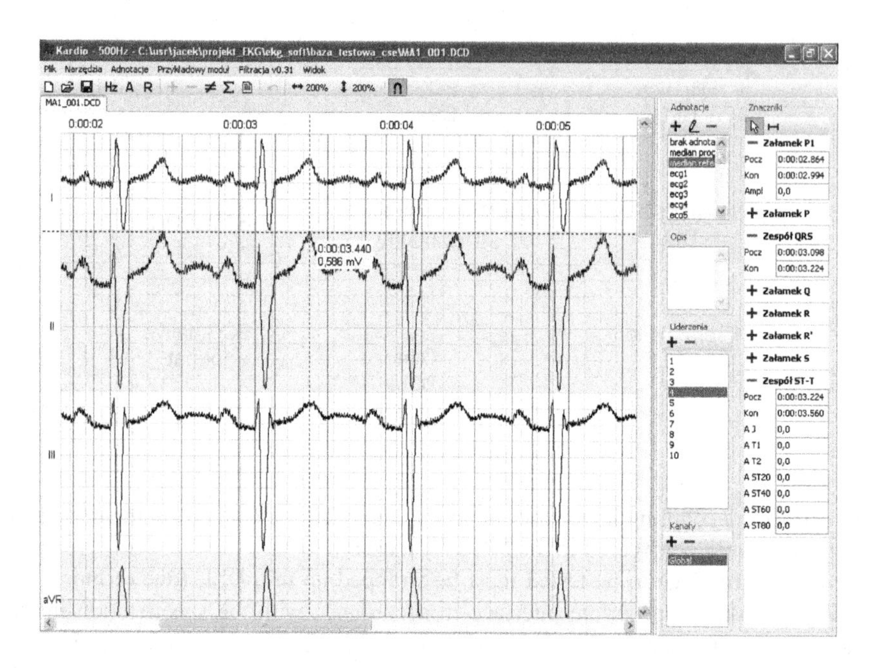

Fig. 6. The GUI layout

Further user's choices depend on the available information (see section 2). If a reference ECG signal is annotated, it is possible to validate analysis algorithm by comparison its results with annotations. The analysis output is then displayed in the signal window. Another option includes batch processing of a number of signals and evaluation of user-defined global quality indexes, which is a standard routine of ECG analysis validation. Missing annotations can be added to the system knowledge base or they can be generated automatically by the system (section 2.2) for separate testing of an interpretation phase with output written in HTML format. The latter is particularly useful when some pathological cases are missing in a reference data base.

5 Conclusion

In this paper we have outlined the features of the CARDIO computer system which is a flexible environment for processing, analysis and interpretation of ECG signals. It can be employed as a computer-aided tool for physicians enhancing their visual assessment of an ECG by improving measurement accuracy, automatic analysis and detection of heart malfunctions. For those designing software embedded in ECG equipment, it allows for using CARDIO as a testing platform. It is also possible to apply CARDIO in education for gaining/testing medical student's skills in visual evaluation of ECG features and diagnostic decision making.

References

1. International Electrotechnical Commission Standard 60601-3-2
2. Willems J.L., et al.: Common Standards for Quantitative Electrocardiography: Goals and Main Results. Meth. Inform. Med. 29, 263–271 (1990); May, P., Ehrlich, H.C., Steinke, T.: ZIB structure prediction pipeline: Composing a complex biological workflow through web services. In: Nagel, W.E., Walter, W.V., Lehner, W. (eds.) Euro-Par 2006. LNCS, vol. 4128, pp. 1148–1158. Springer, Heidelberg (2006)
3. Guglin, M.E., Thatai, D.: Common Errors in Computer Electrocardiogram Interpretation. Int. J. Cardiology 106, 232–237 (2006)
4. Milliken, J.A., Pipberger, H., Pipberger, H.V., et al.: The impact of an ECG computer analysis program on the cardiologist's interpretation. A cooperative study. J. Electrocardiol. 16(2), 141–149 (1983)
5. Endou, K., Miyahara, H., Sato, T.: Clinical usefulness of computer diagnosis in automated electrocardiography. Cardiology 66(3), 174–189 (1980)
6. Willems, J.L., Zywietz, C.: Conformance Testing for Computerized ECG in Conformance Testing and Certification in Information Technology. In: CEN/CENELEC, pp. 307–319. IOS Press, Amsterdam (1990)
7. Zywietz, C.: CTS-ECG Test Atlas. European Pilot Test Center for Computer Electroardiography. Biosignal processing. Medical School, Hannover (1993)
8. ACC/AHA Clinical Competence on Electrocardiography. Journal of American College of Cardiology 38, 2091–2099 (2001)
9. Rautaharju, P., et al.: The Novacode Criteria for Classification of ECG Abnormalities and Their Clinically Significant Progression and Regression. J. Electrocardiology 31, 157–187 (1998)
10. Wagner, G.: Practical Electrocardiography. Williams and Wilkins (1999)
11. Houghton, A., Gray, D.: Making sense of ECG. Arnold Pub. Co. (2003)
12. Chou, T.: Electrocardiography in clinical practice adult and pediatric. W.B. Saunders, Philadelphia (1996)
13. Shah, B., Selvester, R., et al.: Specificity of Electrocardiographic Myocardial Infarction Screening Criteria In Patients with Nonischemic Cardiomiopathies. American Heart J. 136, 314–319 (1998)
14. Warner, R., Yoram, A., et al.: Improved Electrographic Detection of Left Ventricular Hypertrophy. J. Electr. 35(Supp.), 111–115
15. European Standard EN 60601-2-51. Medical electrical equipment. European Committee for Electrotechnical Standarization
16. Czogała, E., Łęski, J.: Application of Entropy and Energy Measures of Fuzziness to Processing of ECG Signal. Fuzzy sets and Systems 97, 9–18 (1998)
17. Pahlm, O., Sornmo, L.: Data Processing of Exercise ECG Signal. IEEE Trans. on Biomed. Eng. 34, 158–165 (1987)
18. Knopfmacher, J.: On Measures of Fuzziness. J. Math. Anal. Appl. 49, 529–534 (1975)

References

Inverse Magnetic Modeling in Computer Tomography

Marek Rudnicki[1,2]

[1] The College of Computer Science, Faculty of Computer Science, Rzgowska 17a, Łódź
[2] Technical University of Lodz, Institute of Computer Science, Wólczańska 215, Łódź

Abstract. Magnetic Resonance Imaging (MRI) technique is widely used for medical diagnostics of human body interior enabling high quality images to be produced. The MRI technique is based on Nuclear Magnetic Resonance (NMR) principle elaborated by Bloch and Purcell in early fifties of 20-th century. Nowadays, NMR is applied in computer tomography devices. In the paper, the problem of optimizing the magnetic field gradients required for NMR tomography is considered. In particular, a double magnetic quadrupole made of inner and outer parts which is intended for producing a magnetic gradient of given distribution is analyzed. The strict requirements on the magnetic field distribution: non-purity and non-linearity related to the quality of tomographic images are taken into account.

Keywords: MRI, NMR, computer tomography, magnetic field gradients, magnetic quadruple.

1 Introduction

Magnetic field gradients are used for getting required field distribution in a diagnostic region. There are two magnetic fields required for NMR: a strong, uniform one appropriately directed along say z-axis and the weak gradient field is excited by means of the magnetic quadruple which changes linearly along y axis. To this end, we need gradient coils. The optimization problem is that of design gradient coils configuration to achieve extremely uniform magnetic field. The problem is formulated in terms of inverse magnetic modeling. The objective is to recover the configuration of the magnetic circuit (quadrupole) given required magnetic field distribution. This is a synthesis problem for which we search for a cause responsible for the result. In the previous papers we have solved the problem using deterministic optimization of the first order [3, 4]. In the present paper we report the optimization results achieved by evolutionary algorithms. Our aim was to design a simple magnetic circuit of highest quality measured with the aid of magnetic field non-purity and non-linearity criteria. However, the main goal is to test an evolutionary optimizer, and not to present a novel configuration for gradient and magnet coils.

1.1 Gradient Coils

The system we study is the gradient system for the whole-body air-core electromagnet which has been presented by Bangert and Mansfield [2]. A gradient in the y direction

E. Kącki, M. Rudnicki, J. Stempczyńska (Eds.): Computers in Medical Activity, AISC 65, pp. 147–153.
springerlink.com

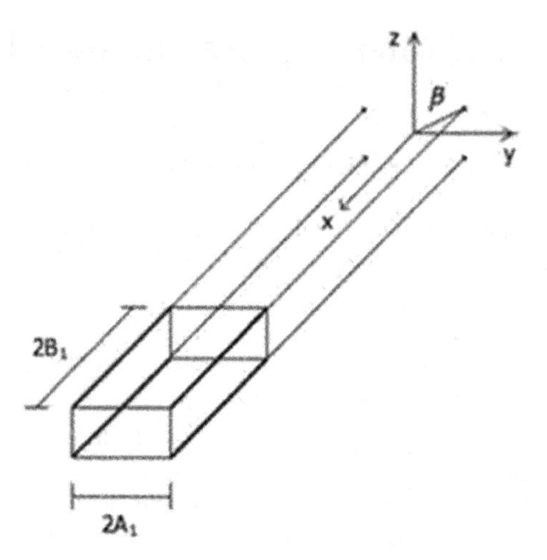

Fig. 1. Inner magnetic quadrupole

B_{zy} may be generated by a quadrupole (a set of four wires) $2B_1$ in length, parallel to the x-axis and running along the edges of the parallelogram (Fig. 1).

The return currents are provided by an outer quadrupole. The inner and outer quadrupole are connected by oblique wires making the angle α with the yz-plane. The full circuit for generation of the y-gradient is shown in Fig. 2.

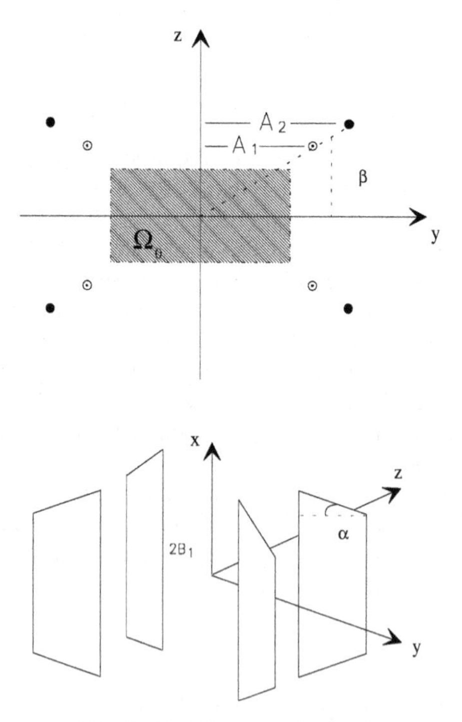

Fig. 2. The full magnetic circuit

Our goal is to design a geometry of the circuit such as to achieve a required distribution of the B_z gradient in the so-called synthesis controlled region (a region of interest). The B_z is, for the double quadrupole, the resultant field of sixteen wires. We assume that the angles α, β are identical for all wires.

1.2 Shape Optimization

The design variables of our problem are geometrical and angular parameters describing the circuit: $A_1, A_2, B_1, \alpha, \beta$ which, together with the current I constitute the design vector. Making use of the explicit expressions for the field $B_z(r)$ given in [3] we can calculate the actual distribution of the $B_z(r)$ over a region in the *yz*-plane. The shape optimization may be formulated as a nonlinear least squares problem. To this end we define an objective function describing the discrepancy between the prescribed field $P(x,r)$ and the actual one $B_z(x,r)$ where x stands for the design vector. Precisely, we require $B_z(x,r)$ to be constant along x and z and it varies linearly along y in a specified controlled sub-region. The objective function to be minimized is given by the formula:

$$F(x) = \sum_{i=1}^{N} E_i^2(x) = \sum_{i=1}^{N} \left[B_z(x_i) - P_z(x_i) \right]^2 \tag{1}$$

where $P_z(x_i)$ is the prescribed, linear with respect to the *y*-axis, distribution of the flux density and $\boldsymbol{x} = (A_1, A_2, B_1, \alpha, \beta, I)$ is the design vector. The above discrepancy is sampled over a set of N=36 points evenly distributed in one quadrant of the region of interest dotted in Fig. 3

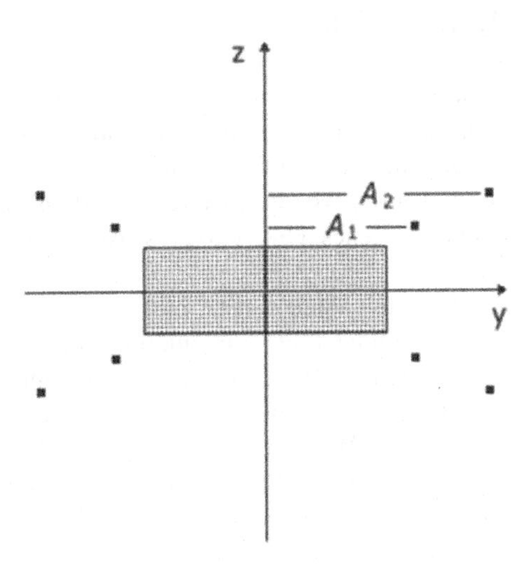

Fig. 3. Projection in the *yz*-plane of the circuit

1.3 Deterministic Optimization

The unconstrained minimization of the objective function (1) was performed with the aid of the Levenberg-Marquardt algorithm with safe-guard step length calculation. Since the objective function was highly multimodal the algorithm converged to different solution depending on the starting point. To constrain the optimization feasible region (volume of the circuit) we have performed as well constrained optimization using a sequential linear programming optimizer with move limits (see [2,3] for the details). The field quality was assessed using the following field estimators:

- a nonlinearity function

$$NL(y,z)=\frac{B_{xy}(y,z)}{B_{zy}(0,0)}-1$$

- a nonpurity function

$$NP(y,z)=\frac{B_{zz}(y,z)}{B_{zy}(0,0)}$$

- an efficiency function (gradient generated by a unit current)
- a maximum and average distortion of magnetic field

Starting from a reasonable set of initial values which did not result in a satisfactory field distribution we arrived at optimal solutions. The numerical results are given in [2,3].

2 Evolutionary Optimization

Contrary to standard genetic algorithms, messy genetic algorithms (mGAs) handle populations of individuals represented by strings of characters of variable length. In nature individuals carry redundant or duplicate information, such as multiple copies of genes, or paired chromosomes. Messy genetic algorithms mimic this, allowing redundant or even contradictory genes. Only two crossover operators are required: cut and splice.

A messy genetic algorithm has three stages: initialization, primordial phase and juxtaposition phase During initialization, a population containing one copy of all substrings of given length is created. We expect that the recombination will find the suitable building blocks (BBs) to assemble them into a good solution structures of virtual objects [5]. A process of BBs filtering takes place after the initialization is completed. BBs are selected and filtrated to, if necessary, shrink chromosomes. Selection is performed in order to increase the number of chromosomes with good evaluation. Afterwards, a random gene deletion is performed to reduce chromosome size to BB size k followed by juxtaposition phase. The advantage of fast messy genetic algorithms (fmGA) is the relatively small population size compared to mGAs. In fact, fmGA was designed to copy with the problem of large population size used by mGAs. A genetic algorithm is likely to converge well if the optimization task can be divided into several short building blocks. What happens if the coding is chosen such that couplings occur between distant genes? Messy genetic algorithms handle this difficulty by using a variable-length, position-independent coding. The key idea is to append an index to each gene which allows identifying its position. As a result, underspecified and over specified individuals may appear in the population. To enhance the BB's propagation rate from one generation to another, a template individual is used. A template is a source of genetic information for underspecified individuals. While messy GAs usually work with a mutation operator similar to that of simple GAs (every allele is altered with a low probability), the crossover operator is replaced by a more general cut and splice operator which also allows to mate parents with different lengths. The above methodology was applied for the solution of the problem.

3 The Results

Generally, the same constrained optimum as the one quoted in [2] was arrived at. It is worthwhile mentioning that similar solutions have been found in many runs of the messy genetic optimizer. Below, the magnetic field estimators are shown for the best initial and final magnetic field distributions Figs [4-7].

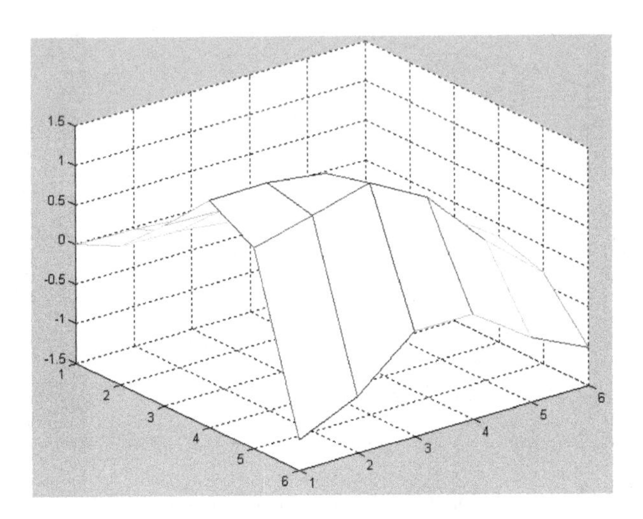

Fig. 4. Initial nonlinearity function

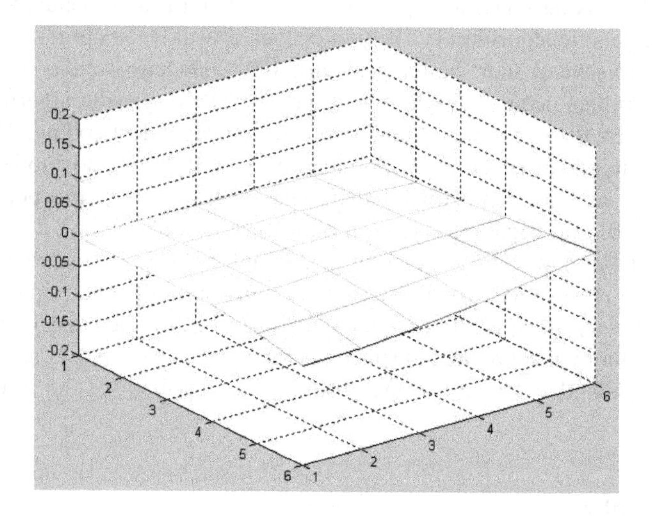

Fig. 5. Final nonlinearity function

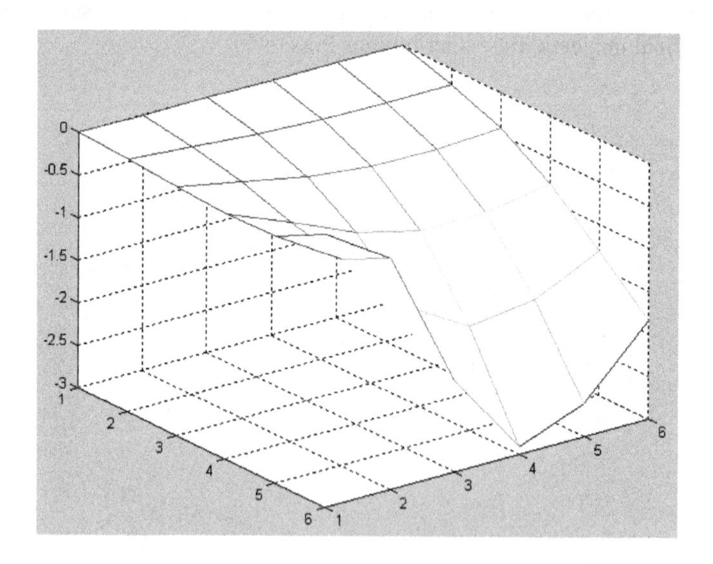

Fig. 6. Initial non-purity function

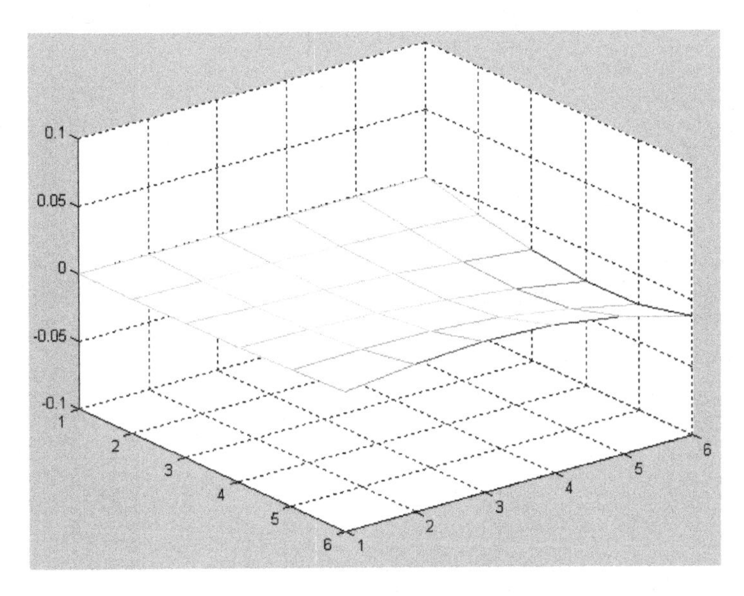

Fig. 7. Final non-purity function

4 Conclusion

The fast messy genetic algorithms appeared to be a reliable tool for optimization of real life magnetic circuits. Even if the initial population size (500 individuals) grows up to 5000 during duplication phase, a few iterations are later needed to arrive at an optimal solution.

References

1. Rudnicki, M.: Application of optimal synthesis methodology in producing gradient magnetic fields for computer tomography. Archiwum Elektrotechniki 1, 63–65 (1991) (in Polish)
2. Mustarelli, P., Rudnicki, M., Savini, A., Savoldi, F., Villa, M.: Synthesis of magnetic gradients for NMR tomography. Magnetic Resonance Imaging 8, 101–105 (1990)
3. Neittaanmäki, P., Rudnicki, M., Savini, A.: Inverse problems and optimal design in electricity and magnestism. Clarendon Press, Oxford (1996)
4. Rudnicki, M., Wiak, S. (eds.): Optimization and Inverse Problems In Electromagnetism. Kluwer Academic Publisher, Dordrecht (2003)
5. Kusztelak, G., Rudnicki, M., Wiak, S.: Propagation of Building Blocks in SGA and MPGA. In: Rutkowski, L., Siekmann, J.H., Tadeusiewicz, R., Zadeh, L.A. (eds.) ICAISC 2004. LNCS (LNAI), vol. 3070, pp. 438–443. Springer, Heidelberg (2004)

Novel CMOS Analog Pulse Shaping Filter for Solid-State X-Ray Sensors in Medical Imaging Systems

Rafał Długosz[1,2,3,*] and Ryszard Wojtyna[3,4]

[1] University of Neuchâtel, Institute of Microtechnology, Rue A.-L. Breguet 2, CH-2000, Neuchâtel, Switzerland
[2] University of Alberta, Department of Electrical and Computer Engineering 114 St – 89 Ave, Edmonton Alberta, T6G 2V4, Canada
[3] The College of Computer Science in Łódź, Poland, Department in Bydgoszcz, ul. Fordońska 246, 85-766, Bydgoszcz, Poland
[4] University of Technology and Life Sciences, Faculty of Telecommunication and Electrical Engineering, ul. Kaliskiego 7, 85-791 Bydgoszcz, Poland
rdlugosz@ualberta.ca, woj@mail.utp.edu.pl

Abstract. A new idea as well as CMOS implementation of a pulse-shaping filter useful in nuclear medicine to realize a multi-element detection by means of a multi-channel readout front-end ASIC have been presented. The filter changes the shape of pulses delivered by a charge amplifier in order to increase the detection speed and robustness. By canceling falling edges of the pulses, a significant increase in the pulse counting rate has been reached (between 3 and 10 MSps in a single channel). The filter takes advantage of a RESET function that is controlled by an asynchronous multiplexer. Including only two resistors, two capacitors and four configuration transistors, it is simpler than other solutions reported to overcome this problem. The proposed shaper together with a peak detector, that receives the shaper signals, dissipates a small amount of power (about 80 μW) for 1V supply voltage. When being inactive, i.e. waiting for the next pulse, the circuit consumes only 200 nW of power.

Keywords: Medical imaging, pulse shaping filter, nuclear medicine.

1 Introduction

Specialized integrated circuits (ASIC) are important part of modern apparatus used in medical imaging. Nuclear medicine techniques use pharmaceuticals that have been labeled with radionuclides and introduced to the patient's body. The role of imaging devices is to detect the emitted X or gamma rays and convert it to an eletrical voltage signal. In most of existing imaging devices, data conversion consists of several steps. First, the X or gamma photons are converted into the visible light using the scintillator and then the light is transformed, using photomultiplier, to a burst of electrons. Multi-step data conversion in such systems is a source of errors, which in practice limit the image resolution.

* Fellow of the EU Marie Curie International Outgoing Fellowship.

E. Kącki, M. Rudnicki, J. Stempczyńska (Eds.): Computers in Medical Activity, AISC 65, pp. 155–165.
springerlink.com

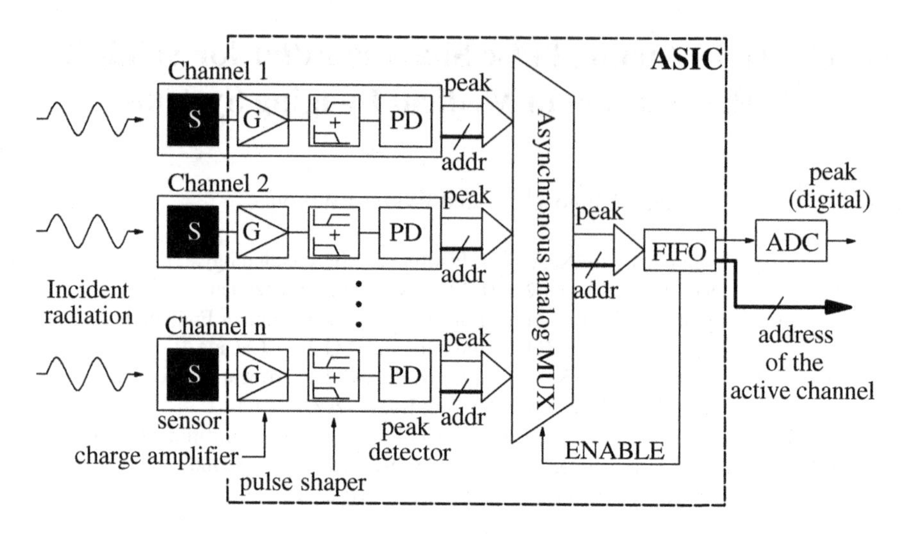

Fig. 1. General block diagram of a typical multi-channel front-end ASIC for multi-element detection systems [3]

In solid-state detectors that recently have been introduced to the market, the X or gamma photons absorbed by an array of sensors are directly converted into an equivalent charge pulses, which may be then processed using the readout multi-channel detecting system [1]. Such diagnostic tools allow for creating medical images of the human body for different clinical purposes.

Front-end readout ASICs, being core circuits in such systems, are subject of research efforts since many years [2, 3]. The observed development in this area is possible due to a continuous progress in microelectronics but also due to development of new circuit solutions, which minimize both chip area and power dissipation, thus allowing for increasing a number of channels integrated in a single chip. In current systems of this type, the number of channels varies between several dozen to several hundreds. Each channel usually contains a charge amplifier (CHA), a pulse shaper (PS) and a peak detector (PD) as show in Fig. 1 [2]. The signal processing scheme in each channel relies on detection of an incident radiation by an associated sensor, which generates an equivalent amount of charge. This charge usually is very small [4] (several dozen aC for 1 keV X-rays) and exhibits random distribution over time for particular events. The task of the CHA circuit is to amplify this charge and store it in a capacitor, generating a voltage proportional to the charge amount for a given radiation event. When this process is quick enough, the PS block gets the signal that can be modeled as a Haeviside step function. The shaper is in practice a band-pass filter, which converts the input step function into a pulse of a given peaking time and amplitude which is proportional to the step value. The role of the PD block (next circuit in the chain) is to store the amplitude in a memory element and set up the flag signal.

2 Proposed Pulse Shaping Band-Pass Filter

For particular radiation events, the CHA circuit generates signals that can be modeled as a Haeviside step function, which in the subsequent PS circuit is converted into a corresponding appropriately shaped impulse, whose amplitude is proportional to the value of this step.

There are several problems encountered in the shaping operation [4]. In real electronic systems, the useful signal is accompanied by a noise, which in this case alters the peak amplitude, introducing a random error to each impulse. To limit the noise spectrum, the useful signal bandwidth at the PS output should be as narrow as possible. Unfortunately, in this case the impulse peak is wide. Although wide peaks simplify the structure of the PD circuit, giving more time for detection and data storage, it decreases the maximal count rate of the channel.

An example implementation of the PS block that overcomes this problem has been described in [4]. In [4], to form wide peaks with short falling edges, the PS block has been realized as a serial connection of passive CR and RC filters, with amplifiers inserted between particular filters to correct the signal amplitude. In this solution, the first block is a band-pass filter shown in Figure 2, while in the next stages additional low-pass RC filters are used.

The first part of our CR-RC circuit is a high-pass filter (R_1C_1), often referred to as a differentiator [4]. To be more precise, this is a differentiator with some inertia mechanism. A "pure" differentiator could not be used in this application as its output amplitude does not depend on the input amplitude, but only on raising time (slope) of the input step function. The problem is that it is not possible to ensure equal rising times at the CHA output because charge impulses received from the sensor have random distributions over time. They can be, for instance, wide and fuzzy or high and narrow. Using a differentiator with an inertia makes the problem insignificant provided that the filter decay time constant is sufficiently large compared to raising time of the input step signals.

The second subcircuit shown in Figure 2 is a low-pass filter (R_2C_2), which is often referred to as an integrator [4]. In fact, this is an inertia circuit whose behavior at higher frequencies is similar to the integrator. For an input signal defined as a step function, the entire CR-RC block operates as a second order inertia circuit excited by a Dirac's delta function. In this case, peaking time of the resultant impulse is constant for a wide amplitude range of the input step function.

Notice that the shaping operation is only possible in the presence of inertia in both the C_1R_1 and R_2C_2 filters. Time constant of the C_1R_1 high-pass filter sets up the width of the impulse. This parameter must be matched to the worst case scenario, i.e. when

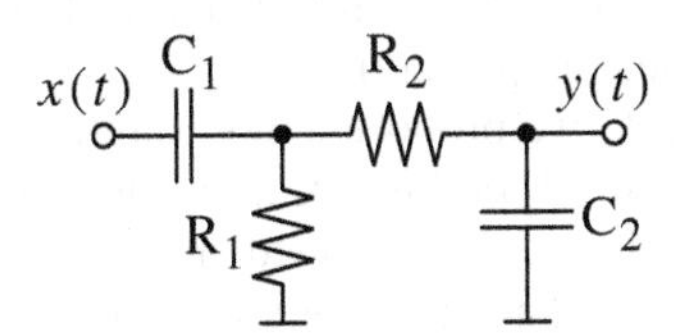

Fig. 2. Simplified electrical scheme of the CR-RC band-pass pulse shaping filter [4]. The amplifiers used to the amplitude correction are not presented in the figure.

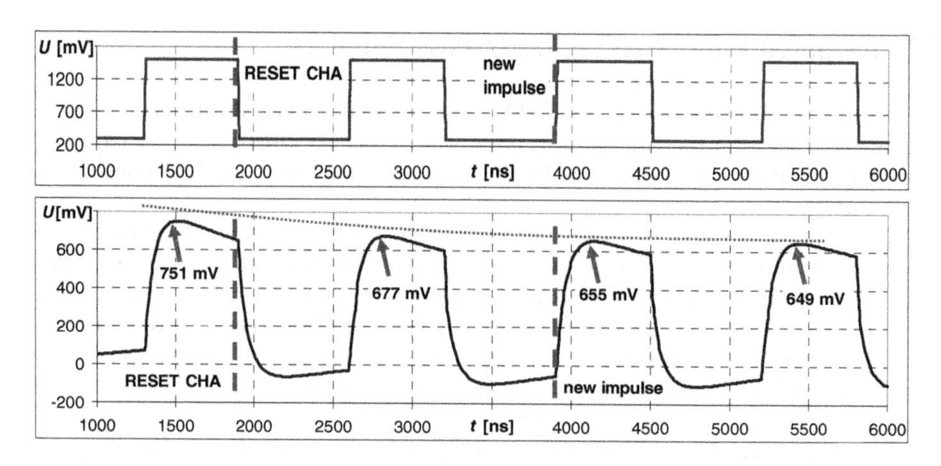

Fig. 3. Input (upper) and output (lower) signals of the pulse shaping filter shown in Fig. 2 in case when input events occur too frequently and pulses overlap each other

the raising time of the input step function is the longest. Increasing this parameter makes shaper's output insensitive to the raising time of the input step function, but this limits the count rate of the channel. The time constant of the R_2C_2 low-pass filter influences both raising time and amplitude of the output signal.

The other important problem related to the pulse shaping is overlapping of adjacent pulses, resulting from long falling edges. Theoretically, the falling edges never vanish, but in practice, when a sufficiently long time is allocated then impulses can be assumed to be independent events. When this time is to short, a new event triggers the transition state with non-zero initial conditions, which introduce additional errors to the output signal. The additional problem is that resetting the CHA circuit means a negative step function at the PS input. This starts a new transition state with non-zero initial conditions, which is illustrated in Figure 3. Note that adjacent impulses occur too frequently causing random errors of the impulse amplitudes.

Key parameter of the detection system is peaking time. Therefore, the impulse falling edge can be considered as a parasitic effect that must be optimized to increase capacity of the channel. Using many CR and RC filters in the shaper described in [4] allows for increasing the decay time constant, but this solution is not optimal due to several reasons. When the number of low-pass filters in the chain increases, a performance improvement resulting from additional stages is smaller and smaller with an increase of stages. For example, adding only one low-pass filter to an existing one brings a better improvement than adding additional four filters to existing four [4]. The problem is that each additional RC filter enlarges both the chip area and power consumption (due to additional amplifiers).

To eliminate this drawback, we propose a new solution, shown in Figure 4, where only a single CR-RC filter is used. In this circuit, a naturally long decay time has been shortened using a RESET signal. The applied mechanism quickly discharges both capacitors (C_1 and C_2) and the channel is ready for a new shaping operation with zero initial conditions. This is illustrated in Figure 5. The shaper is excited by the same input signal like in the experiment shown in Figure 3.

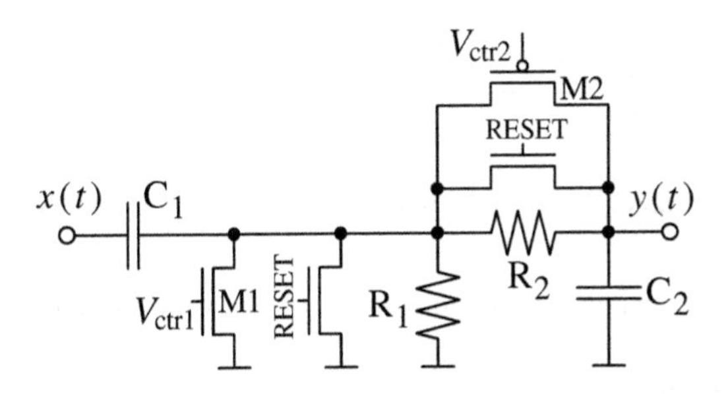

Fig. 4. The proposed pulse shaping filter with built-in RESET and programming functions

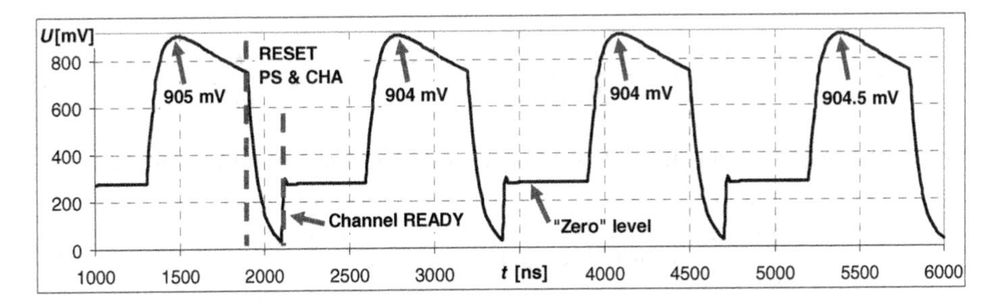

Fig. 5. Output signal of the proposed pulse shaping filter shown in Figure 4

The proposed solution possesses several important advantages. First, the circuit chip area is relatively small (equal to 0.005 mm^2) because of the shaper simplicity (only four passive elements, i.e. C_1=1.7pF, C_2=0.8pF, R_1=500k, R_2=100k). This is important in detecting systems with many channels, where each channel must include the shaper. Another advantage is a very low power consumption of the filter as no correction amplifiers are needed.

2.1 The Shaper Adjusting Capabilities

One of our objectives was to realize a shaping filter that enables controlling both the peaking time and amplitude of the obtained impulse. *S*-domain block diagram of the shaper of Figure 4 is shown in Figure. 6. Its input signal, $X(s)$, is assumed to be a Haeviside step-function voltage, while $Y(s)$ is output voltage of the filter.

Neglecting in Figure 4 the presence of the transistors, the shaper output signal is described by:

$$Y(s) = H(s)X(s) = A\frac{R_1C_1}{s^2R_1R_2C_1C_2 + s(R_1C_1 + R_2C_2 + R_1C_2) + 1} \tag{1}$$

Assuming that R_1 and R_2 as well as C_1 and C_2 are linearly related, i.e:

$$R_2 = aR_1 \text{ and } C_2 = bC_1, \tag{2}$$

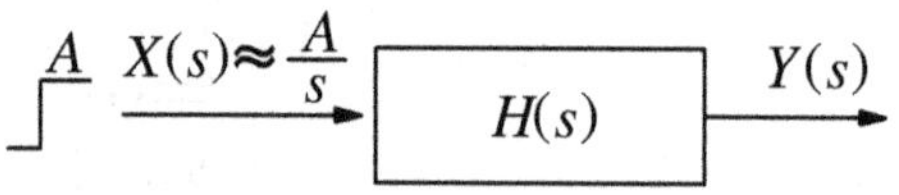

A $X(s) \approx \frac{A}{s}$ $H(s)$ $Y(s)$

Fig. 6. Block diagram of the pulse shaper in s-domain

where: a and b are constant coefficients. Poles of (1), s_1 and s_2, can be expressed as:

$$s_1 = \frac{-(1+ab+b)-\sqrt{1+a^2b^2+b^2+2b+2ab^2-2ab}}{2abR_1C_1} = \frac{k_1}{R_1C_1} \tag{3}$$

$$s_2 = \frac{-(1+ab+b)+\sqrt{1+a^2b^2+b^2+2b+2ab^2-2ab}}{2abR_1C_1} = \frac{k_2}{R_1C_1} \tag{4}$$

Finally, the shaper output signal described in s and time domains takes to forms:

$$Y(s) = A\frac{1}{abR_1C_1(s_2-s_1)}\left(\frac{1}{s-s_2}-\frac{1}{s-s_1}\right) \tag{5}$$

$$y(t) = \frac{1}{\sqrt{1+a^2b^2+b^2+2b+2ab^2-2ab}}\left(e^{s_2t}-e^{s_1t}\right) \tag{6}$$

From (6) it is seen that amplitude of the output signal (peak value) remains unchanged as long as relations between the R_1 and R_2 are kept constant as well as that between C_1 and C_2, i.e. when the dimensionless parameters, a, b, k_1, k_2, in (3), (4) and (6) remain unchanged. As a consequence, by proper varying values of R_1, C_1, R_2, C_2, we can influence only the pole values (s_1 and s_2) and control only peaking time, causing no variations in amplitude of the output signal, which is shown in Figure 7 (MATLAB simulation results). As can be seen from Figure 7, for $R_1/R_2 = 10$ the amplitude is approximately equal to 0.6V and for $R_1/R_2 = 2.5$ equal to about 0.5V.

To make the circuit to be useful in practice, two transistors marked in Figure 4 as M1 and M2 have been added to our filter. These transistors are controlled by means of two biasing voltages V_{ctr1} and V_{ctr2}. Being connected in parallel with R_1 and R_2, respectively, they enable reducing the $R1$ and $R2$ values and varying in this way the R_1C_1 and R_2C_2 time constants of the filter and its output impulse shape. This allows us to perform wider laboratory tests of the system. Example impulses obtained for the same input step function but different values of the bias voltages V_{ctr1} and V_{ctr2} are illustrated in Figure 8. The five curves plotted in Figure 8 correspond to the points A, B, C, D, F in Figure 9, where the horizontal axis represents the V_{ctr1} and the vertical one the V_{ctr2} biasing voltages. In this example, the longest peaking time (Δt =190 ns) is approximately 3 times bigger than the shortest one (Δt = 60 ns).

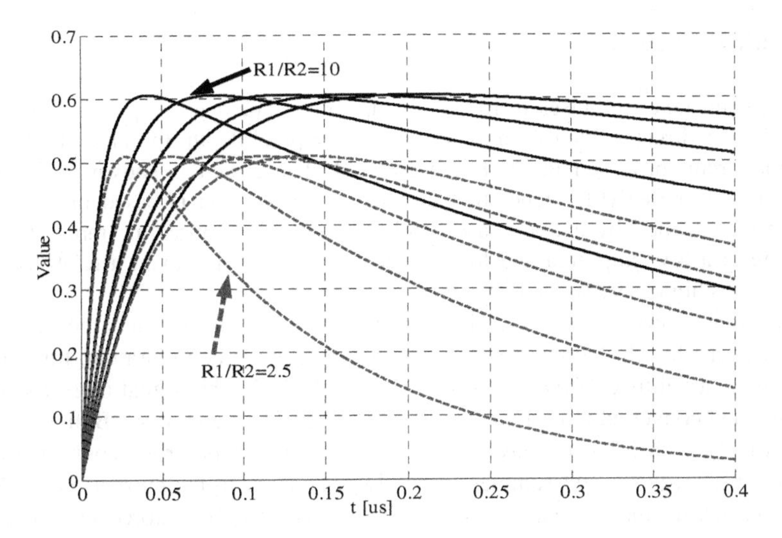

Fig. 7. Theoretical curves of the pulse shaping filter for selected values of passive elements and constant a and b coefficients

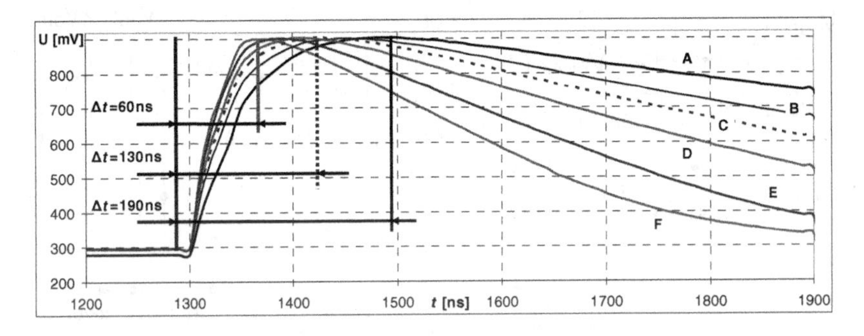

Fig. 8. Output signal of PS for different values of the biasing V_{ctr1} and V_{ctr2} voltages

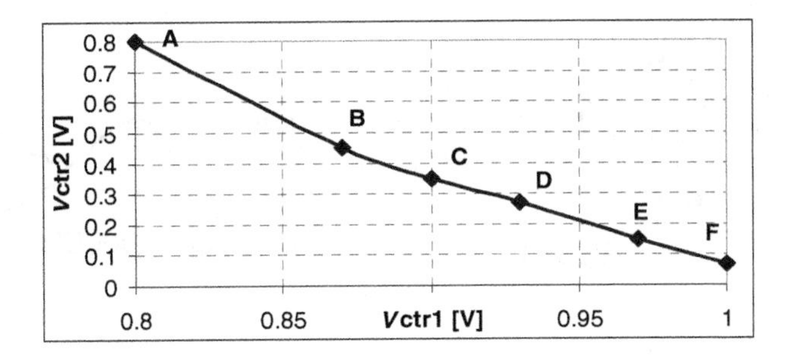

Fig. 9. Values of the V_{ctr1} and V_{ctr2} biasing voltages used in HSPICE simulations of Figure 8

3 Peak Detector

Peak detector takes impulses from the shaping filter. The detector precision is essential and has a direct influence on the output-image pixel-depth. In our studies, a peak detector circuit proposed in [5] has been used. The circuit is shown in Figure 10 together with a flag (FL) generation circuitry. Its operation is based on two delay elements controlled by a two-phase clock. The circuit features a simple structure, resulting in a low chip area and low power dissipation. Moreover, a relatively high precision (as high as 99 %) can be achieved.

This circuit works as follows. The $V_{in}(t)$ input voltage signal enters the C_{st} capacitor as well as the MN1 transistor that operates in a diode configuration, limiting the input signal amplitude of the transistors MN2 and MN3. This signal is next sampled and held and converted to currents that flow through MN2 and MN3. Both capacitors at the MN2 and MN3 gates have values of 20 fF. The appropriate configuration of switches causes the recent samples to be always copied to the current mirror MP1-MP2 and then to the comparator as a positive value. Samples stored previously are transferred to the current mirror MP3-MP4 and then to the comparator as a negative value, using the current mirror MN4-MN5. As a result, when the input signal is rising,

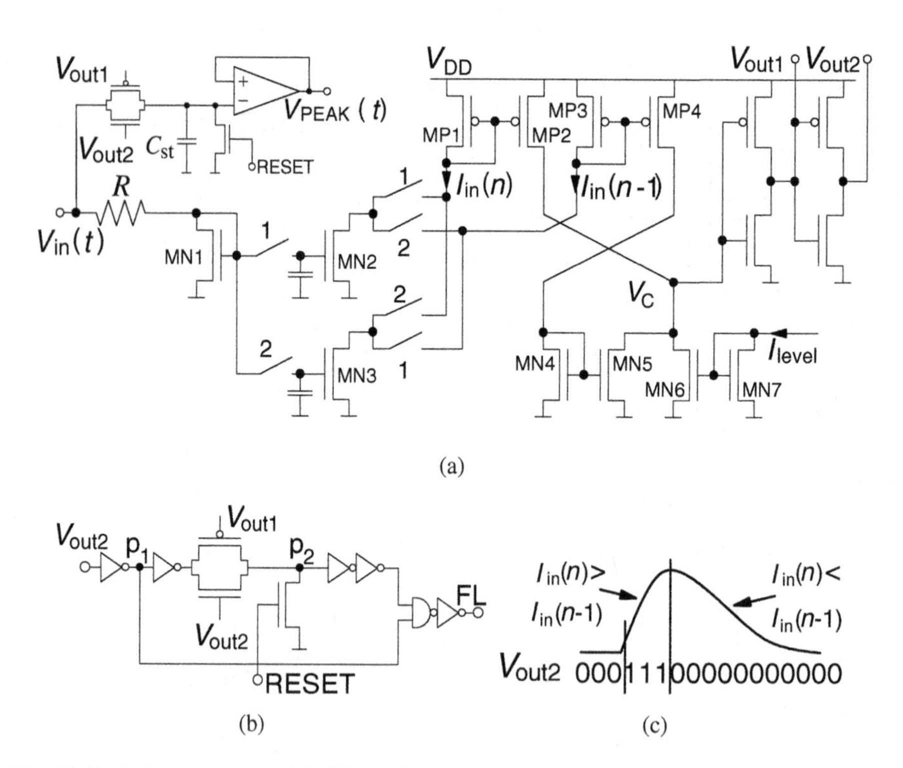

Fig. 10. Peak detector reported in [5]: (a) latching circuit with a switched current circular delay line and a voltage-mode sample-and-hold element, (b) flag generation circuitry, (c) the latch circuit principle of operation

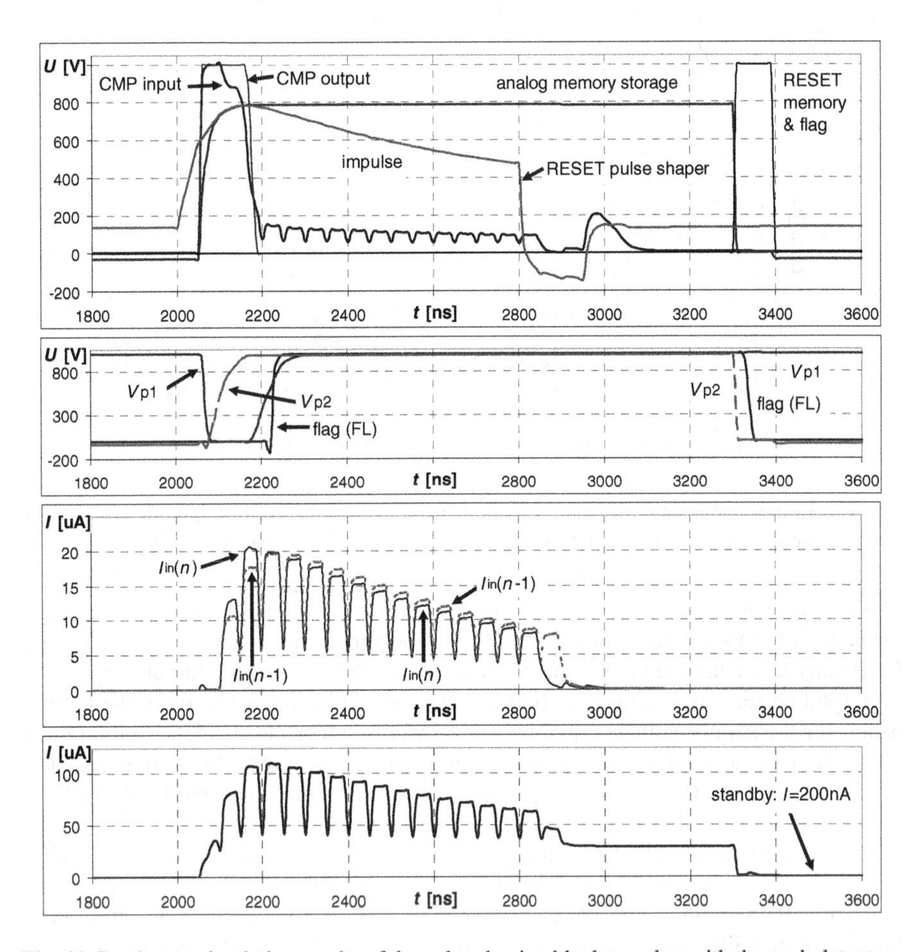

Fig. 11. Postlayout simulation results of the pulse shaping block together with the peak detector

$I_{in}(n)$ is larger than $I_{in}(n\text{-}1)$ and the comparator output enables tracking the input signal of the S&H element shown in the upper left corner of Figure 10 (a). When both signals became equal, i.e. when a peak is reached, the S&H element latches the peak value across the capacitor C_{st} and sets the FL signal to logical "1" by means of the circuit shown in Fig. 10 (b). The detector operation principle is illustrated in Figure 10 (c). Experimental results presented in [5] concern a PD block operating as a separate block, with the input sinus signal applied. In this paper, we present simulation results of an entire channel, where both the proposed PS and PD blocks are joined together.

Postlayout simulation results are shown in Figure 11. Operation of the main (latching) block is presented in the upper panel. The waveforms of the flag generation circuit are shown in the second panel. Note that the FL signal is set up only when the impulse is already stored and the comparator output becomes logical "0" [5]. This allows for reading out this data by an MUX circuit just after the signal fully settles in the PD analog memory.

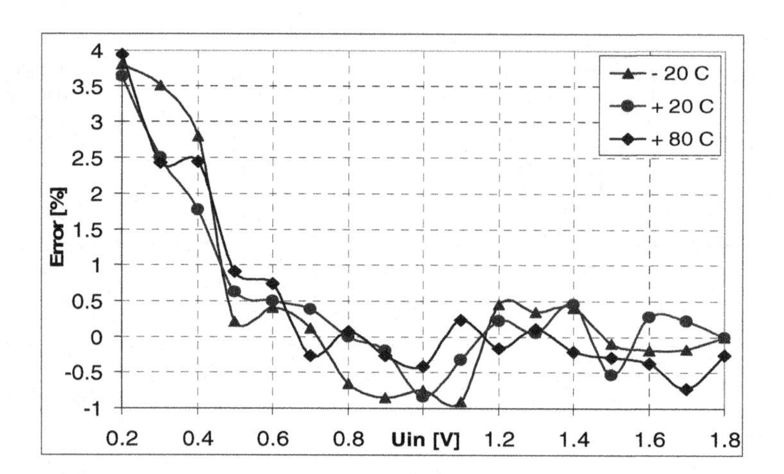

Fig. 12. Accuracy of a single channel (PS and PD blocks), expressed by amplitude error versus the input step voltage in a wide temperature range for standard 1.8 V supply voltage

The third panel illustrates operation of the delay line. When the input signal is rising then $I_{in}(n)$ is greater than $I_{in}(n\text{-}1)$. When the input signal reaches the peak, the $I_{in}(n)$ current becomes smaller, which switches over the comparator output.

A total current consumption in both the PS and PD blocks is shown in the bottom panel, for the supply voltage equal to 1.1 V. After reading out the data, both circuits are reset and channel goes to a power-down mode, where power dissipation becomes small and is below 0.5 μW. This is a very important feature, as both the PS and PD blocks are used in a large number of the system channels.

Accuracy of the PS-PD pair, illustrated in Figure 12, was tested in a wide temperature range, using transistor models related to a standard TSMC CMOS 0.18 μm process. The obtained amplitude error is kept below 1 % in a wide range of amplitudes. For small amplitudes this error raises up reaching the value of about 4 % for $A = 0.2$V. This is not a serious problem, as the error is of systematic nature and can be easily corrected after the analog to digital output data conversion. After the error compensation, the resultant system accuracy at the level of 99.5 % is achievable.

4 Conclusions

This paper presents a new analog-digital CMOS circuit suitable to play a role of pulse shaping band-pass filter in medical imaging systems that take advantage of multi-element detection. Multi-channel readout ASIC's, where our circuit is to be included, are used as front-end blocks in such systems. Development of modern analog-digital ASIC's is associated, among others, with miniaturization of particular building blocks and optimization of their electrical schemes, which allows for enlarging the number of channels implemented on a single chip.

Our filter exhibits important advantages compared to other techniques applied for the pulse shaping purposes. Including only two resistors, two capacitors and four MOS transistors it occupies only 0.005 mm^2 of chip for a standard TSMC 0.18 μm

CMOS process. It is also effective in solving the problem of overlapping two adjacent impulses. The pulse overlapping problem degrades detection precision and speed considerably. Previous attempts to solve this problem were not fully satisfactory as regards power and area consumption. In our filter, the overlapping effect has been defeated without power and area enlargement, by applying a proper filter concept with a simple reset technique and proper designing its element values. This has lead to narrowing the impulses provided to the peak detector. As a result, the obtained impulses have the required width and peaking time can be retuned by means of two biasing voltages in the range from 60ns to 200 ns. The applied RESET function allows for canceling the impulse falling edge just after the data has been read out and the channel is immediately ready to process a new impulse. Not taking into account the input charge amplifier, a single channel in the readout ASIC dissipates during the data acquisition an average power of 80 μW from 1 V supply voltage. When awaiting a new impulse, the PS and PD blocks are in the power-down mode, dissipating only 200 nW. The circuit works properly in a wide range of supplies from 0.8 to 1.8 V.

References

1. Knoll, G.: Radiation Detection and Measurements. Wiley, Chichester (2000)
2. De Geronimo, G., O'Connor, P., Grosholz, J.: A generation of CMOS readout ASIC's for CZT detectors. IEEE Transactions Nuclear Science 47, 1857–1867 (2000)
3. Anghinolfi, F., Dabrowski, W., Delasgnes, E., Kaplon, J., Koetz, U., Jarron, P., Lugiez, F., Posch, C., Roe, S., Weilhammer, P.: CTA-a rad-hard BiCMOS analogue readout ASIC for the ATLAS semiconductor tracker. In: IEEE Nuclear Science Symposium, Conference Record, November 2-9, vol. 1, pp. 46–50 (1996)
4. Spieler, H.: Semiconductor Detector Systems. Oxford University Press, Oxford (2005)
5. Długosz, R., Iniewski, K.: High precision analog peak detector for X-ray imaging applications. Electronic Letters (2007)
6. Długosz, R., Iniewski, K.: Synchronous and Asynchronous Multiplexer Circuits for Medical Imaging Realized in CMOS 0.18um Technology. In: SPIE International Symposium on Microtechnologies for the New Millennium, Gran Canaria, Spain (May 2007)
7. Długosz, R., Iniewski, K.: Hierarchical Asynchronous Multiplexer for Readout front-end ASIC for multi-element detectors in medical imaging. In: International Conference Mixed Design of Integrated Circuits and Systems (MIXDES), Poland (June 2007)

Laser Beam Properties

H. Małecki, W. Gryglewicz-Kacerka, and J. Kacerka

The College of Computer Science in Lodz, 93-008 Łódź, Rzgowska Str. 17a
Technical University of Lodz, 90-924 Lodz, Zeromskiego 116
wkacerka@ics.p.lodz.pl, kacerka@p.lodz.pl

Abstract. A stimulated emission of radiation is possible only in media where a population inversion occurs. The change of a particle energy from a higher-energy state to a lower-energy state is a result of an electron moving to a lower orbital. The laser phenomenon is interesting due to the specific light it emits. It is a well focused monochromatic beam, it has a well-defined wavelength and high energy density. Laser light is very useful in many areas (medicine) because it is monochrome, focused and because of its coherence and very high power density.

The foundation of laser operation is well defined by the compound term for which LASER is an acronym: Light Amplification by Stimulated Emission of Radiation. A stimulated emission of radiation is possible only in media where a population inversion occurs, i.e. a phenomenon very rare in nature may be observed: the population of a higher-energy state exceeds that of a lower-energy state for a relatively long period of time.

The change of a particle energy from a higher-energy state to a lower-energy state is a result of an electron moving to a lower orbital. If the electron moves from a higher-energy orbital E_2 to a lower-energy orbital E_1 the emitted photon contains the energy equal to the difference of energies of the orbitals:

$$h\nu = E_2 - E_1 \tag{1}$$

h=6,62 10^{-34} Js, ν - frequency

Emission of a photon may be spontaneous or stimulated by another photon of the same energy $h\nu$. In the latter case a laser beam is emitted (fig.1).

The laser phenomenon is interesting not because of its complicated construction or method of operation, but due to the specific light it emits. It is a well focused monochromatic beam, i.e. it has a well-defined wavelength (frequency) and high energy density.

The most fundamental properties of a laser beam are that it is: monochromatic, coherent and has a well focused beam of high energy density. The idea of laser construction includes a stimulating source of energy, i.e. a pump source, and a gain medium – a resonator (fig.2).

E. Kącki, M. Rudnicki, J. Stempczyńska (Eds.): Computers in Medical Activity, AISC 65, pp. 167–171.
springerlink.com

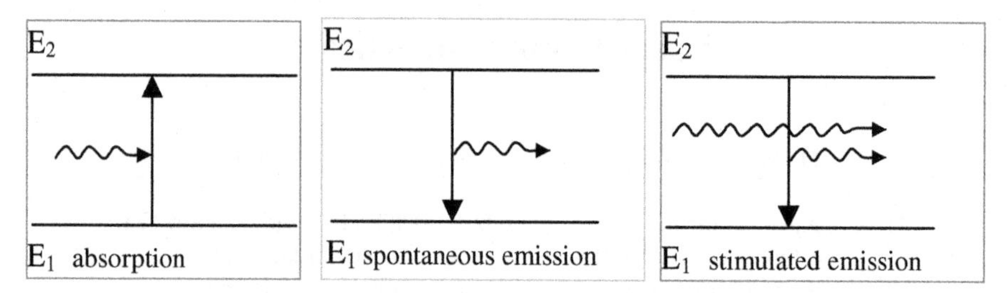

Fig. 1. Interaction between a particle and radiation

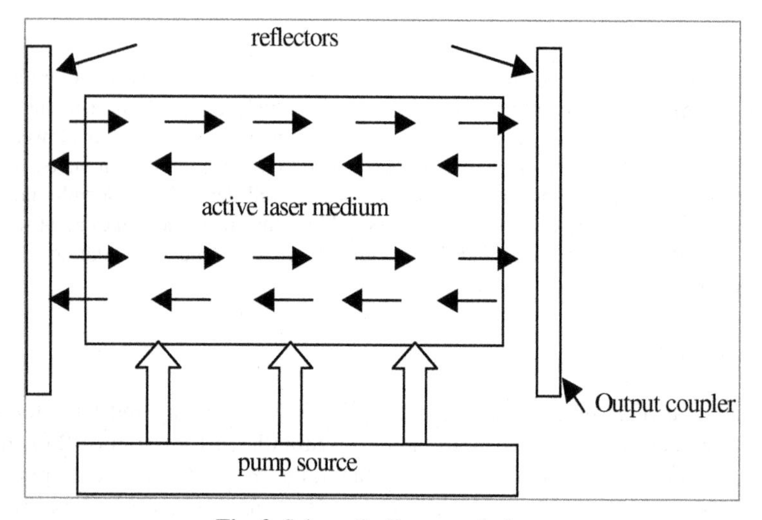

Fig. 2. Schematic diagram of a laser

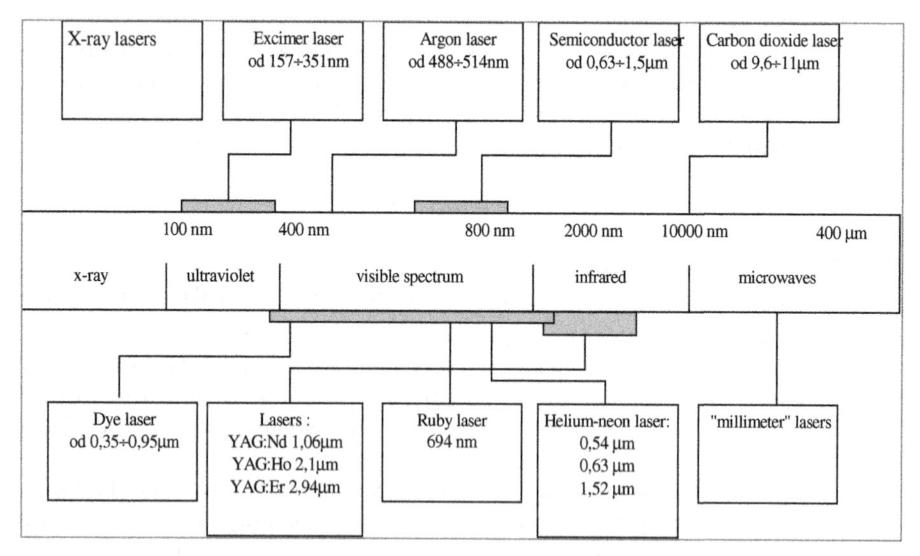

Fig. 3. Laser types and groups and their spectral output

Lasers differ in construction and performance, but are connected by certain properties of their radiation. The output power varies from 10^{-6} W to 10^{9} W, the radiation frequency spectrum spreads from X-ray to microwave [1] (fig. 3).

Talking about electromagnetic waves, radiation or laser beams is virtually talking about the same phenomenon – mostly due to the wave-particle duality of electromagnetic radiation. The photon energy depends on its frequency and is described by the equation (1).

$$E = h\nu \quad (2)$$

where: h– Planck's constant, υ – frequency

Sources of finite dimensions may radiate waves in a certain solid angle or isotropically – equal in all directions. However they may not produce a flat wave, i.e. a wave which traverses the whole space and has one particular property – at any point along the direction of propagation the density of radiation power and scattering is constant. Hence in an empty space the radiation power density at a larger distance from the source is not equal to that at a smaller distance. The power density changes with the distance *r* at the rate:

$$\frac{1}{r^2} \quad (3)$$

The power density distribution across a laser beam – i.e. in the axis perpendicular to the beam – is described by a Gaussian bell-curve, fig. 4a. The beam divergence is defined as a angle of flare of a cone circumscribed on the power density equal to e^{-1} of the maximal value (36.8%). The angle of divergence of a beam passed through a circular hole with equal phase and amplitude is given by (2) (fig.4b)

$$\Theta = \frac{1,22\lambda}{D} \quad (4)$$

where D – radiation source diameter, λ - wavelength.

According to the equation (4) the beam divergence angle – with constant hole diameter – increases with increasing wavelength. A low beam divergence allows for pointing almost whole generated radiation energy in the desired direction (ignoring the losses in transmission medium).

Monochromatic laser beam may be converged (even using a single lens) to a spot of a few μm in diameter (fig.5a). The diameter is given by (5)

$$d = 2\Theta f = \frac{2,44\lambda}{D} f \quad (5)$$

where f – focal length of the focusing lens system,

Non-monochromatic light (white light) may not be focused to such little spots (fig. 5b). By focusing a laser beam into a spot of diameter *d* given by (5) the beam power density is increased.

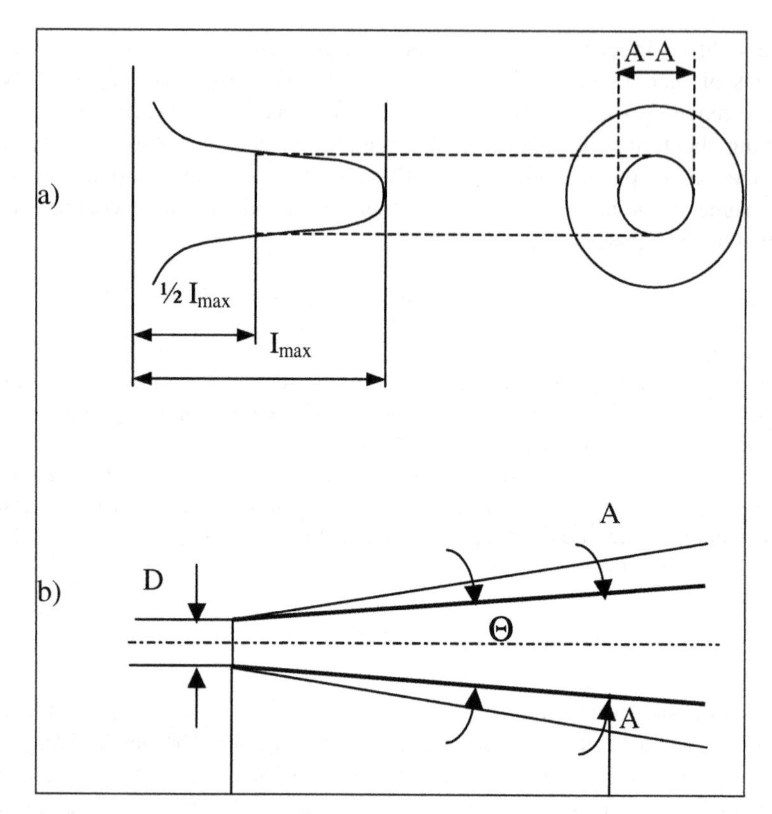

Fig. 4. Lase beam divergence

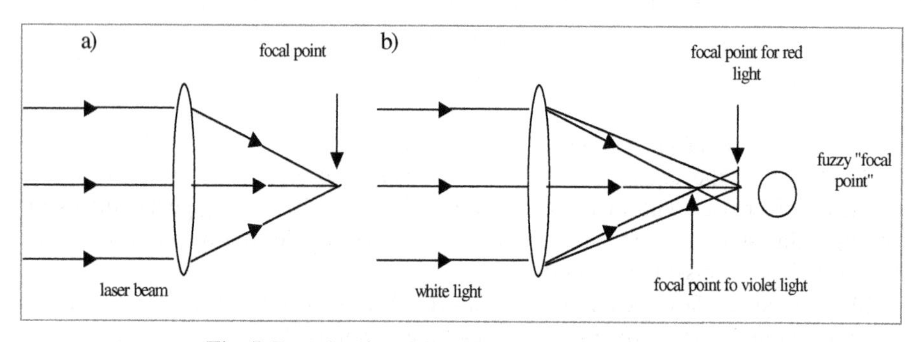

Fig. 5. Focusing for: a) laser beam, b) white light beam

Assuming the power of laser beam equal to 1kW the power of density in a 50μm spot would equal approximately 10^9W/cm^2, i.e. an energy of 10^9J passing through an area of 1 cm^2 in one second. It should be noted, that the power density of sunlight is approximately $7 \cdot 10^3$W/cm^2 - six orders of magnitude less powerful than the beam in the example above. For a laser beam having wavelength of 514 nm (Argon) the energy of photons would equal $E=3{,}8 \cdot 10^{-19}$J (72eV), and the number of photons passing through a surface of 1 cm^2 in 1 second is approximately $2{,}6 \cdot 10^{27}$.

Laser light is very useful in many areas because it is monochrome, focused and because of its coherence and very high power density. Very few other discoveries in the history of science have so many applications.

The application of lasers in medicine is possible also because laser beam photons have relatively low energy and thus do not cause ionisation of the atoms while passing through matter, unlike photons of Roentgen or gamma radiation.

Notwithstanding the wide application of laser radiation in technology and medicine one should always remember that the laser radiation is hazardous to human eyesight. Eye is a very sensitive biological structure. Laser radiation, characterized by high density of power is particularly dangerous for eyes. In the range of wavelengths from 400 nm (ultraviolet) to 1400 nm (infra-red) the retina is the most exposed, as the cornea, lens, aqueous humour and vitreous humour are transparent for the radiation [2],[3].

Laser beam may achieve substantial density of power when focused on the eye retina. The power density occurring at the retina depends on the type of laser, its power and the degree of beam coherence. The gain of radiation due to passing through the lens and focusing is approximately equal to the ratio of pupil area to the area of image focused on the retina. Assuming that the maximal diameter of the pupil is about 7 mm, the image on the retina may have a diameter of 10-20μm. The increase of radiation power between the cornea and the retina may be approximated between $2 \cdot 10^5 W/m^2$ and $5 \cdot 10^5 W/m^2$ [1], [4].

Bibliography

[1] Owczarek, G.: PhD thesis – Central Institute for Labour Protection. Warszawa (2000)

[2] PN-83/T-01028. lasers. Terms and definitions

[3] PN-EN 207. Individual eye protection, means of eye protection, filters protecting eyes from laser radiation

[4] Mizerski, W.: Chemical tables. Wydawnictwo Adamantan. Warszawa (1997)

Computer Aiding and Virtual Integration of the Medical Activities

Zbigniew Kierzkowski and Piotr Tarlowski

Networked Virtual Activities Organization Laboratories: Lodz-Olsztyn-Polkowice-Poznan, The College of Computer Science in Lodz & Poznan University of Technology

Abstract. Within the healthcare reform, it is necessary to fulfill a lot of conditions, amongst which the important role plays elaborations of information systems directed on consideration rationalization of medical care, medical personnel works, availability of modern equipment, medical apparatus and data about human wellbeing state. In new solutions we have to do with computer integrated activities organization in the environment of structures of mutual data exchange and the problem domain. There are created computer oriented healthcare systems. Computer aiding includes bigger and bigger range of routine medical activities and is adjusted in bigger and bigger degree to ways of doctor's process. There are observed consolidation of functions and tasks of computer integration and virtual medical activities organization with functions and tasks of computer aiding integration and virtual medical activities organization systems where the result is co-operation organization process of doctors and the healthcare institution.

Keywords: computer integrated activities organization – CIAO, computer integrated medical activities organization – CIMAO, computer medical activities aiding – CMAA, computer integrated medical activities – CIMA, virtual medical activities organization – VMAO, information processes in the health care systems.

1 Basic Concepts

Observed processes of structural changes of activities organization is progress implication of computer science and applied informatics in mutually connected spaces: (a) computer and information systems engineering, (b) computer networks and co-operative information systems engineering, (c) information and communication technology – I&CT and cooperation technology within arising the new structures of the activities organization – information society technology – IST. These processes are also sequence of appearing newer and newer concepts of computer integrated activities organization – CIAO, or information and organization integration of the activities.

One can talk about information and organization foundations of structural changes of various real systems taking out from the progress in the development of methods and informatics applications and from the development of CIAO methods.

E. Kącki, M. Rudnicki, J. Stempczyńska (Eds.): Computers in Medical Activity, AISC 65, pp. 173–188.
springerlink.com

Initial CIAO concepts rely on structural modeling of data organization and computer aided activities – CAA. CAA conception expansion in CIAO is methodology of functional modeling of data organization and computer integrated activities – CIA. Cap of CIAO conception is process modeling of data organization and virtual activities organization – VAO in enterprises (institutions) cooperation and human collaboration.

CAA methodology based on the computer knowledge representation about problem domain – PD and realization in human-computer interaction. Problem domain – PD or domain space, fragment of real world, objects system, is set of facts about material and abstract subjects and their properties as well as connections which are interesting from the point of view of various classes of creating information systems and domain computer applications. PD can be treated as separate fragment of real world or can be artificially created i.e. realistic in the form of certain programs system, data, and knowledge. PD presentation using formalized characters system can be its model. The data processing organization in CAA systems are loose connected (subject) schemas of calculations.

CIA includes examining activities in the environment of network aggregated resources aiding. The information environment model of CIA is functional activities organization and application integration. Solutions characterize dispersal, changes dynamics in short time, big resources aggregation with determined access modes to various data. The data processing organization in CIA systems is the scheme about large scale of integration.

VAO notion hails only from computer aiding and computer activities integration (consolidation of information and organizational elements of CAA and CIA systems), and also from transparent pointed out tasks of CIAO users: co-operating organization and human collaboration. In VAO we take into consideration activities allocation and resources consolidation. Resources consolidation relies on the dynamic exchange of documents in the digital form; it represents the problem knowledge – PK (knowledge process organization about PD) mutual (interactive) exchanging within the structures of common (co-operative) solving multitask problems. Data processing organization in VAO systems is the structure about large scale of integration in processes of mutual data exchange representing PK sin the direct interactive communication.

To organizational foundations of structural changes of real systems we include:

- Structural modeling of data organization and activities,
- Functional modeling of data organization and co-operation activities,
- Process modeling of data organization within the virtual information environment and enterprises co-operation and human collaboration.

However structures of mutual (interactive) data exchange and the problem domain using nested structures of distributed and transaction information systems are the information environment of structural changes of the real systems. In building computer aiding systems of integration and virtual activities organization we have to do with hierarchy of mutual connected models of information supporting of human activities and organization co-operation. In virtual information environment there consolidated levels of problem domains, interoperability of federal systems and co-operation coordination within mutual executing multitasking problems of real systems.

Each model in hierarchy models of virtual information environment should have features, which determine the name of internal and external features. Through internal features we understand assurance of confidence, cohesion, minority, efficiency. Confidence is related to the degree of the realization of functions, tasks, problems in the organization model. Cohesion (consistency) refers checking of possible conflicts and unconformity between elements of the system; we take care about protection prior to creating information and activities not compliant with the model of the real system. Points of minority allow to counter redundant redundancy in information modeling of the system. Efficiency depends on implementation efficiency achievement and utility of the information system. There also appears some external features of information system elements. They enable realization of connections and answers forwards and backwards in the hierarchy of information system elements. We take care that in the case of structural changes of the organization model and resulting changes of information system elements one can propagate these changes up and down in the effective and coherent means.

2 Information Aiding and Process Medical Activities Organization

Methods and technologies of development CIAO systems – since 25 years – are the subject of medicine interests. Topicality of this problem presently enriches facing elaboration of computer medical activities aiding systems – CMAA within works upon building new information systems for reforming the healthcare.

At first CMAA systems are built in scientific centers, next computer integrated and virtual medical activities organization systems - VMAO. In building systems for aims of computer aiding and next computer integrated and virtual activities organization, we take into account:

- Utility (useful properties) of building systems,
- Description of activities (activity processes) and synthesis of computer aiding resources,
- Synthesis of storing and integrating digital resources in structures of services of the information flow co-ordination.

First conditions concern the role of human-computer system and structural and functional elements of building systems. Structural elements determine resources and ways of their storing, required in aiding however functional properties determine data conversion ways corresponding needs of users. Next conditions result from the aiding aim resulting from activities character amongst which one can separate routine activities and next corresponding intelligent behavior. Because activities comprise on complex information-decision processes in which activities grokly (difficult for formalization) resulting from qualifications and experiences, interlace with activities of routine processes so based on methods giving formalization. Computer aiding is based on composing methods and resources to behavior creative character of activities (intuition, qualifications, expert experiences) at simultaneous interception by built systems of full service of routine activities. Succeeding conditions concern synthesis of co-operative network information environment giving possible organization and co-operation aiding (of the group work).

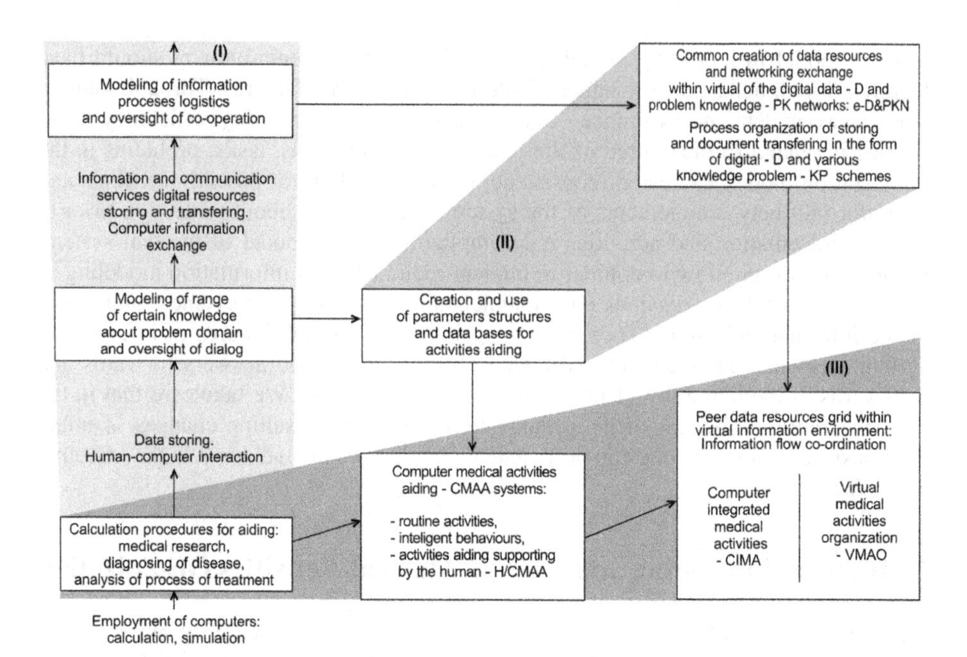

Fig. 1. Analysis of main functions (I) and elements of models (II) of computer aiding and integration and virtual medical aiding organization systems (III)

The condition analysis allows to separate elements of computer aiding and medical activities integration foundations and also creating instrumental means of well treatment of building particular systems (Fig. 1).

The analysis consists of:

- Conceptualization of computer aiding and activities integration what includes: modeling and settlement of system classes described by similar features, structural and functional properties,
- Separation of main functions, what includes: settlement of new aiding aims on the basis abstraction from features and properties of built and used systems and focusing required new functions,
- Practical realization of main functions, what includes substantiation ways of new functions; there are settled succeeding elements of systems models computer integrated medical activities organization – CIMAO, next consolidated with function models of previous solutions.

In building at first, mainly in different scientific centers, computer medical activities aiding systems – CMAA, include inter alia computer aiding for example clinical investigations, aiding of treatment analysis in the clinic process, scruds recognition etc in these solutions we have used various processes of statistical inferring, computer representation or clinic problems and laboratory experience analysis. One can take into consideration the expert approach for illness recognition in aiding clinic process.

In succeeding solutions we observe aggregation of CMAA methods with their computer integration. There are appeared network, distributed, medical information systems. Co-operating activities are represented i.e. computer medical activities aiding and process organization of health state investigation and treatment service of patients. Aggregation of CMAA problems with process oriented organization of health state investigation and the treatment service of patients leads to structural changes of the healthcare, directed on virtual medical activities organization. Structural changes are not only directed on computer aiding of various medical activities but also on widespread computer aiding more numerous activities of healthcare workers and appearing new co-operation forms of various organization: cutting loose outpatient clinic, hospitals, pharmaceutical and manager companies etc. We have to do with virtual medical activities organization – VMAO, realized in the environment of storing systems and transferring data resources and the problem domain, in the environment of virtual data networks and the medical problem domain: e-D&(Medical)PKN.

In structures of computer aiding and integration medical activities systems one can separate the following chains of main functions, their models and technical solutions.

In the chain of main functions we separate: representation of some knowledge range about the problem domain – PD and supervision over dialogue, logics representation of information processes of the healthcare system and supervision over co-operation. Main function results from possibilities of computer services of storing data and the human-computer interaction and using different modes of computer information exchange and utilizing information and communication services in building storing and transferring resources systems.

The chain of elements of main function models includes: creating and utilizing program and parameter structures and data bases for aiding activities, common creating resources and network their exchange, process organization of storing source documents in the digital notion – D and their transferring in created various schemas of the problem domain. In the chain of technical solutions we separate solid systems CMAA, CIMA and VMAO. The practical realization of computer integration aiding and virtual medical activities organization requires creating partner structures of data resources and mechanisms of information flow co-ordination for settlement of the range of information aiding of process organization of doctor's co-operation and co-operation of various healthcare institution.

3 Evolution and Integration of Computer Aided Medical Activities Systems

Ways led for better recognition of scruds as well as pathogenesis as treatment to clinical and laboratory experiences and statistical examinations. The most important works enabling aiding of experience analysis, already from many years are based on using computers and organizing registration, storing information and using systems development for their aims.

Computer aiding, as well as routine activities as aiding activities in more and more degree adapted ways of doctor's behavior what is the result of general using of computers in the range of: (1) filing system and seeking information for statistical inferring about effects of medical procedures in treatment, (2) storing data of aiding diagnosing processes for elaborating patterns of wellbeing evaluation of patients, (3) creating intelligent systems of aiding diagnosis, connecting with finding doctor's action in the treatment process.

In building systems of computer aiding activities we have to do with development and integration of functions and tasks servicing medical activities. They are the result of computer services development including: calculations, simulations, data storing and human-computer interaction.

Development of aiding ranges in succeeding generations of practical solutions results from analysis of foundations of building particular information systems.

Development of medical activities aiding ranges accompanies the function integration of previous solutions with aiding models of succeeding functions in systems of next generation.

The escape point is aiding of routine activities and statistical inferring. We use structures of built banks of medical data and statistical inferring. The result of inferring is the presentation of facts describing models of various elements of medical problem domain.

Exemplary solution is the structure of computer aiding of investigations lead over efficacy for example clinical treatment of patients (fig. 2), what applied in statistical analysis of operational operative treatment of retinal detachment. In the clinical database there is stored information about patients. Statistical analysis programs allowed to analyze clinical problems as elements of knowledge about efficacy of the operative treatment in procedure in retinal detachment.

Next one uses integration management what enriches the aiding model of medical activities. Result of these activities is storing data allowing creating bases of cases and bases of information about patients. Using information of patients enables, on the base of enriched inferring, better recognition of scruds and taking out of facts and further elements of medical problem knowledge.

Interaction management enriches the aiding model of clinical investigations. The structure of computer aiding of investigation descriptions and the process of patient's hospitalization (fig. 3) is the example of this solution.

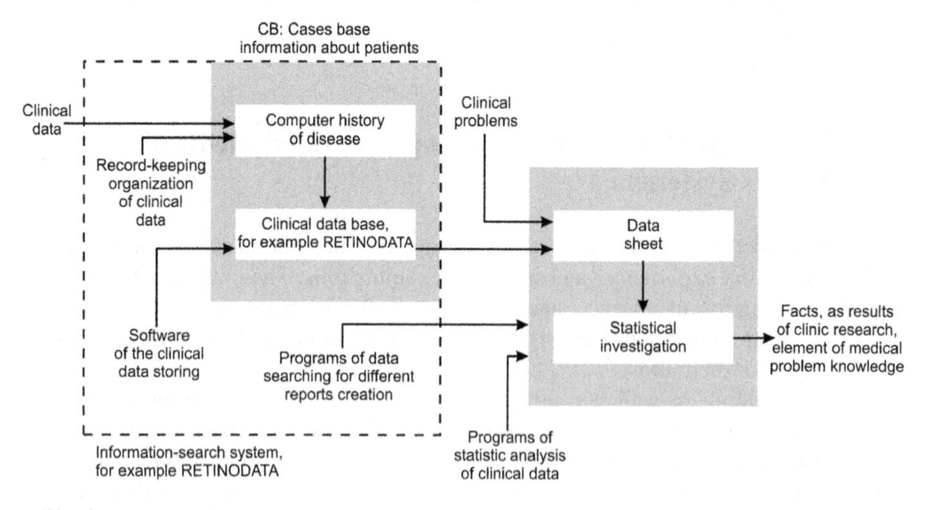

Fig. 2. Structure of exemplary aiding computer system of statistical analysis of clinical data

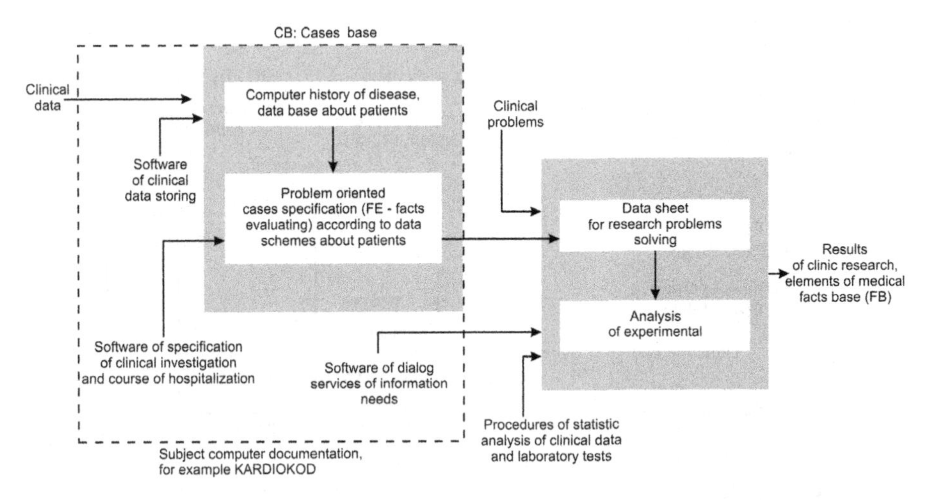

Fig. 3. Structure of computer registration and data analysis for aiding activities in treatment of patients

Storing clinical data allows creating cases bases (CB), information bases about patients. Using this information about patients makes possible, on the basis of enriched inferring, better knowing of scruds and derivation of facts (facts base – FB), for example about retinal detachment and clinical cardiologist problems.

Further increasing from the aiding range of medical activities includes succeeding activities of the treatment process and well treatment of inferring based on medical experiences on the base of expert solutions. So it appears possibility of aiding of doctor's behavior in the treatment process.

It is possible to connect problems of data registration about patients and their treatment process with illness recognition elements (fig. 4).

In computer aiding of illness recognition there are appeared additional information making possible leading processes of inferring. One uses databases about patients, facts description consists of expert knowledge and elaborated schema inferring. In the structure of computer scruds recognition aiding system in aiding one uses the description of doctor's activities in the clinic (routine) process, completed the description of activities supported by expert' knowledge (patterns of scruds descriptions), and also description of inferring processes on the basis of clinic experiences completed about descriptions of the case delivered by the DS system. Computer aiding includes some range of routine activities. Computer aiding is adapted in a bigger degree to doctor's expectation, what was checked in solutions of using computers for aiding illness recognition of nervous system.

Elements of the expert system CMAA are: cases base – CB, domain description in the form of facts base describing the case – FB and inferring representation base – IRB. Existing elements CB and FB on account of their specification and function, one can organize as databases elements. Element IRB enlarges functions CMAA. IRB functions are as follows: (1) schemas of inferring processes on the basis of register facts in CB, (2) inferring schemas on the basis of CB and results of earlier inferring. One can usually base on CB. It is necessary to verify IRB contents. More often one

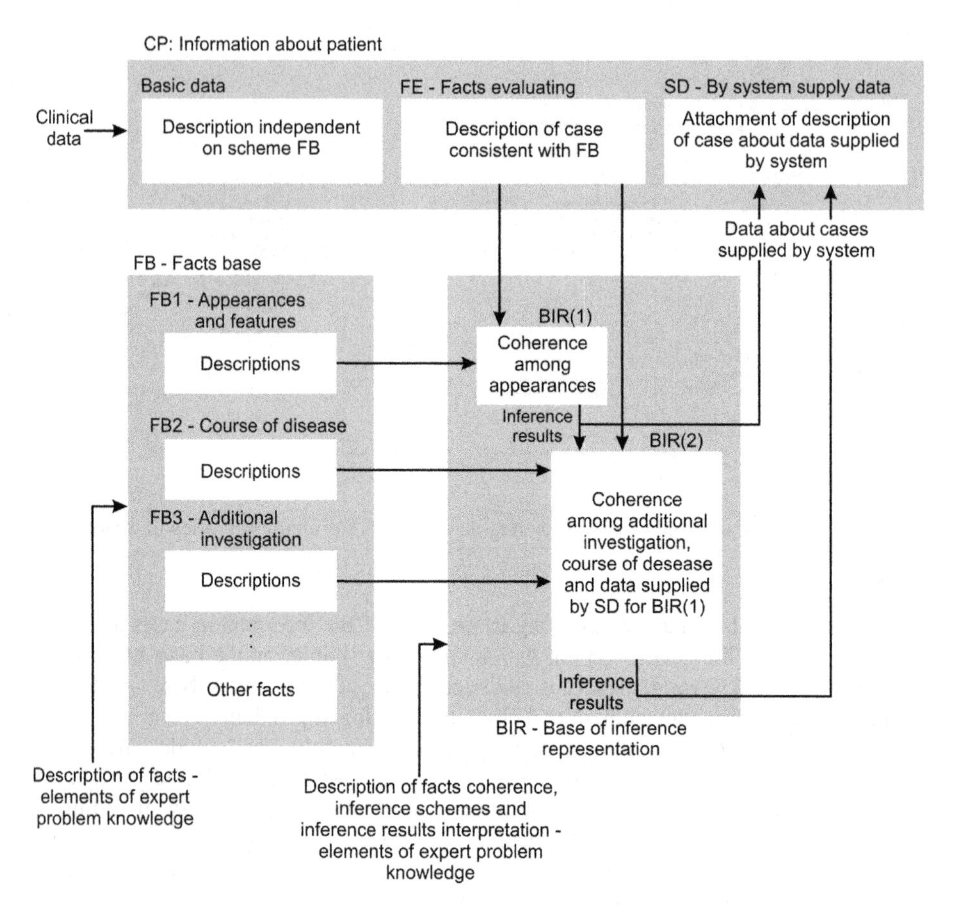

Fig. 4. Structure of exemplary aiding computer system of diagnosing of disease – NEURODIAG system

refers to contemporary knowledge i.e. results of investigations in the problem domain, which includes functions and tasks of solid CMAA system. In exemplary CMAA solution referring to neurological scruds, the system includes interactive using of information registered in mentioned bases of casus, facto and solutions.

4 Towards Virtual Medical Activities Organization Based on Network Services

Virtual activities organization – VAO is the base of creating effective organization structures and changes of structural activities organization in the service environment of global information systems. The VAO notion takes from the consolidation of three information and organizational elements of computer aided activities systems – CAA and computer activities integration – CAI.

First element is associated with the computer representation of the problem domain (PD) and knowledge domain (KD). Representation is concerned with creating resources, and next with creating configurations of the integrated information exchange, intelligent systems of the access and exchange for searching and gaining information in bases and data-bases, treated as the information media. Second element concerns creating structures of the human – computer interaction. Interaction structures are created on the base of linking the dialogue interface in aiding (including building aiding means on computer stations), with elements of the co-operative function implementation (integrated activities aiding) and with elements of the co-ordination function implementation, partnership of users in the group-work. Third main element includes the organization modeling. In VAO problems it is visible to use the structural, functional and process approaches in the organization modeling.

Virtuality depends on this, that real systems are represented by abstraction with which information bytes (objects) are created. They are freely moved, distributed and aggregated in the information space. They have certain access to information resources for computer aiding and activities integration. Operations on executed on objects, are realized in the centralized way, and are initiated asynchronously by different users. Each user perceives as well objects as operations in the proper way for realized partial tasks. It has the virtual screen of activities realized in the real system. Knowledge about entity, globalize screen of activities is multi-aspectness represented in the conceptual scheme of the real system and is contained in distributed, intelligent systems controlled by the process of activities realization.

VAO meanings results from the range and sense of notions: virtual, virtual organization, activities. Virtual means such which is not settled in a rigid way, that functions dynamically and the integration of its elements does not follow through the structure but through realized functions. The virtual organization is virtual organizing way i.e. through co-operation in information space. The place in which participants act, is not valid and each element is valid as a producer (source) and a consumer (receiver) of information and as a decision maker. Activities are actions in the information space. They respond to activities in the real systems. The real systems are the source (of activities) and the subject on which activities are directed and are their substance and final verifier.

It is seen that virtual organizing way i.e. creating VAO systems, depends on the representation of "real world" structures in the information space – in structures of the "information beings world" in I&CT services environment.

Creating VAO systems requires common information space what realizes various functions in the organization and human co-operation structures. It concerns with creating VAO systems depending on solving organizing problems and using common information space (fig. 5).

The process of common information space forming is based on third dimensions: R, S, C. First dimension – R is results from creating data resources – D ways. They consist in applying determined methods of creating source documents in the form of computer files and different access modes to these sources (computer reading out, reading out with possibilities of implementing changes). Second dimension – S determines communication procedures transferring and mutual exchange of the resources. It relies on software implementation of the runtime application, destined for the service information needs in problem knowledge – PK schemas. They are being

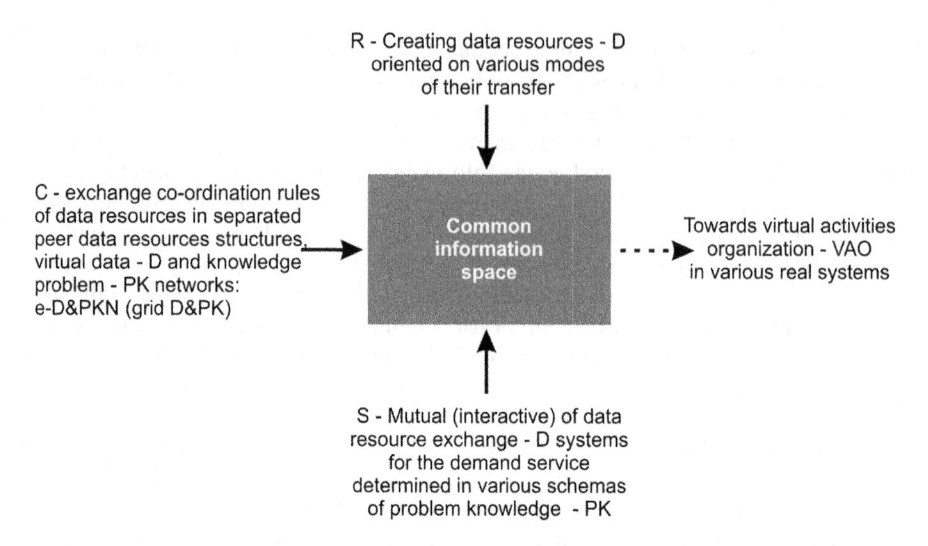

Fig. 5. Main factors of forming information environment for creating virtual activities organization systems

established by participants of VMAO structures. Third dimension – C is being conditioned by principles of cooperating, e.g. enterprises cooperation and human collaboration within information environment VMAO structures. There is a need to establish coordination of the exchange rules. It relies on creation of peer resources D&PK within common information space for aiding function task and problems of the VMAO.

Development of methods of computer aiding, integration and virtual medical activities organization is the sequence of using traditional computer services and contemporary trends in integration of data resources and synthesis of services of network connections.

Main factor – new qualifiedly – becomes integration of traditional computer services with services of network connections. So it appears possibility of services synthesis for exchange of information resources and creating systems used for cooperating aiding of (joint) medical solving problems.

Data resources and applications of computer aiding systems, integration and virtual medical activities organization begin to form sui generis common information space of structural changes of healthcare systems. There is appeared the global environment of computer integrated medical activities organization – CIMAO.

Factors of forming the common information space are as follows: physical integration of data resources, application integration of information systems, process integration of participants of virtual medical activities organization as well as medical organization co-operation as personal co-operation of partners in the treatment process which are doctor-patient. In consolidation concerning integration of different CIMAO levels, that is information integration of activities organization, we aim to create solid systems for all integration needs.

Facts of non-procedure specification of these needs according to contemporary trends of computer science, take into account automatic choice of proper methods or method combinations in problem solving (services of patients in complex environment of mutual connected healthcare organization).

Problems of computer aiding and medical activities integration, we can count to basic factors of forming new orderliness in the healthcare organization. It concerns with new virtual systems of the healthcare with participation of many medical services (doctor, out-patient clinic, hospital organizations, pharmaceutical companies, finance management organization), what depends on internal and external organizational changes conditioned accessibility to information and communication technologies (fig. 6).

The process of creating virtual organization is based on third dimensions: X, Y, Z. First dimension – X determines internal changes. They depend on activities organization and resources for structure works rationalization of the healthcare, out-patient clinics, hospitals, pharmaceutical companies, finance administration etc.. Second dimension – Y determines external changes. They depend on the communication organization (integrality) in co-operation at spaces: doctor-patient, out-patient clinics, hospitals-patients, healthcare organization-pharmaceutical companies and also their connections with finance management. Third dimension – Z, conditioning forming new orderliness, what results from the participation of CMAA, CMAI and VMAO results from the participation of CMAA, CMAI and VMAO in creating common information space, necessary in the process organization of patients' service.

Organization problems and using common information space we can notch to basic factors of creating VMAO systems. In common information space it is possible to use

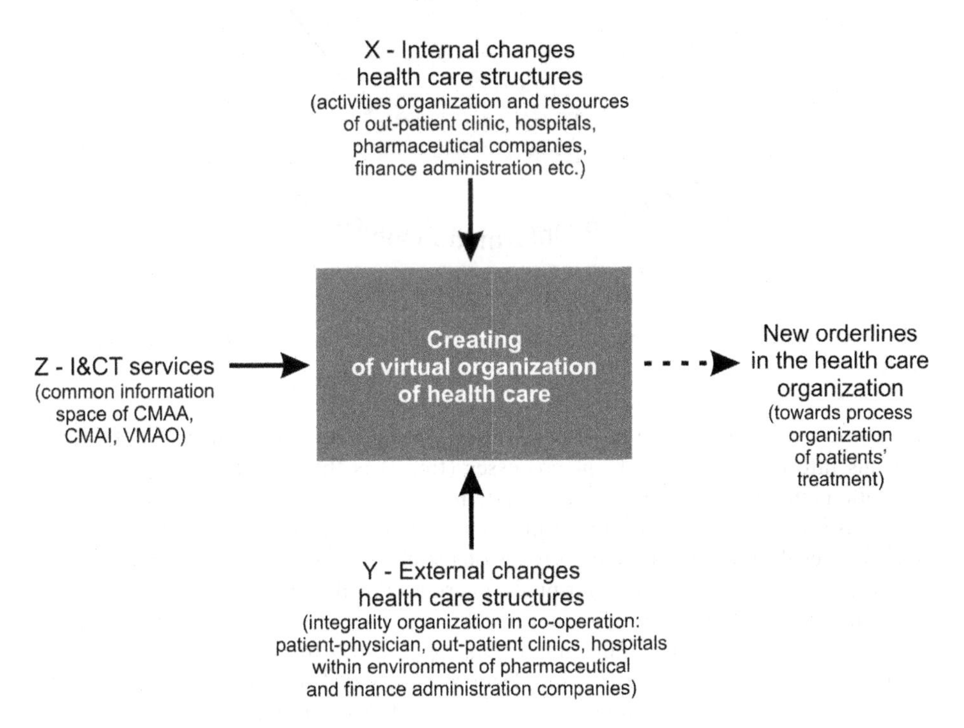

Fig. 6. Organization and information factors of health care structural transformation

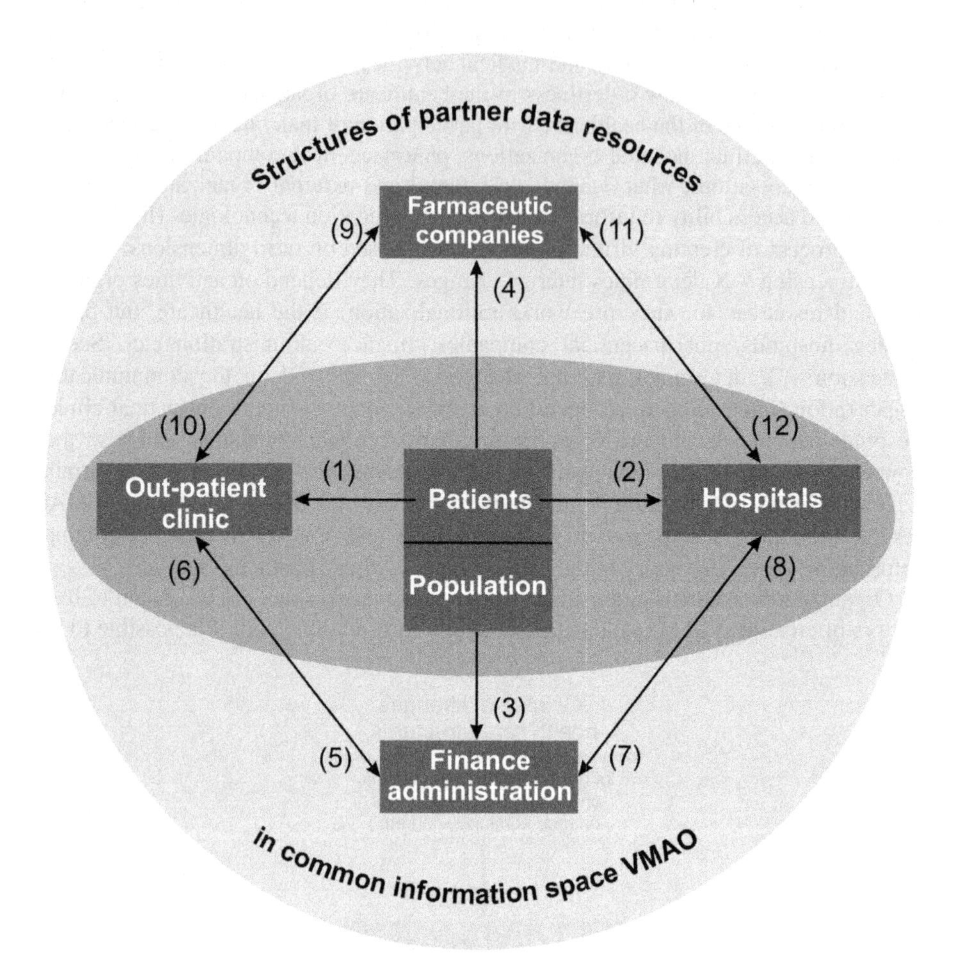

Fig. 7. General logistic structure of the management information processes in the health care systems

the co-operation integration process of various medical service organization. Logic of various information management processes (fig. 7) is the model of the process co-operation integration in the healthcare system.

Logistics results from the shit of thematic models of data processing processes for the service of common problem solving of patients' treatment by mutual connected structures of out-patient clinics, hospitals, pharmaceutical companies and organizations engaging finance management.

Meaning of 1-12 arches of the graph from fig. 7 results from the service of different thematic problems of data processing. Data resources and service procedures of tasks (1-9) allow to model composed grid of data D and problem domain PD, used for information aiding of functions, tasks and problem solving in VMAO systems, so in the composed healthcare system. The substantive co-ordination of finance management plays the special role because it closely combines with all problems of healthcare organization integration.

Common information space of VAO systems and solid data networks D&WP form files exchange methods inspired by applications of the P2P architecture to resources integration. It concerns with the data exchange organization consolidating creation and exchange procedures of source documents in WP schemas of particular VAO partners. The P2P architecture renders accessible distributed mechanisms of data exchange with marking representations between chosen resources of other partners resulting with meaning of partnership, i.e. neighborhood or clouts. In the P2P architecture the schema of the global resources description does not exists. Groups of partners can create networks for solving various tasks for example a group working patients' registration or servicing the diagnosing process, treatment etc.

In the P2P architecture partners exchange commands between themselves, realize these ones and servers fulfill the role of central catalogues and aiding of searching information partners. The principle of the network operation depends on that, that all partners are included in the process of files exchange. The file is usually divided into fragments being exchange units. It is necessary to control authenticity of these fragments.

In the P2P architecture there are represented data exchange processes. P2P consists of the open network of distributed applications of peers, where each application can exchange data and services with the file of other application, creating the file of its acquaintances. It is assumed that applications are in full autonomous in the choice of their acquaintances. Furthermore it is assumed that there is no control in the form of global registers, services or global resources management.

Data are stored in different data bases and can have its semantics. These relations can be expressed using coordinated formulas determining the way of application relations with their acquaintances. The application (service) of home doctor and pharmacy service are the example of these relations. These services can coordinate information about the patient, received by him prescriptions and bought drugs. The result of this coordination is mutual assignment information ourselves and in the simplest case assignment of updating to relation "Prescription and Drug" existing in both bases. One can also consider more complicated case of the realization of queries (services) requiring decomposition of commands and reference to succeeding acquaintances.

Coordinated formulas enforce data cohesion and propagation of updating. Additionally applications require acquaintances of the exchange protocol and settlement of the coordination level between them. The coordination level should be dynamic what means that the set of coordinating rules can change depending whether connections between pairs are slack or in general closed down (due to changes of interests and tasks of particular applications).

So at such dynamic changes one can not assume existing of the global schema for data resources in the P2P network, or even for all partners of data resources. What more, these changes mean, that partners should hale possibility of mutual integration at minimal human intervention.

We have to do with dynamic and extended environment. Partners can go in and out from the system. The partner entering the system, inputs his data, schemas or representations between them and his partners. In this way it forms the network, creating different ways of connected systems co-operating in integration processes and data exchange. Data exchange between partners connects with co-ordination problems of this exchange and data integration in the exchange process.

5 Conclusion

Analysis of notion models of using computer and communication services in development and integration of computer integrated medical activities organization systems – CIMAO allows settling works directions over building healthcare information systems. This development considers on the basis of analysis of first solutions of using CMAA methods to clinic investigations. We take into consideration contemporary trends of using information and communication services, causing system changes of the healthcare, utilizing information environment of computer medical activities integration and virtual medical activities organization.

In CMAA there are stored fact graphic data (aimed to computer record of illness history using database technique), what leads to the progress in computer instrumentalization for aiding routine medical activities. In CMAA it is possible representation of didactic medical inferring what enriches aiding medical activities fulfilling expectation of doctors.

Development and integration of CIMAO is the sequence of using computer and communication services for storing and processing medical data. Development of activities aiding range accompanies integration of functions of previous solutions representing more and more activities in doctor's process. Therefore process in CMAA development conditions first of all investigations over computer oriented medical activities methodology, so over computer medical knowledge representation and doctor's behavior in recognition and treatment of illness.

In notion models development of systems of medical computer aiding activities one appears presently new elements, resulting from using network information and communication services. A lot of new points result from contemporary trends of systems development of computer integrated activities organization for which completion is virtual activities organization.

In building systems of medical virtual organization activities we have to do with connection of aiding of doctor's function and data registration about the patient. One can take a gander at points of medical information structuralization next represented in network storing resources of digital data including different ways of the access to information being data interpretation. It also appears possibility of network services synthesis which is designated for information aiding of behavior in the treatment process, not only doctors, and also for determination of advices directed for patients.

Building systems of medical virtual organization activities are based on co-ordination of storing resources and information exchange. Co-ordination problems result from logistics of semi-using network processes of partnership digital resources, representing function consolidation and tasks of partners participating in the organization of medical activities: doctors, patients, out-patient clinic and hospitals, organizations of medicine-care.

The escape point of building medical virtual activities systems is structuralization of network digital data storing treated as partnership digital resources, as well as synthesis of co-ordination services and their exchange.

In the information environment of virtual medical services we model co-ordination processes of resources exchange. It becomes establishment of partnership in co-operation, what results from semi-joint co-ordination rules of partnership resources of digital data (peer digital data resources).

Structuralization of digital resources storing and co-ordination processes of their exchange is a base of building medical virtual activities organization about different range. Examples are as follows: (1) network out-patient clinic service, as well doctor as registration of patients, connected with organizations of hospital and pharmacy medicine (2) building systems of health protection, environmental, countrywide, or regional, including different world parts.

References

1. Kierzkowski, Z.: Medyczne systemy informatyczne i komputerowo integrowana organizacja działań badawczych, [W]; Komputery w medycynie (red. E. Kącki). t. II, Łódź, s.257–s.262 (1994)
2. Kierzkowski, Z.: Computer Integrated and Information Aided Investigation Activities. In: 14th International CODATA Conference: Data and Knowledge in a Changing World, Chambery, France (1994); In: Dubois, J.E., Gershon, N.D. (eds.) Modeling Complex Data for Creating Information, pp. 95–104. Springer, Heidelberg (1996)
3. Kierzkowski, Z.: Infosfera komunikowania bezpośredniego i organizacja telepracy, [W]: Konferencja "Telemedycyna" (red.: E. Kącki), Wyższa Szkoła Informatyki, Łódź, s.155–s.158 (2000)
4. Kierzkowski, Z., N'sir, M.: Wymiana danych poprzez standardową reprezentację w projektowaniu multimedialnych centrów informacyjnych – MCI, Konferencja "Telemedycyna" (red.: E. Kącki), Wyższa Szkoła Informatyki, Łódź, s.127–s.131 (2000)
5. Kierzkowski, Z.: Zarządzanie danymi w organizacji telepracy, [W]: Materiały Konferencji: Telemedycyna II (red. E. Kącki). Wyższa Szkoła Informatyki, Łódź, s.167–s.170 (2001)
6. Kierzkowski, Z., Kluska-Nawarecka, St., Sielicki, A. (red): Wymiana informacji i interaktywne komunikowanie medialne, Polskie Towarzystwo Informacji Naukowej, Wydawnictwo SORUS, Poznań (2003)
7. Kierzkowski, Z. (red): Inteligentne metody komputerowe dla nauki, technologii i gospodarki, Polski Komitet Narodowy CODATA przy Prezydium PAN, Wydawnictwo SORUS, Warszawa-Poznań (2004)
8. Kierzkowski, Z.: Correctness of co-operative activities in the arising virtual information environment. In: 19th CODATA International Conference – The Information Society: New Horizons for Science, Book of Abstracts, Berlin, Germany (2004)
9. Tarłowski, P., Pankowski, T.: Koordynacja wymiany danych w środowisku P2P, [W]: Bazy Danych: Struktury, Algorytmy, Metody (red.: S. Kozielski, B. Małysiak, P. Kasprowski, D. Mrozek), Wydawnictwo Komunikacji i Łączności, Warszawa, pp. s.37–s.45 (2006)
10. Tarłowski, P., Sikorski, A.: Zarządzanie współbieżnością w systemie integrowania informacji z uwzględnieniem uzgadniania i tolerowania sprzeczności, [W]: Bazy Danych - Struktury, Algorytmy, Metody; Wydawnictwo Komunikacji i Łączności, Warszawa, s.91–s.102 (2007)

11. Kierzkowski, Z.: Evolution and integration of computer aided medical activities systems. In: Proceedings of International Conference: Computers in Medical Activity, Polish Society of Medical Informatics & The College of Computer Science, Łódź, September 19-21, pp. 47–48 (2007)
12. Kierzkowski, Z., Tarłowski, P.: Virtual medical activities organization based on network services. In: Proceedings of International Conference: Computers in Medical Activity, Polish Society of Medical Informatics & The College of Computer Science, Łódź, September 19-21, p. 49 (2007)
13. Kierzkowski, Z.: Virtual Activities Organization within Information Society Structures. In: 21st International CODATA Conference: Scientific Information for Society – from Today to the Future, Abstracts, Kyiv, Ukraine, October 5-8, pp. 81–82 (2008)
14. Kierzkowski, Z., N'sir, M., Polkowski, Z., Tarlowski, P.: Data and Problem Knowledge Environment within Co-operation Structures. In: 21st International CODATA Conference: Scientific Information for Society – from Today to the Future, Abstracts, Kyiv, Ukraine, October 5-8, pp. 54–55 (2008)
15. Pankowski, T.: Query Propagation in a P2P Data Integration System in the Presence of Schema Constraints. In: Hameurlain, A. (ed.) Globe 2008. LNCS, vol. 5187, pp. 46–57. Springer, Heidelberg (2008)

Expert Systems in the Medical Insurance Industry

Liliana Byczkowska-Lipińska[1], Mariusz Szydło[2], and Piotr Lipiński[3]

[1] Technical University of Lodz, Institute of Computer Science,
ul. Wólczańska 215, 90-924 Łódź, Poland
lilip@ics.p.lodz.pl

[2] The College of Computer Science,
ul. Rzgowska 17a, 93-008 Łódź, Poland
szydlo@wsinf.edu.pl

[3] Division of Computer Networks, Technical University of Lodz,
ul. Stefanowskiego 18/22, 90-537, Łódź, Poland
piter@amuz.lodz.pl

Abstract. Here we have described the expert system for the medical insurance industry which has been developed at the Collage of Computer Science in co-operation with Technical University of Lodz. The system has been implemented and tested in an insurance company. The system reduces resources, costs and improves reliability of the insurance decision-making process. The time required to insure a customer has been reduced by eight times. The system is an ideal teacher for beginners, and can be used when educating new employees.

1 Introduction

Expert systems are a developing branch of artificial intelligence [1,2]. They are divided into advisor systems, critic systems and decision-making systems [3,4]. An important application of expert systems is to make observations and test them against various constraints. Their tasks include interpreting, prediction, repairing and monitoring of an object's behavior basing on experts' knowledge implemented in knowledge base [5,6,7]. Experts' knowledge is provided by a human expert or a group of experts (private knowledge), but it can also be gained from books, catalogs, factory information files etc (public knowledge). The key to a successful expert system is the ability to build a knowledge base [8]. Here we introduce a complete expert system for insurance industry which has a knowledge base which has been developed upon knowledge of experts in insurance industry as well as medical experts and public knowledge.

2 Insureance Process Scheme before the Expert Sytem Creation

Here we describe the information flow in the insurance company before the expert system creation. This is important because the expert system reflect this information flow. Before the expert system was created every customer was assisted by an

E. Kącki, M. Rudnicki, J. Stempczyńska (Eds.): Computers in Medical Activity, AISC 65, pp. 189–199.
springerlink.com

insurance agent, who was chosen according to the place of living or preferences of the customer. The task of the insurance agent was to present to the customer the simulation of his life insurance and familiarize him with all the legal and financial aspects of signing an insurance policy. On the basis of data provided by the actuaries, the insurance agent estimated the amount of coverage, which is the premium multiplied by the index and frequency of payment. With the help of an insurance agent, the customer was filling in an application form and was choosing the options (products) that he was fining best [9,10,11,12]. The application was passed on to the insurance company and constituted the basis for risk evaluation and insurance policy formulation. Information gained in this way was sent to the underwriting department [13,14,15,16]. Often supported by additional research, it was thoroughly analyzed by the experts who were assisted by medical specialists. The decision was recorded in customer data base, and the customer was informed about it by a customer service worker (or the agent). Every customer received also a reply in a written form. Fig. 1 illustrates an example of insurance process scheme.

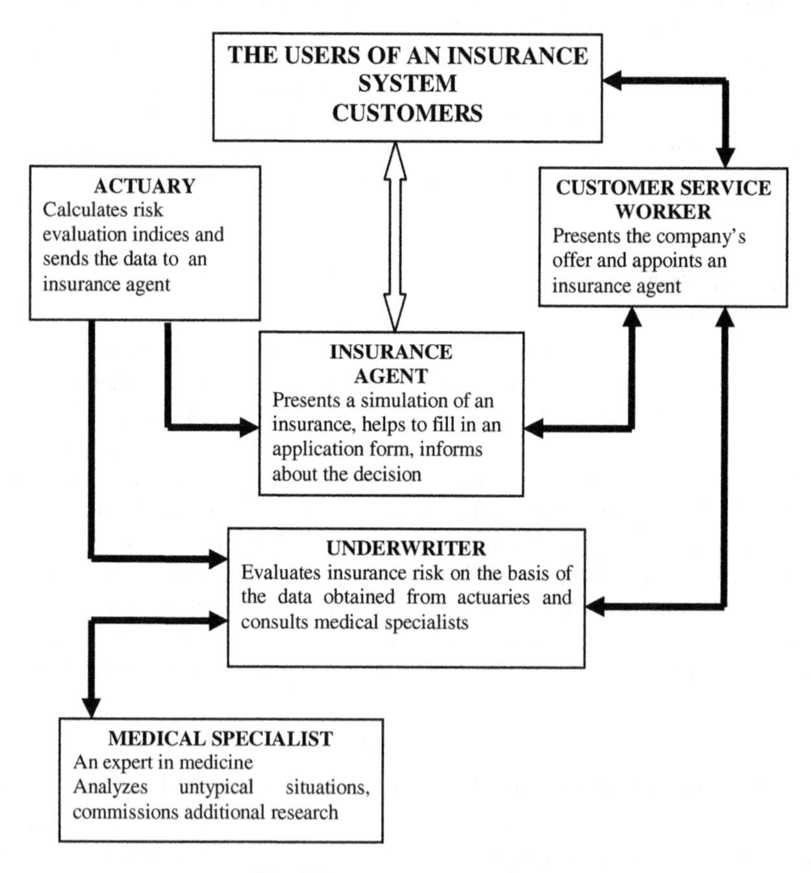

Fig. 1. Insurance process scheme

3 Expert System Considerations

The expert system which was developed aims at replacing work of medical specialist, underwriter and actuary, and allows an insurance agent to perform a complete proces shown in fig. 1. We developed the expert system assuming that it should provide:

- Reliability - it must give reliable answers basing on knowledge gathered in knowledge base.
- Efficiency – the final answer must be given based on the minimum possible parameters which involves examination heuristic, probabilistic, experimental dependencies, to reduce the time required to insure a custormer.
- The knowledge should be accessed through a dialog with a computer.

The typical structure of an expert system is depicted in fig. 2. We can see that it includes:

- Two databases:
  - Constant database, which is used to store constant parameters, eg. insurance premium,
  - Variable database, which is used to store variables, such as customer's blood pressure etc.,
- Knowledge base, which includes inference rules, knowledge in the domain and set of rules which are used to compose the answer to a question
- Inference procedures, which are executed to obtain knowledge from the knowledge base.
- Dialog control procedures, which control the communication between the user and inference procedures and translates them into human readable form
- Explanation procedures, which give the answer to the user, based on dialog control procedures

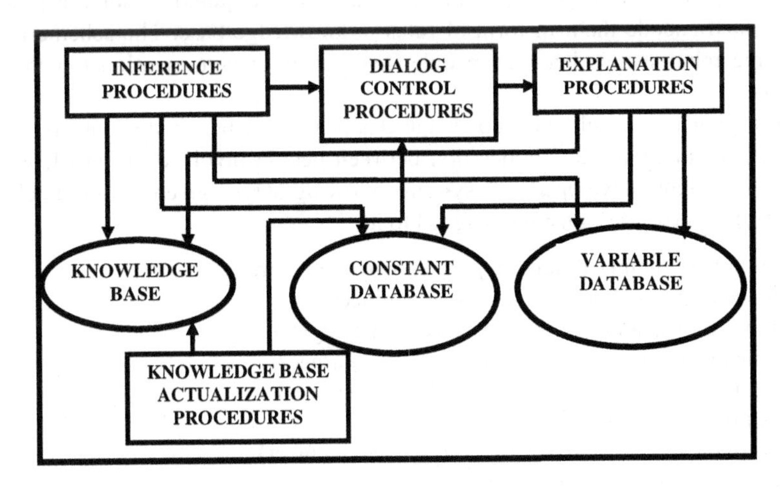

Fig. 2. Block diagram of an expert system

An expert system creation involves development of all abovementioned elements. As a result the project implementation and testing of an expert sytem is expensive. Therefore, expert systems should be developed only when they are planed to be employed by many users for a long period of time, which takes place in our case, as the system can be used by a number of insurance agents. Moreover, it leads to severe cost reductions, because reduces overall employment in the insurance process, as it replaces underwriter, actuary and medical specialist and reduces the time required to give a final decision.

4 Knowledge Acquisition and the Process of Building an Expert System

The design of reliable knowledge base is work- and time-consuming. This is because it should incorporate the knowledge obtained from many experts. In the seventies, it was observed that the power of the systems lies in the knowledge encoded in the system, not in the type of inference process applied. Thus, it can be said that the more complete the knowledge, the more reliable and more quickly obtained the solution. Knowledge base creation requires information to be collected and evaluated. Next, it requires implementation of numerous basic algorithms, integration and verification. This is not an easy task, as it requires intensive work from a team of information technology researchers, knowledge engineers and experts in a given domain. The key to a successful expert system is the ability to build a knowledge base. This task belongs to a specialist called knowledge engineer. The knowledge engineer is an indirect link between knowledge sources and the expert system. He is an information technology specialist or a related software expert, who should not only be a skillful programmer but he should also possess reporter skills and general knowledge in a given domain, so as to be able to assist the programmer and expert in a domain to obtain from them the most important facts and rules required to solve a particular problem and encode them in form of rules in knowledge base. The scheme in fig 3 shows the relationships between people involved in system creation together with their roles.

The design of the reliable knowledge databease can be divided into the stages. Those stages facilitate the cooperation between people involved in knowledge base creation. We have developed our system following stages given below. Each stage have had the person responsible assigned to it:

- Preliminary inquiry (client, expert, knowledge engineer)
- Choice of methodology (knowledge engineer)
- Knowledge acquisition (expert, knowledge engineer)
- Formal record of knowledge (knowledge engineer)
- Creation of knowledge base (knowledge engineer)
- Testing of knowledge base (expert)
- Improving of knowledge base (knowledge engineer)
- The use of an expert system (user)

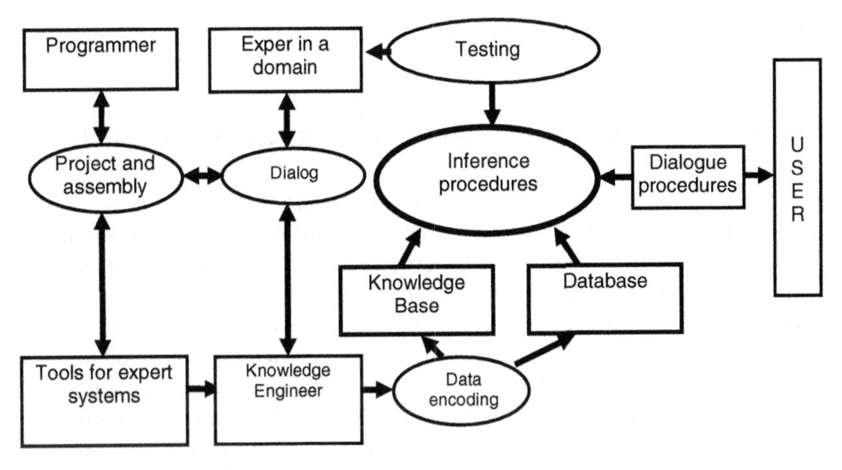

Fig. 3. The relationships between specialists involved in system creation together with their roles

5 The Tools for Creating an Expert System

Before starting implementing an expert system, the creator of an expert system decides about the type of system he wants to build, so that it would meet user expectations. According to those expectations a knowledge engineer must decide if he wants to build a dedicated system or use an available system shell together with artificial intelligence languages. Dedicated systems are created from scratch by a knowledge engineer (in cooperation with an information technology specialist). A dedicated system can be created with the majority of programming languages available at present. This solution is the most flexible, but also the most complicated, time consuming and most expensive. Another method of creating an expert system is by the use of expert system languages (CLIPS) or artificial intelligence languages (LISP, PROLOG) together with system shells. System shells are expert systems with an empty knowledge base. In this case, the creating of an expert system is shorter, the only requirement being the acquisition of knowledge and its appropriate implementation in the system. System shells possess built-in inference mechanisms and procedures that enable the creating of an interface and dialog options. Examples of such a program are PC-Shell and EMYCIN.

6 Choosing a Tool for Building an Expert System

Our initial plan involved the development of dedicated expert system written in Borland C++ language. However, this task was not realized because the insurance company refused to provide access to the clients' data and did not consent to its processing, even if anonymous. Instead, the complete rules and procedures that govern life insurance decisions were made available by the insurance company. Thus, it was more convenient to build an expert system using shell. Aitech SPHINX package (PC-Shell) turned out to be ideal for this purpose. It allowed building many knowledge bases and interface for consulting the user, using built-in inference mechanisms, and provided the possibility to translate decisions.

7 The Architecture of an Expert System Based on PC-Shell

After establishing input and output data, receiving information about the whole risk evaluation process, knowing the procedures for awarding insurance, insurance products and the specific character of an expert's work, a PC-Shell-based expert system was built. Fig 4 shows the architecture of the AITECH system shell. It describes the relationships between knowledge sources and internal parts of the PC-Shell.

Thanks to the file interface, the master program, activated by PC-Shell application, can refer to many knowledge sources. The knowledge sources are separate files that include the list of facts and rules on the basis of which the main program infers a specific decision. The role of the control module is to coordinate all the processes of PC-Shell. One of its tasks is to communicate with the user by a user interface. The interface works in text mode and has been developed in such a way as to show the user a set of alternative actions to be performed in a given context, so that the user does not have to memorize them. The expert knowledge is inserted in the knowledge base with knowledge base description language in PC-Shell. The description of a database can be made and stored in disk memory using any text editor. The task of database description language translator is to read the disk file containing database description, translate, and key in an appropriate code to the base of PC-Shell, the whole of which is located in the computer's operating memory. The inference module solves problems using data contained in the knowledge base. This is performed using appropriate inference (chaining) procedures, in this case – backward chaining.

PC-Shell was used to build an expert system with particular elements of the program, compatible with insurance guidelines. Before starting to build the system, it

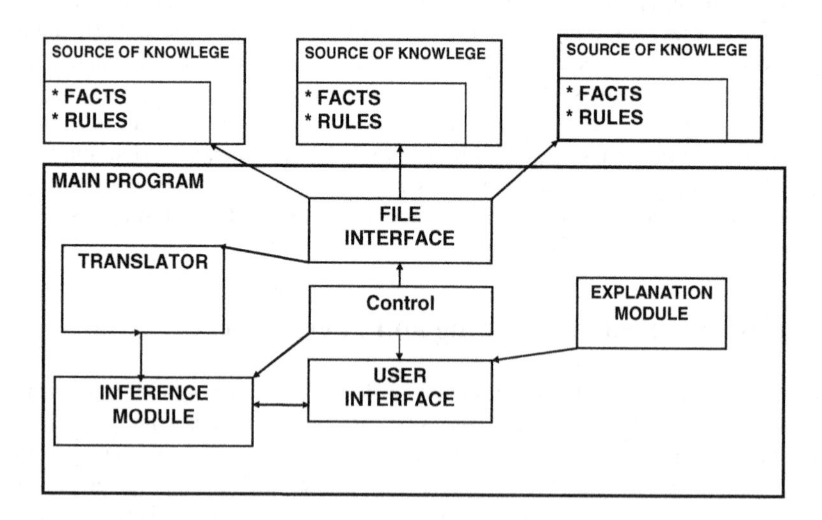

Fig. 4. PC-SHELL – architecture

was necessary to consider the process of data acquisition and the way of data storage. System PC-Shell could refer to knowledge sources, but what was necessary for the expert system to work properly, was one complex model with all the data about life insurance risk evaluation. Those data came from an insurance guide, but also from procedures, insurance tables, and medical literature. Although there were many knowledge sources, all of them led to a common result, that is the decision. It was sufficient to collect all the data and record them appropriately. For data acquisition and rules generation Microsoft Excel was used. It helped to make secondary decisions, but it was not enough to make the main decision. For this purpose, a subprogram which is a part of the expert system was developed. It enabled making the main decision on the basis of constituent decisions. The constituent decisions are evaluated and constitute a basis for making the main decision. In practice, this program is a base that can be used as a batch file to Detreex, which is a part of SPHINX package. The combination of decision-making algorithm (Borland C++) and the logical abilities of Detreex (SPHINX) produced very satisfactory results while building knowledge sources.

8 Inference Stages

The expert system developed on the basis of all the input information gained from the specialists enables subsequent reasoning stages. The main decision depends on constituent decisions, which in turn depend on other constituent decisions. The diagram in figure 5 illustrates the classification of decisions according to the type of input data.

The main decision in the system is made on the basis of the decisions about health condition, job and hobby. In turn, the decision about health condition is made on the basis of the decision about disease, build and physical condition. The decision about build results from the decisions about age, height and weight, and the decision about physical condition results from the decisions connected with blood pressure, nicotine and cholesterol. A decision diagram created in this way was very helpful in developing and proper organizing of the inference mechanism (fig. 5).

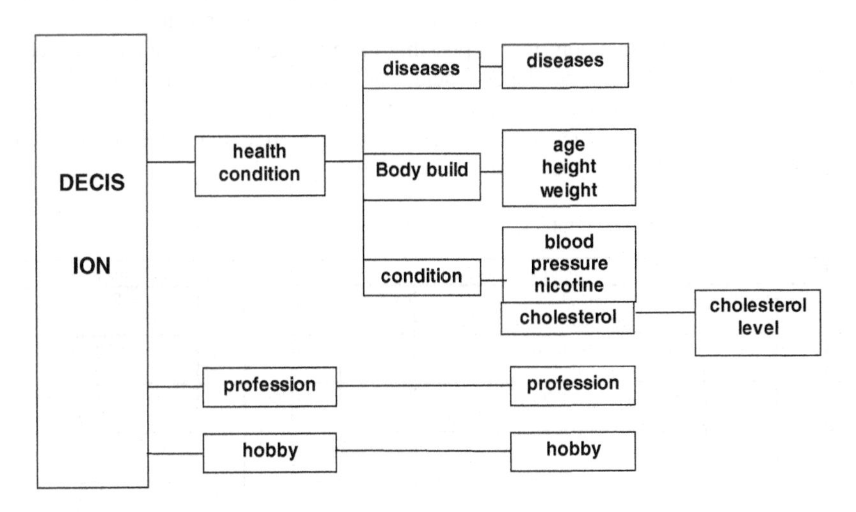

Fig. 5. Classification of decisions according to input data

Table 1. Shows 3 classes of decisions together with their significance (with the highest risk on the left)

We do not insure		We may insure		We insure				
refuse	Postpone decision	Extra medical consultation required	Master of your choice	Excluded	300%	200%	150%	standard

While solving the problems connected with taking insurance risk, one has to analyze thoroughly input data. As an expert system is to make an unquestionable insurance decision, without high risk, it must know the significance of each constituent decision. After careful analysis, an additional division of decisions was introduced. They were classified into 3 groups:

- We insure
- We may insure
- We do not insure

Standard insurance risk is connected with the obligation to pay standard insurance premium. The premium can increase, due to risk increase. It may even amount to 150%, 200%, or even 300% of the standard premium. The insurance procedure may also indicate "the necessity to postpone the decision" i.e. the delay of signing an insurance policy. In other words, the applicant does not qualify for insurance, because the risk is too high, but there is a possibility that the disadvantageous agent will be reduced after some time, and the application may be reconsidered. In case of drastic risk growth, the insurance company rejects the application for insurance. As for untypical cases requiring medical advice, it is advisable to consult a medicine specialist. It is also often the case that there are no definite procedures for risk evaluation. The information at your own discretion (table 1) means that the case under consideration oscillates between two classes (most often refusal or insurance on very high premium terms). In such cases it is the expert who makes the decision. The last possible decision type is the clause excluded. It is employed by the insurance company when the client practices a dangerous sport or has a risky hobby. The company agrees to issue a policy provided that it does not cover sport-related damages or injuries.

Owing to this classification, it was possible to introduce the so called significance mechanism that specified the dependencies and interrelations between constituent decisions and conclusion. Table 2 shows five exemplary situations involving different constituent decisions together with the conclusion. Notice that in most cases the conclusion reflects the most risky partial decision.

Table 2. Exemplary constituent decisions and their results

case	Partial decisions								conclusion
1	refuse	postpone	Medical consultation required	Your choice	Excluded	300%	200%	150%	Refuse
2		postpone	Medical consultation required	Your choice	Excluded	300%	200%	150%	postpone
3			Medical consultation required	Your choice	Excluded	300%	200%	150%	Medical consultation required
4				Your choice	Excluded	300%	200%	150%	Your choice
5					Excluded	300%	200%	150%	Excluded Premium 300%

9 Insurance Options

A very important aspect of insurance expert systems is the choice of insurance options. As far as the risk evaluation is concerned, the most problematic options for the experts are:

- ADB (Accidental Death Benefit),
- TPD (Total and Permanent Disability),
- DI (Disability Income).

Each of the insurance option must be considered separately and the whole inference procedure must be done separately for each insurance option. Every insurance option results in different final decision. Therefore, in the expert system one chooses the insurance option at very beginning and performs separate inference procedure for each insurance option. The user indicates the insurance option for a particular client and in the following steps verifies if the client can be insured on considered bases. The final decision concerning particular option is artificially decomposed into minor, constituent decisions, thanks to which every problem can be considered separately.

10 The Expert System

The sample window of the expert system is given in fig. 6. It shows the consultation window concerning hobby risk evaluation. We can see the hobby selection combo

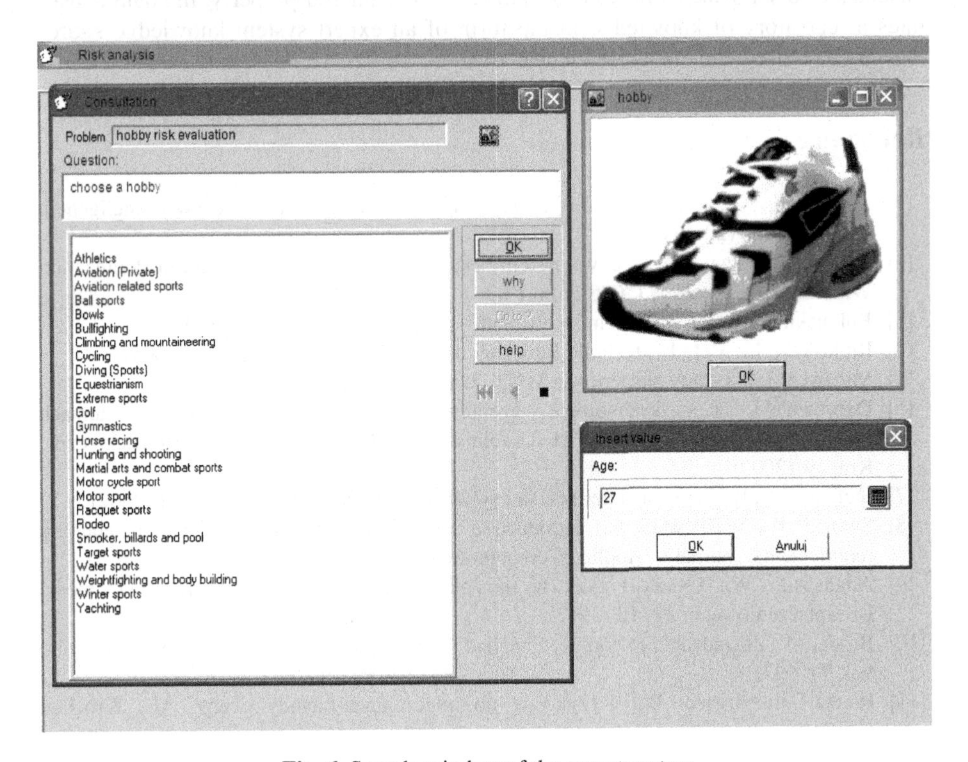

Fig. 6. Sample window of the expert system

box. Other partial decisions are calculated based on the analogous selection lists. Numerical parameters are inserted through the dialog box shown in the bottom right corner of the fig. 6.

11 Summary

Here we have described the expert system for the medical insurance industry which has been developed and implemented in an insurance company. The system uses decision-making algorithms on the basis of constituent decision (Borland C++), decision tree (DETREEX) and inference (PC-Shell). The system reduces resources, costs and improves reliability of the insurance process (the time required to insure a customer has been reduced by eight times). The system is an ideal teacher for beginners, and can be used when educating new employees. A complete inference translating module provides great possibilities for testing and comparison of results. The expert system in question makes it possible to analyze almost 2500 disease symptoms, over 3000 sport-related options, 1600 jobs and many rules that enable quick, accurate, clear and unquestionable health insurance decision-making.

While discussing the advantages and disadvantages of the expert system, one should also mention some of its drawbacks. First, data collecting may be very time-consuming. Second, when many knowledge sources are taken into consideration, mistakes or discrepancies may occur. However, if gathered properly, the data constitutes a repository of knowledge in the form of an expert system knowledge source that can be reused and elaborated repeatedly.

References

[1] Greenspan, S.I., Benderly, B.L.: Rozwój umysłu. Emocjonalne podstawy inteligencji. Rebis, Poznań (2000)
[2] Grzech, A.: Inżynieria wiedzy i systemy ekspertowe. Oficyna Wydawnicza Politechniki Wrocławskiej, Wrocław (2006); tom 1 i 2
[3] Bubnicki, Z.: Wstęp do systemów ekspertowych. PWN, Warszawa (1990)
[4] Rutkowski, L.: Metody i techniki sztucznej inteligencji. PWN, Warszawa (2005)
[5] Mulawka, J.: Systemy ekspertowe. WNT, Warszawa (1996)
[6] Dobrowolski, G.: Technologie agentowe w zdecentralizowanych systemach informacyjno-decyzyjnych. AGH Uczelniane Wydawnictwo Naukowo-Dydaktyczne, Kraków (2002)
[7] Stefanowicz, B.: Sztuczna inteligencja i systemy eksperckie. Warszawa SGH (2002)
[8] Swirski, K., Wasilewski, R.: Introduction to gathering, documenting and maintaining requirements. Journal of Applied Computer Science 14(2) (2006)
[9] Adamczuk, W.: Ocena ryzyka w ubezpieczeniach na życie (cz. I), Wiadomości Ubezpieczeniowe, nr 11, 12 (1997)
[10] Broda, M.: Zarządzanie ryzykiem, Przegląd Ubezpieczeń Społecznych i Gospodarczych, vol. 9 (1997)
[11] Ronka-Chmielowiec, W.: Ryzyko w ubezpieczeniach-metody oceny. AE, Wrocław (1997)

[12] Ciszek, W.: Risk management, moda czy konieczność. Wiadomości Ubezpieczeniowe, vol. 4, 5, 6 (1995)
[13] Jamrozy, W.: Underwriting w ubezpieczeniach na życie. Wiadomości Ubezpieczeniowe, vol. 4, 5, 6 (1996)
[14] Jamrozy, W.: Underwriting w ubezpieczeniach życiowych. Prawo Asekuracyjne, vol. 2 (1996)
[15] Luffrum, G.G.: Life underwriting. Institute of Actuaries. Alden Press, Oxford (1990)
[16] Swiss, R.: Life Underwriting: Rating Guidelines (1982)

Cost-Effectiveness Analysis of Transferring Medical Data over P2P Network

Beata M. Jankowska[1], Krzysztof T. Zwierzyński[1], and Magdalena Szymkowiak[2]

[1] Poznan University of Technology, Institute of Control and Information Engineering
pl. M. Skłodowskiej-Curie 5, 60-965 Poznań, Poland
{beata.jankowska, krzysztof.zwierzynski}@put.poznan.pl
[2] Poznan University of Technology, Institute of Mathematics
ul. Piotrowo 3a, 60-965 Poznań, Poland
mszymkow@amu.edu.pl

Abstract. In the paper, a transfer of medical data over P2P network is considered. The data are homogenous, of textual type. They are transferred between the nodes representing medical systems, along transmission lines. Although only some of the nodes can produce, process or integrate data, all of the nodes are able to propagate them to their neighbours. The costs of building the transmission lines are high, so an optimum network topology is being searched. The random graphs with bounded degree are used for modelling of such networks. The process of transferring data over network is examined by means of the original algorithm RST for searching rooted spanning trees.

Keywords: medical data transfer, P2P network, random graph model.

1 Introduction

Considering the fast growth in storing as well as distributing of electronic medical evidence, we have to think about medical data exchange and integration. The works should be performed on a large scale [1, 10]. The data exchange results not only in a greater knowledge everywhere the data come up but also – due to replication – in a better data protection against undesired modification or loss. Next, the medical data integration makes it possible to obtain the collective medical evidence that can be the base for designing reliable diagnostic and therapeutic rules [7]. Such the evidence makes it easier to design and implement medical expert systems aiding both clinicians and general practitioners in their work.

The matter of data integration [6] is beyond the limits of this paper. Instead, we will examine the problem of medical data transfer in a network. There are two main network architectures: centralized and with distributed control. Each one has its own strengths and weaknesses. In the case of a centralized solution, the main pro is easiness of nodes synchronization, while the main cons are: a low network capacity (an overworked server becomes a bottleneck of the network) and long periods of network inactivity (due to the server inaccessibility). A good example of a network with distributed control is a P2P network [11, 12, 5]. Although this network is more resistant to node inaccessibility, it has difficulty with keeping the data coherent when

E. Kącki, M. Rudnicki, J. Stempczyńska (Eds.): Computers in Medical Activity, AISC 65, pp. 201–210.
springerlink.com

often updates. However, it cannot be denied that the importance and the number of P2P networks is growing more and more each day.

In the paper we will focus our attention on medical P2P networks. We will assume that network's nodes represent medical systems cooperating one with another. They produce, exchange and integrate data, and also protect them against any change or undesired access. The main goal of the research is to find a suboptimum topology of a medical P2P. This topology is to guarantee transferring data in a time that is short enough (according to the constraints assumed). We mean here transferring the data both to all the nodes (broadcasting) and to some chosen nodes (routing) of the network. In addition, the way of network functioning should secure its resistance to various disturbances, as well intentional (medical spying) as accidental (disasters, injuries).

We propose the algorithm $G(n, f, p)$ for modelling of such networks. In this model we can set both the number of network nodes and the maximum number of node's neighbours. Also, we can influence the density of network connections. The model will let us examine the network's behaviour for its various possible configurations.

2 Topology and Functionality of P2P Medical Network

Let us make some essential assumptions about the network's topology and functioning. First of all, we will consider only the network whose topology is assumed to be static over time. It means that the number and character of the network nodes as well as of the connections between the nodes are fixed. Thus, we do not take into account either the possibility of connecting new nodes to the network or the possibility of disconnecting any of them. This simplification does not affect the essence of our considerations since we assume that the accessibility of each network node is dynamic over time (the node can be in two states: active or passive). Simultaneously, the average accessibility of a node can be described by means of a certain statistical distribution.

All network nodes can be divided into two categories: ordinary nodes and super nodes, also called repositories (Fig. 1). In the network, the number of the first type nodes should be significantly bigger than the number of the second type nodes.

Each network node can be characterised by the list of its functionalities. Namely, the node has an optional ability of data generation. We can distinguish the ability of textual (D_1) and multimedial data generation (D_2). Producing the data, both textual

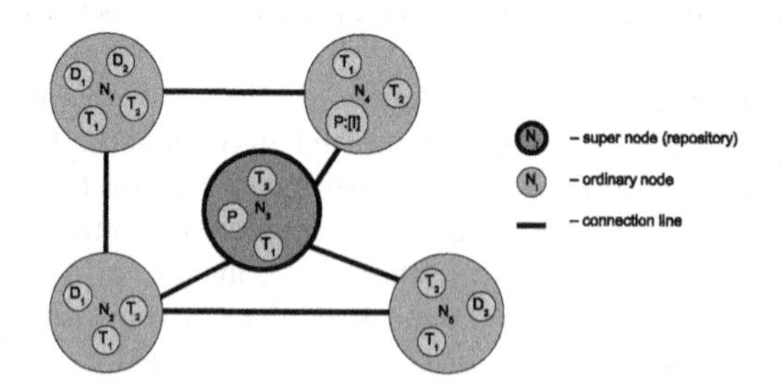

Fig. 1. Topology and functionality of medical P2P network

and multimedial, proceeds in time according to certain, characteristic for the node, statistical distributions. It takes place simultaneously in all (active) network nodes. Also the sizes of textual data units and multimedial data units can be characterised by means of statistical distributions. However, these are the same for all nodes.

Each node can propagate (generated by itself or obtained) data to the other nodes. The ability of textual (T_1) as well as multimedial data propagation (T_2) is an obligatory feature of all nodes, which guarantees proper functioning of P2P network. Here, we shall assume that each textual data produced must be placed – by means of propagation – in all network nodes, and each multimedial data produced – in at least two repositories. Moreover, the textual data can be propagated on demand, that means to some chosen ordinary nodes only.

The last, optional functionality of nodes consists in the ability of data processing (P), including – data integration (I). It does not depend either on the ability of data generating or, even more, on the ability of data transferring. The data processing can take place in ordinary nodes as well as in repositories.

The above statements give us an approximate description of a medical P2P network. In order to examine the network efficiency, we will subject it to a thorough procedure of several stages. To this end, at the beginning, we will set up a number of constraints on topology and functioning of the network. Next, step by step, we will eliminate most of the constraints. Necessarily, at each stage of the procedure, the speed of data transmission is assumed to be fixed. It does not depend either on data format or on network nodes that participate in transmission process. Also, we will assume that the time needed for linking one node to another can be ignored.

Each network node will be defined by means of the values of its three attributes: efficiency, capacity and accessibility. We will assume that all nodes have the same efficiency, it means that they need the same amount of time to do the same job. The capacity of node is related to the size of its memory. We assume that node's memory is enough to store any number of textual data. Memory limit can be only considered for multimedial data storing. However, it is the case of ordinary nodes: repositories should be seen as nodes with unlimited memory. It is natural in large networks that nodes are sometimes not available. The accessibility is a ratio between time when the node is working and communicating with other nodes and the global time of network activity. This attribute's value is also related to the type of the node. We assume that ordinary nodes have small accessibility in opposite to super nodes.

3 Modelling of Simple P2P Network

In the simplest model of P2P network we have only ordinary nodes, of the functionalities D_1 and T_1. All the textual data produced have the same size and their generation in time is according to the Poisson distribution. At any unit of time, a node can communicate with at most one of the other network nodes and no one elementary transmission between two nodes can be broken.

For the investigation purpose, a simulation model of the P2P has been designed. In this model, the network is represented by a graph $G = (V, E)$, where V is the set of vertices of G and E is the set of edges. Vertices of G correspond to nodes of the network and edges to transmission lines. Every vertex has its own attributes: c - capacity, a - accessibility, and λ - the parameter of the Poisson distribution.

The structure of the network will be modelled by random graphs with bounded degree [2]. The proposed model is called $G(n, f, p)$, where n is the number of vertices, f is the maximum vertex degree ($3 \leq f \leq n - 2$), and p is the edge probability. In this model, a random graph G has vertices of degree not greater than f. Two vertices i, j are joined by the edge $\{i, j\}$ with probability p, provided the degree of these vertices is smaller than f. The generated graph G has to be connected (there is a path from a vertex to any other vertex in G).

There are at least two reasons why the limitations of vertices degree should be considered. The first one results from impossibility of implementing a great number of connections at a node. The second one is related to (economic) costs of maintaining network connections. Note, that the global maximum number of connections depends on f, being equal to $\lfloor n \cdot f / 2 \rfloor$.

Obtaining of the considered graph is by means of the following algorithm GNFP, being a modified version of the known algorithm of Kennedy and Quintas [8]:

Algorithm 1 (GNFP)

Input: n – the number of vertices, f – the maximum degree of vertex, p – the edge probability.

Output: G – the graph of the type $G(n, f, p)$.

Method:

1. Create a basic table (E) with all possible pairs of vertices $e = \{i, j\}$, and an additional table (D) with current degrees of vertices, initialized with zeros.
2. Randomly change the order of elements in E.
3. For each $e \in E$, if current degree of corresponding vertices is less than f, and a random value from interval $<0, 1>$ is greater or equal than p, then mark this pair as an actual edge in G and update the table D.

4 Simulations of Data Transfer in the Network

Using the above graph model, we carried out an experiment broadcasting of a single (textual) data unit in a network with a fixed number of nodes. We examined the functional dependence of time interval needed to broadcast data unit upon the maximum node degree. The size of data unit was fixed and it had no influence on the results obtained. Additionally, we assumed that while the experiment was running, all the network nodes were available.

In our graph model, the described above process of data propagating corresponds with searching a random spanning rooted tree. The height of such a tree will be proportional to the time of propagating data over the whole network.

An example of a graph G and its spanning trees is shown in Figure 2. The arrows point to the roots of spanning trees. The graph's edges are marked with labels corresponding to the time intervals in which transmission has been done. As we shall see, propagation times can differ one from another. As an instance, for the first and second spanning trees, the times of propagating the data generated in the top vertex, differ by one.

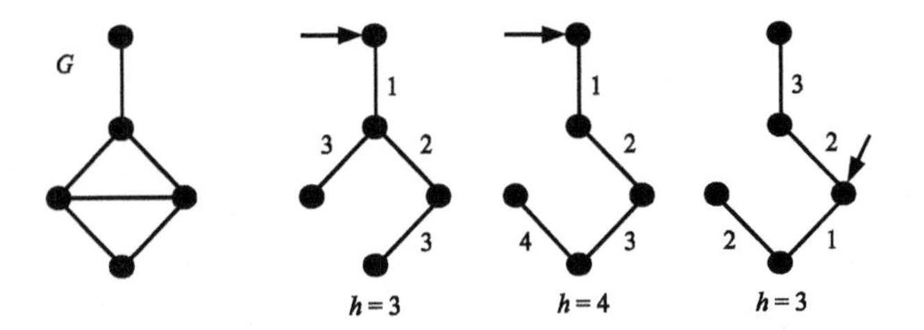

Fig. 2. Graph G and some of its spanning trees

Searching of minimum height spanning trees is by means of the known algorithm BFS [3]. However, let us remark that, for simulation purposes, spanning trees do not necessarily have minimum heights. What is more, randomly built spanning trees will better model the way of data propagating in P2P networks. That is why we propose the following algorithm RST for generating of random Rooted Spanning Trees.

Algorithm 2 (RST)

Input: G – the graph, v – the root vertex.

Output: T – a random rooted spanning tree and its height h.

Method: We assume the graph G to be connected. Let S denote the set of vertices that have been already visited.

1. Add the vertex v to the empty set S; h:=1.
2. Find all the neighbours of the vertices from S in the set V/S. Mark them as "free".
3. Randomly, for each vertex from S, choose one of its "free" neighbours and mark it as "busy".
4. Increment h by 1.
5. Add each "busy" vertex to the set S. If the set V/S is empty then stop, else return to the step 2.

By means of the given algorithm RST, we will simulate the way of functioning a medical P2P network in which textual data can be produced once for a long time or repeatedly, in quick succession, in many nodes simultaneously. We will measure the period of time between the moment when a new data unit is produced and the moment when – after having been broadcasted or routed – it reaches the last node of the network. We will examine how the time depends on the global number of nodes and the maximum number of connections leaving a node (the maximum node degree).

5 Experiments – Course and Results

At the beginning, the simple experiment was carried out in order to check how quickly a textual data is transferred from one node to all the nodes of the network. To this end, a set of connected graphs was generated by means of the algorithm GNFP. The input parameters were as follows: n = 10, 20, …, 150, f = 3, 4, …, 9 and p = 0.5, 1.0. For any combination of the values mentioned above, the algorithm RST was called and, as a result, an average height of spanning trees was obtained.

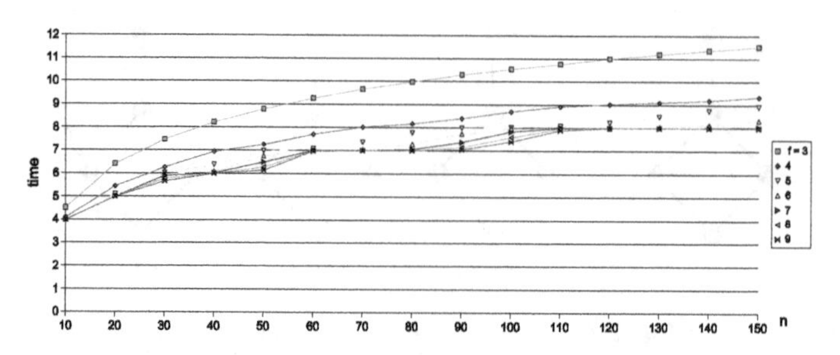

Fig. 3. Propagating of an individual data over the network – dependency of time on the number of network nodes and the maximum degree

The diagram in Figure 3 represents results for a fixed value of $p = 0.5$. The experiment has proved that minimum time needed for building a rooted spanning tree grows monotonically with the global number of vertices. While fixing this number, the greater the maximum vertex degree, the shorter the time necessary for building of a spanning tree. However, let us remark, although there is a quite big difference in time for the cases of $f = 3$ and $f = 4$, the continuation of increasing f only weakly influences the time.

The case of $p = 1.0$ is very similar to this one mentioned above and it does not cause any change in the interpretation of experiment's results. After considering the similarity of the results, we realized that the network capacity depends not on the global number of connections but on the possible number of simultaneous transmissions. Let us remark that, at any moment, only $n/2$ transmissions can be carried out simultaneously.

The conclusion from the first experiment is the following: while designing a medical P2P network that will be never overworked, it is sufficient to connect nodes at degree not greater than 4. The higher maximum node degree, the higher cost of network installation and maintenance. At the same time, a decrease in time of data propagating is just to ignore.

In the second experiment, we analyzed the time of transferring textual data, which were generated simultaneously in many nodes. To this end, by means of the algorithm GNFP, we built a random connected graph, and later, for each vertex of this graph, we generated a certain number of textual data units destined for broadcasting in the network being modeled. The generation proceeded according to the Poisson distribution with a fixed value $\lambda = 2$. The experiment was carried out for the graphs with a number of vertices $n = 10, 20, \ldots, 100$ and the maximum vertex degree $f = 2, 3, \ldots, 9$. The sample size was set at $s = 1000$. In the subsequent steps of the simulation, particular data were propagated to these and only these vertices to which they had not come earlier.

The result of the above experiment is shown in Figure 4. Let us notice that, for each tested network, the global number of generated data units generated was proportional to the number of nodes in the network and it was approximately $\lambda{\cdot}n$. The experiment finished at the moment in which the data reached all the network nodes. According to the expectations, it appeared that the time needed for data broadcasting reduces along with the increase of the maximum node degree. However, even if these differences were significant before f reached the degree 4, any further increase of the

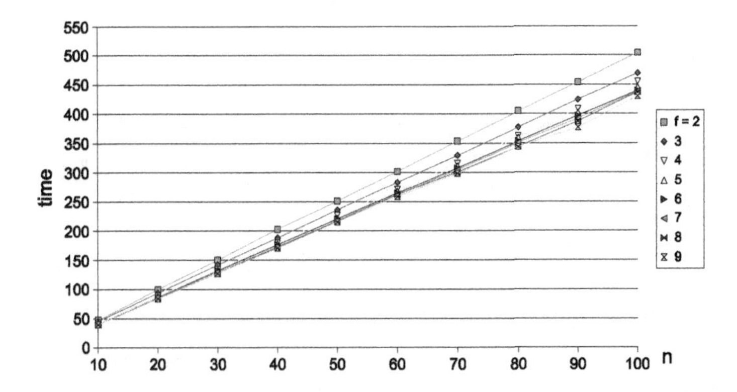

Fig. 4. Propagating of multiple data over the network – dependency of time on the number of network nodes and the maximum degree

maximum node degree had a slight influence on the time needed for data propagation. The second, quite unexpected result of the experiment was finding a linear dependency between the number of network nodes and the time of data transfer at a fixed degree f.

The experiment described above confirms our conviction that, also in case when the network is intensively used (intensive movement of data in the network), it is sufficient to connect nodes at the degree not greater than 4. It is also worthwhile to balance the pros and cons of building big networks. In some cases, an apparently better solution is building a few local networks than a central, huge one.

In the last, third experiment, we assumed that textual data generated are propagated only to some chosen nodes of the network. Like in the previous cases, a set of connected graphs was generated by means of the algorithm GNFP, with a number of vertices n = 10, 20, ..., 100. This time, however, each graph had the same, fixed maximum node degree $f = 4$. Next, for each node of the graph, a certain number of textual data units was generated which were destined for transferring to 10, 25, 50 and 100 per cent of nodes from their global number n. Generating the data units proceeded according to the Poisson distribution with a fixed value $\lambda = 2$, whereas generating the list of nodes, which were the data receivers, proceeded totally at random, from the full set of graph nodes n, reduced by the node – a data producer. The size of each random sample was set to $s = 1000$. The aim of the experiment was to test the time of propagating the textual data generated to all of their receivers.

The presented in Figure 5 experiment result shows that the time of data propagating to the randomly chosen fixed part of nodes depends mainly on the total number of network nodes, and not on the maximum node degree, nor even – contrary to our expectations – on the number of data receivers. For the fixed node degree and the fixed number/percentage of the receivers, this time depends linearly on the total number of network nodes.

In the light of our experiment results, we become convinced that in case of the expected medium or highly intensive data movement in the network, it seems to be reasonable to build a few local networks rather than a huge, global one.

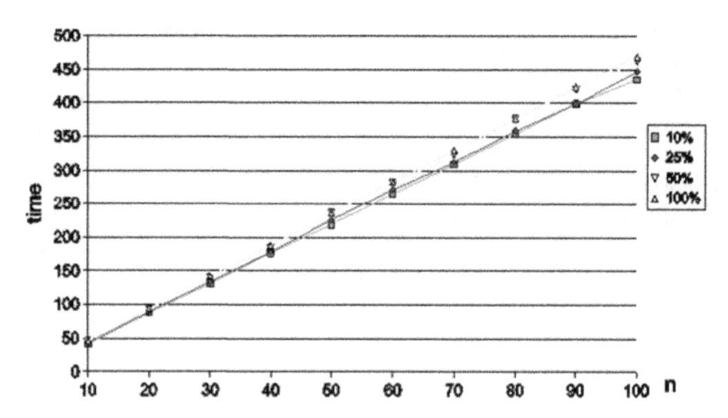

Fig. 5. Routing of data over the network – dependency of time on global number of nodes and number of data receivers

6 Concluding Remarks

The problem of an effective data transfer in the network has been very often discussed. As a result of the research, different algorithms of routing and broadcasting were proposed [4]. The specificity of network problems that we consider is connected with the use of P2P network in medicine. In the medical network, the nodes – representing medical systems – generate and exchange the data of two categories: textual (personal data of patients, laboratory test results, short reports on the hospitalization course or the visit in a doctor's surgery, short diagnostic and therapeutic conclusions), as well as multimedial data (mainly – the image documentation of specialist medical tests). The nodes can be ordinary (a vast majority, generating a great number of textual data and a slight number of multimedial data) or super (a few repositories, mainly used for storing the multimedial data). Until now, we considered only the homogenous networks, built with the ordinary nodes.

As regards the transferred textual data, it is worth noticing that, in general, their sizes only slightly differ from each other. Therefore, without any loss for the generality of our considerations, in the experiments we assumed a fixed size of the textual data unit. By means of appropriately built graph models, we carried out simulations in which we tested the dependencies of the time of broadcasting and routing textual data on the network topology. On this basis we can draw the following conclusions:

- The time of data broadcasting (or routing) increases in proportion to the increase of the number of network nodes (in case of medium or highly intensive data movement - even linearly); in such a situation, the purposefulness of building a big network should be considered;
- Because of the broadcasting, both in case of an expected slow and intensive data movement, it is worthwhile to build such a network in which the degrees of particular nodes are similar to each other and they are equal to 3 - 4;
- With the used, flooding algorithm of data transfer, an average time of propagating the data to randomly chosen receivers, is linearly dependent on the total number of

network nodes; obviously, the shorter list of data receivers, the shorter time of data transfer, but the differences in time are quite small; also the level of the maximum node degree has only slight influence on the time of the transfer considered.

Taking into account the importance of multimedial data, more and more used on a large scale in many medical specializations (e.g. the sophifisticated image documentation concerning glaucoma [9, 13]), we will carry out further simulations in order to:

- Analyze the behaviour of a homogenous network, in which the textual and multimedial data are generated and transferred (we will take into account various multimedial data sizes, and various proportions between the number of textual data and the number of multimedial data transferred);
- Test the influence of super nodes existing in the network (we will consider various "behaviours" of repositories and various proportions between the number of ordinary nodes and repositories).

Finally, we will simulate the incidence of potential transmission mistakes and analyze their influence on the data transfer durations.

Acknowledgments. Partial support of this work was provided by the research grant from Poznan University of Technology BW45-087/2009. Some computations were done at the Poznan Supercomputing and Networking Center.

References

1. About HL7, `http://www.hl7.org/`
2. Balińska, K.T., Quintas, L.V.: Random Graphs with Bounded Degree. Publishing House of Poznan University of Technology, Poznań (2006)
3. Cormen, H.T., Leiserson, C.E., Rivest, R.L., Stein, C.: Introduction to Algorithms. The MIT Press, Cambridge (2001)
4. D'Alberto, P., Nicolau, A.: R-Kleene: A High-Performance Divide- and Conquer Algorithm for the All-Pair Shortest Path for Densely Connected Networks. Algorithmica 47(2), 203–213 (2007)
5. Fischbach, K., Schmitt, C., Schoder, D.: Core Concepts in Peer-to-Peer (P2P) Networking. In: Subramanian, R., Goodman, B. (eds.) P2P Computing: The Evolution of a Disruptive Technology. Idea Group Inc., Hershey (2005)
6. Jankowska, B.M.: On Efficient Methods of Medical Data Integration. In: Proc. of XII Int. Conf. on System Modelling and Control SMC 2007, Zakopane, Poland (2007)
7. Jankowska, B.M., Szymkowiak, M.: How to Acquire and Structuralize Knowledge for Medical Rule-Based Systems? In: Kacprzyk, J. (ed.). Studies in Computational Intelligence. Springer, Heidelberg (2007) (to appear)
8. Kennedy, J.W., Quintas, L.V.: Probability models for random f-graphs. Combinatorial Mathematics 555, 248–261 (1989)
9. Niżankowska, M.H.: Jaskra (Glaucoma). In: Basic and Clinical Science Course (BCSC 10), 1st Polish edition, Wrocław (2006)

10. OpenERC,
`http://svn.openehr.org/specification/BRANCHES/Release-1.0.1-candidate/publishing/architecture/overview.pdf`
11. Ripeanu, M.: Peer-to-Peer Architecture Case Study: Gnutella Network. Technical Report. University of Chicago (2001)
12. Steinmetz, R., Wehrle, K. (eds.): Peer-to-Peer Systems and Applications. LNCS, vol. 3485. Springer, Heidelberg (2005)
13. Szymkowiak, M., Jankowska, B.M., Zwierzyński, K.T.: Designing of Medical Rule-Based Systems from Heterogenous Data. In: Proc. of the 5th International Conf. on Computer Methods and Systems, Kraków, pp. 53–58 (2007)

Influence of Upper Respiratory System Disease on the Performance of Automatic Voice Recognition Systems

Jakub Gadek

College of Computer Science in Lodz
ul. Rzgowska 17a, 93-008 Lodz
jgadek@wsinf.edu.pl

Abstract. This article is devoted to the examination of the influence of upper respiratory system disease in humans on the functioning of voice recognition systems. To recognize the speaker by their voice, such systems must be prepared in advance for recognition of the person's voice on the basis of recorded sound samples. Then the recognition system analyzes a new voice sample and verifies whether it has been spoken by the same person. However, often in life there are situations when the human voice is changed. They may be caused by a disease, passage of time, effect of intoxicants or deliberate user action in order to mislead the system. This article is devoted to an analysis of a situation when the speaker's voice has been modified between the system's phase of preparation for recognition, and the actual recognition of the speaker. For the research purposes, the focus has been restricted to voice deformation of Polish speaking persons, caused by an acute disease of the upper respiratory system.

1 Introduction

To recognize the speaker by their voice, recognition system must be prepared in advance for recognition of the person's voice on the basis of recorded sound samples. Then such a system analyzes a new voice sample and verifies whether it has been spoken by the same person. However, often in life there are situations when the human voice is changed. Changes can be temporary or permanent. They may be caused by a disease, passage of time, effect of intoxicants or deliberate user action in order to mislead the system. An example of such action can be impersonating a user who is already registered in access control systems or such modification of one's voice as not to be recognized by the system used for purposes of the police. This paper is devoted to an analysis of a situation when the speaker's voice has been modified between the system's phase of preparation for recognition, and the actual recognition of the speaker. For the research purposes, the focus has been restricted to voice deformation of Polish speaking persons, caused by an acute disease of the upper respiratory system.

For testing, a dedicated database of sound phrases was created, containing both fragments of text spoken in a normal way and modified fragments. Because of difficulties associated with the acquisition of recordings of voice modified in the natural way, in most cases, speakers were asked to deliberately modify their voice to imitate the disease.

E. Kącki, M. Rudnicki, J. Stempczyńska (Eds.): Computers in Medical Activity, AISC 65, pp. 211–221.
springerlink.com

The tests were made using the developed experimental system. This system has been created on the basis of "Open Source" software and is available along with the source code. All basic elements have been written in C/C++ language. The system has been implemented in the UNIX® FreeBSD operating system. Also, elements written in Perl language and UNIX® Bash shell scripts have been used.This is an example of how your paper is to be prepared according to the instructions. When numbering equations enclose the number in parentheses and place it flush with the right hand margin as shown below.

2 Speech Database

One of the major problems in the testing process of the speaker and speaker's voice recognition applications is lack of available, free of charge samples of voices recorded in different languages. The "BaFra" Project designed in The College of Computer Science in Lodz, Poland will cover this gap.

Under the supervision of the author of the article the structure of the database has been worked out containing speech samples spoken in polish language. It concerns mainly tests of speaker recognition applications although the structure had been prepared in such a way that it is possible to rebuild it in the future and use it for tests of speech and emotions spoken by the speaker.

The "BaFra" Project has been designed in order to create the polish speech corpus specialized in testing speaker recognition applications. The Corpus contains the phrases spoken by the speakers in a normal way as well as phrases spoken in a modified way. Those modifications was the result of changes caused by an illness, especially by upper respiratory system disease, although in the database most of the speakers change their voices consciously simulating the natural changes. Such a language base permits to make algorithms resistance-tests which are responsible for speaker recognition being based on changes accruing in the voice.

3 Experimental System for Executing the Research

In order to undertake experiments on the text independent voice recognition a described corpus has been executed within the College of Computer Science in Lodz. More comprehensive description of the system can be fond at [2].

3.1 Construction of the System

Created software has the modular construction what enables to modify and adjust to the needs of a concrete experiment more easily. All algorithms are written in C/C++ language. Particular elements of the system are small, self – contained, executive programmes. Those elements are induced by the outer programmes written in Perl language, while the whole is steerable by generated script for a particular experiment, written in Bash shell language. Figure 1 presents the block scheme of the system.

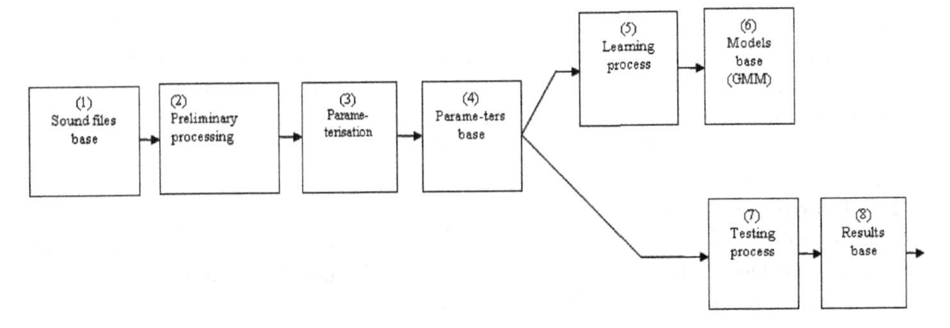

Fig. 1. Block scheme of the system

3.1.1 Sound Files Base

The initial element of each experiment is the base of samples sound – recording conducted on a certain group of people assigned for the experiment. It is compulsory that its structure is precisely specified. It has been assumed, that the recording of one speaker should appear in one catalogue while sessions recordings should appear in sub- catalogues. All the recordings should remain in one format concerning a particular experiment; it means that the recording format and the recording process parameters such as sampling frequency should be the same. In the following experiment, a different base can be implemented with different parameters of the record.

3.1.2 Preliminary Processing

At this stage, optionally, the preliminary processing of the sound can be executed before establishing the parameters. This processing can include sound digital processing of every kind. At the time being, only the algorithm of automatic removal the spaces that do not contain speech signals based on the mean (average) height of the amplitude within the certain sample space, has been implemented.

3.1.3 Signal Parameterisation

Signal parameterisation is based on interchange sample signal for the adequate set of vector parameters and is has been the key – element of the whole processing. For each file of the sound sample complies with a new file of corresponding set of vector parameters. The possible kinds of vectors are as follows: LPC, the coefficient of linear predicate, LPREF, reflection coefficients, cepstrum coefficients, MFCC coefficients. Precise description of presented kinds of parameters are shown in [3]. Additionally, they can be connected with differential parameters (the first, the second, the third) and measure energy as well as they can change vector magnitudes. Within one experiment one must decide on a concrete set of parameters which means, that each induced file with parameters should contain the same set. Within the next experiment a different set can be used.

3.1.4 Parameters Base

During establishing the parameters the set of files is being produced containing parameters vectors corresponding with sound samples derived from the sound files database. For each file containing a sample sound in the wav format, a file containing an adequate set of vector parameters comes into being. As the result of such interchange a new base is formed, containing files with parameters of the same structure as the one described in point 2.1. All further operations are executed on the parameters' base but not on sound files.

3.1.5 Learning Process

Learning process is based on creating GMM models (Gaussian Mixture Model) on the grounds of previously prepared part of staff from the database of parameters for each speaker being present in the database.

3.1.6 GMM Models

Gausian density mixture is a weighted sum of density components M, as it has been shown on Fig. 2 and forms the following equation (1)

$$p(\vec{x}|X) = \sum_{i=1}^{M} p_i b_i(\vec{x}) \tag{1}$$

where $\overset{\rho}{x}$ is random, D – dimensional vector, $b_i(\overset{\rho}{x}), i = 1,...M$, are the density elements, and $l = 1,...,M$, are weights of particular elements of the mixture. Each density element is an equation (2)

$$b_i(\vec{x}) = \frac{1}{(2\pi)^{D/2}|\Sigma_i|^{1/2}} \exp\left\{-\frac{1}{2}(\vec{x}-\vec{\mu}_i)'\Sigma_i^{-1}(\vec{x}-\vec{\mu}_i)\right\} \tag{2}$$

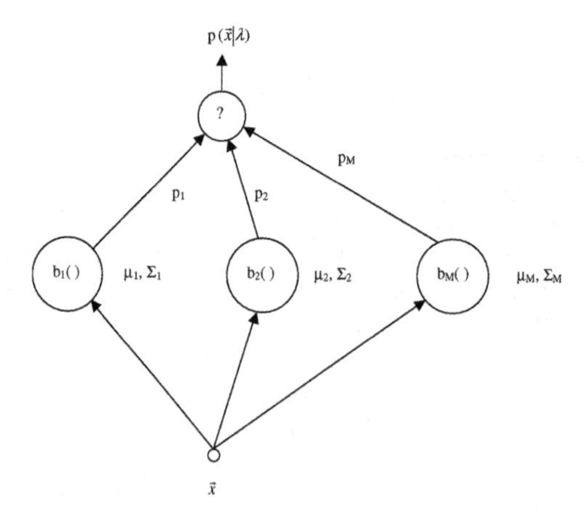

Fig. 2. Scheme of M components of density Gausian mixture. Density Gausian mixture is the weighted sum of Gausian density, where pi, i,...,M, are weights and $b_i(), i = 1,..., M$, are Gausian components.

with the mean vector value $\vec{\mu}_i$ and the covariance matrix $\sum_i$. The weights of mixture perform the following constraint $\sum_{i=1}^{M} P_i = 1$.

A complete density of Gausian model (set) has been parameterised through mean vectors' values, covariance matrixes and weights. Those parameters are represented by the record:

$$\lambda = \{p_i, \vec{\mu}_i, \sum_i \} i = 1,...,M \tag{3}$$

For identification each speaker is represented by GMM model through set of λ parameters.

GMM can appear under a few, different forms depending on the choice of covariance matrix. The model can posses one covariance matrix oriented for Gausian component as in (3) (nodal covariance), one covariance matrix for all components in the speaker model (grand covariance) or a single covariance matrix, common for all speaker models (global covariance). The covariance matrix can also appear as overall or diagonal. In this course, nodal and diagonal covariance have been used basing on presented research in [1].

3.1.7 Estimation of Model Parameters

There are several available techniques for estimation of parameters GMM [3]. The most popular method is maximum likehood *(Maximum Likehood Parameter Estimation ML).*

The aim of ML estimation is to find model parameters that maximise the GMM likehood basing on database from the test. For sequence of vectors from the test $T, x = \{\vec{x}_1, ... \vec{x}_T\}$, likehood GMM can be presented in the following way:

$$p(X|\lambda) = \prod_{t=1}^{T} p(\vec{x}_t|\lambda) \tag{4}$$

Unfortunately, the equation (4) is a non-linear function of parameters λ and direct maximization is impossible. However, ML parameter can be iteratively obtained through applying a special algorithm occurrence [3] of expected - maximization (EM).

The basic idea of EM algorithm is, starting from the initial model λ, estimation for a new model $\overline{\lambda}$, meaning $p(x|\overline{\lambda}) \geq p(x|\lambda)$. In such a situation, the new model becomes the initial model the following iteration and the process is being repeated till the convergence threshold has been reached. For each EM iteration, the following estimations were used, as the form of guarantee for monotonous growth of likehood model value:

Weights:

$$\overline{p}_i = \frac{1}{T}\sum_{t=1}^{T} p(i|\vec{x}_t, \lambda) \tag{5}$$

Mean values:

$$\bar{\vec{\mu}}_i = \frac{\sum_{t=1}^{T} p(i|\vec{x}_t, \lambda)\vec{x}_t}{\sum_{t=1}^{T} p(i|\vec{x}_t, \lambda)} \tag{6}$$

Variances:

$$\overline{\delta}_i^2 = \frac{\sum_{t=1}^{T} p(i|\vec{x}_t, \lambda)x_t^2}{\sum_{t=1}^{T} p(i|\vec{x}_t, \lambda)} - \overline{\mu}_i^2 \tag{7}$$

Where $\delta_i^2, x_t, and \mu_t$ refer successively to the elements of vectors $\overset{\rho}{\delta}_i^2, \overset{\rho}{x}_t\ and\ \overset{\rho}{\mu}_i$. A posterior probability for the acoustic class i is presented by (8)

$$p(i|\vec{x}_t, \lambda) = \frac{p_i b_i(\vec{x}_t)}{\sum_{k=1}^{M} p_k b_k(\vec{x}_t)} \tag{8}$$

In the course of learning GMM models one should pay attention on two factors which have to be matched. One is the quantity M and the other is the initial initiation of the model [1].

3.1.8 GMM Models Base

This check-up is based on creating a new model GMM for it which is based on sound record not recognised during the learning process in which models are not produced, then, the its identification takes place basing on models that have been in the base. During the configuration of the system we can establish which part of stuff will be taken under consideration in the learning phrase and which [part of research will appear during testing phrase. For the speaker identification we consider the group of speakers S, S={1,2,...,S}, represented by models GMM $\lambda_{1,}\lambda_2,...\lambda_s$. The aim is to find the model of the speaker that possesses maximum a posterior probability for a given observation section.

That is:

$$\hat{S} = \arg\max_{1 \le k \le s} \Pr(\lambda_k | X) = \arg\max \frac{p(X|\lambda_k)\Pr(\lambda_k)}{p(X)} \tag{9}$$

Where the second equation is based on Baye's theory. If we assume that all speakers are equally probable $(\Pr(\lambda_k) = 1/S)$ the classification of the rule is:

$$\hat{S} = \arg\max_{1 \le k \le S} p(X|\lambda_k) \tag{10}$$

Using logarithms and independencies between observations we can count:

$$\hat{S} = \arg\max_{1 \le k \le S} \sum_{t=1}^{T} \log p(\vec{x}_t|\lambda_k) \tag{11}$$

Where $p(\overset{\rho}{x}_t|\lambda_k)$ is described in (1).

More details concerning GMM models can be found in [4].

3.1.9 Results Base

The result of testing phase has been a set of text files containing results of the experiment. Those files contain numerical values adequate to probability in which a particular model has been developed by a particular speaker, having developed comparative identification models. As the result of test a file is being generated by the system enriched with a record of certain activities and their period of time. The module of results analysis defines the programmes set which enables to present tests files in more clear and legible way.

4 Experiments

All studies have been conducted using the above described experimental system with the use of sound material from the "BaFra" database. The purpose of these tests was to check, on the example of some specific experience, the effect of voice modification caused by illness of the upper respiratory system, on the efficacy of automatic identification of a person's voice. As one can guess, such change of voice may not leave the performance of identification system unaffected. Substantial deterioration of the operational effectiveness of the system takes place here.

Each single experiment always proceeded in the same manner. The samples base was replaced with a database of files with appropriate parameter vectors using the appropriate algorithm. Algorithms used to create basic parameter vectors have been described in [3]. Tests were performed for the following parameters: LPC linear prediction coefficients, LPREF reflection coefficients, CEP cepstral coefficients, MFCC coefficients.

For each type of parameters two successive experiments were conducted, marked as BM and ZM. In the first experiment, marked as BM, only phrases without modification were verified, this means that both the models and subsequent tests were created using non-modified phrases. Such experiment emulates the basic situation when no change of voice has occurred in the phase of learning and testing. The test was made on the other 21 samples not used for the development of models. Altogether, throughout the whole BM experiment, 525 checks were performed.

In the second experiment, marked as ZM, only modified phrases were verified, this means that models were generated for non-modified phrases and the test was made for modified phrases. Such experiment emulates the least favourable situation when a major change of voice occurs between the phase of learning and testing. The test was made on 70 modified voice samples, not used for the development of models. Altogether, throughout the whole ZM experiment 1750 checks were performed.

After each experiment, the results were collected, this means the number of correct decisions was calculated in relation to all the decisions made. A correct decision is one when the highest probability has been calculated for the speaker who spoke the given phrase. The highest probability is exactly present when the calculated value is as close to zero as possible. The number of correct decisions in relation to all the decisions made, expressed as percent, was registered as the result of a given experiment. An additional important factor is the duration of the experiment. It was recorded in order to measure how change in the way of parameterisation affects the complexity of calculation. Single recalculation or single model creation time was not recorded, only was the duration of the process consisting in converting "wav" files to parameter collections, and then execution of the two earlier discussed experiments. For the particular type of parameterisation the whole calculation sequence was exactly repeated, the calculations were made in exactly the same conditions, what makes the duration of the whole experiment a good measure of calculation complexity.

For later discussion I introduce the following symbols:

BM - result of the first experiment expressed as percent (learning and tests using phrases without modification),

BMT - quantity of correct decisions in the first experiment (learning and tests using phrases without modification),

BMF - number of incorrect decisions in the first experiment (learning and tests using phrases without modification),

$\mathbf{t_{BM}}$ - duration of the first experiment (learning and tests using phrases without modification),

ZM - result of the second experiment expressed as percent (learning using phrases without modification, tests using modified phrases),

ZMT - number of correct decisions in the second experiment (learning using phrases without modification, tests using modified phrases),

ZMF - quantity of incorrect decisions in the second experiment (learning using phrases without modification, tests using modified phrases),

$\mathbf{t_{ZM}}$ - duration of the second experiment (learning using phrases without modification, tests using modified phrases),

N - number of parameters in one vector.

5 Presentation of Results

Primarily tests were made for basic parameters LPC, LPREF, CEP, MFCC for various N. The results of these tests are shown below.

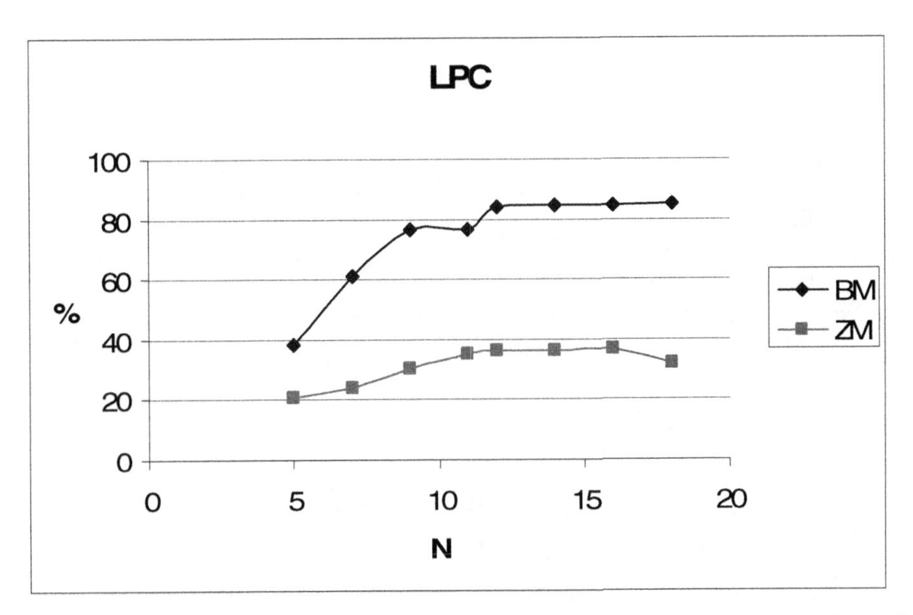

Fig. 3. Graph presenting decision correctness in tests BM and ZM depending on N for LPC parameters

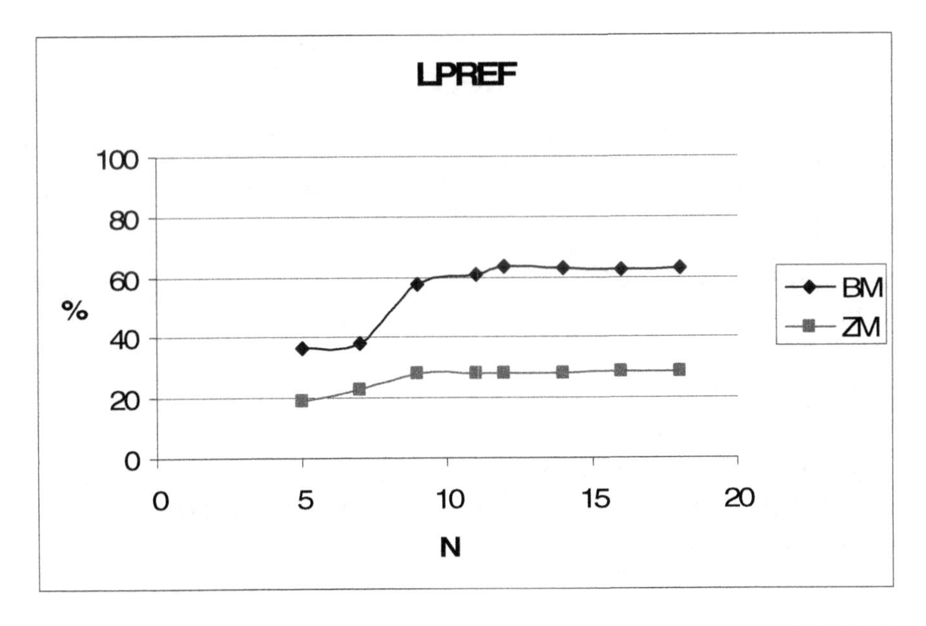

Fig. 4. Graph presenting decision correctness in tests BM and ZM depending on N for LPREF parameters

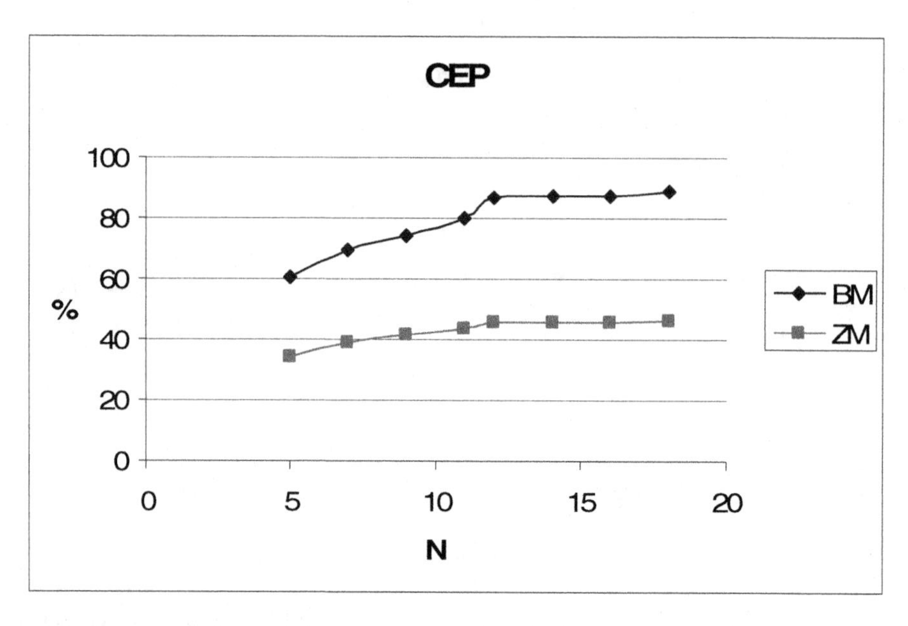

Fig. 5. Graph presenting decision correctness in tests BM and ZM depending on N for CEP parameters

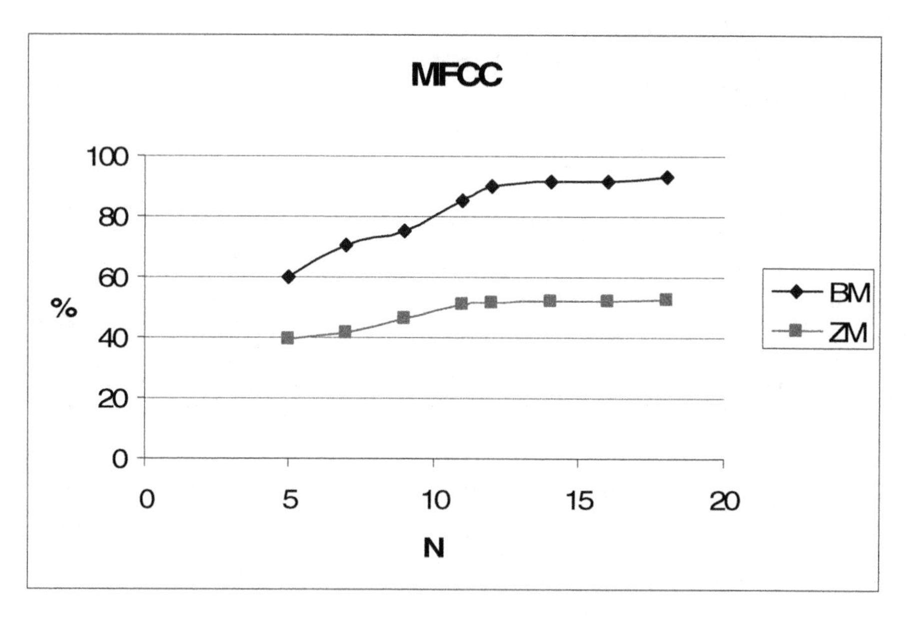

Fig. 6. Graph presenting decision correctness in tests BM and ZM depending on N for MFCC parameters

6 Conclusions

As one can see, on the basis of the above presented test results for all kinds of applied parameters, substantial deterioration occurred in the quality of recognition. MFCC parameters proved relatively best and they will be the basis for further study over system enhancement in order to minimize the effect of changes in voice on the correct operation of the system. I doesn't make sense to increase the parameter vector to more then N=12.

References

[1] Young, S., Everman, G., Kershaw, D., Moore, G., Odell, J., Ollason, D., Povey, D., Valtchev, V., Woodland, P.: The HTK Book. Microsoft Corporation 1999, Cambridge University Engineering Department (2002), http://htk.eng.cam.ac.uk/

[2] Gadek, J.: Experimental system for research of speaker independent voice recognition. Information extraction and processing 23(99), 200, 101–106 (Lvov 2005)

[3] Huang, X., Acero, A., Hsiao-Wuen, H.: Spoken Language Processing. Prentice Hall, Englewood Cliffs (2001)

[4] Reynolds, D.A., Quatieri, T.F., Dunn, R.B.: Speaker verification using adapted Gaussian mixture models. Digital Signal Processing 10, 19–41 (2000)

From the Research on Synthesis of Static Images of Melanocytic Skin Lesions

Zdzisław S. Hippe[1], Jerzy W. Grzymała-Busse[2], and Łukasz Piątek[3]

[1] Department of Expert Systems and Artificial Intelligence, University of Information Technology and Management, 35-225 Rzeszów, Poland
[2] Department of Electrical Engineering and Computer Science, University of Kansas, Lawrence, KS 66045-7621, USA
[3] Department of Distributed Systems, University of Information Technology and Management, 35-225 Rzeszów, Poland
{zhippe,lpiatek}@wsiz.rzeszow.pl, Jerzy@ku.edu

Abstract. Some algorithms to synthesize static images of melanocytic skin lesions are briefly outlined. The key approach in the elaborated synthesis methodology of images is a semantic conversion of textual description of melanocytic skin lesions - by an inhouse developed system - into hybrid (vector-raster) images. It was found, that the developed methodology can be successfully used in the process of teaching of dermatology students and also in training of preferred medical doctors.

Keywords: synthesis of medical images, dynamic generation, melanocytic skin lesions, TDS.

1 Introduction

In the past few years an increasing interest in images of melanocytic skin lesions is observed, what could be treated as a support of the visual, computer-aided diagnosis of malignant melanoma, currently one of the most dangerous type of tumors [1]. On the other hand, the lack of professional computer informational databases containing images of above mentioned lesions is still noticed. This situation inspired us to start the research on the development of algorithms for the synthesis of medical images, specifically for the synthesis of static images of melanocytic skin lesions. It is assumed, that implementation of these algorithms within a special computer program system should allow to create multi-category informational database, containing both synthesized (in other words, artificial) and real images of skin lesions.

2 Methodology of the Research

Our initial research [2] was dealt with the semantic conversion of records from the textual informational database [3] into respective digital images [4]. This source (**textual**) database contains information of **548** real cases of anonymous patients' lesions, confirmed by histopatological tests. According to the methodology described by

E. Kącki, M. Rudnicki, J. Stempczyńska (Eds.): Computers in Medical Activity, AISC 65, pp. 223–229.
springerlink.com

Braun-Falco [5] and Stolz [6], classification of every real case in above mentioned database relies on the application of the **ABCD rule** [3], in which **A** (*Asymmetry*) shows a result of evaluation of lesion's asymmetry, **B** - (*Border*) estimates the character of a rim of the lesion, **C** - (*Color*) identifies number of colors (one or more, from **6** allowed) present in the lesion, and **D** - (*Diversity of structures*) stands for the number of structures (one or more, from **5** allowed). Elements of **ABCD rule** enumerate four main symptoms of an investigated lesion, and at the same time these elements are used to compute the **TDS** (**T**otal **D**ermatoscopy **S**core) parameter [5], using the equation presented below:

$$\mathbf{TDS} = \mathbf{1.3} * Asymmetry + \mathbf{0{,}1} * Border + \mathbf{0{,}5} * \sum Color + \mathbf{0{,}5} * \sum Diversity\ of\ Structure \quad (1)$$

For example, for a case described by a vector:

- *Asymmetry* – **symmetric change**,
- *Border* – **0**,
- *Color* – **four** selected colors present in a lesion,
- *Diversity of Structure* – **four** selected structures present in a lesion,

the value of **TDS** equals to **4.0**:

$$\mathbf{TDS} = \mathbf{1.3} * 0 + \mathbf{0.1} * 0 + \mathbf{0.5} * (0 + 0 + 1 + 1 + 1 + 1) + \mathbf{0.5} * (1 + 0 + 1 + 1 + 1) = \mathbf{4.0} \quad (2)$$

According to **TDS** value, the analyzed lesion could be assigned to one of four accepted categories (classes) of melanocytic skin lesions, namely: *Benign nevus, Blue nevus*, *Suspicious nevus* or *Melanoma malignant.* (see Table 1.)

Table 1. Classification of melanocytic skin lesions in dependence of **TDS**-value

TDS value	Lesion classification
TDS < 4,76 and lack of **color blue**	*Benign nevus*
TDS < 4,76 and **color blue** is present	*Blue nevus*
4,76 <= TDS < 5,45	*Suspicious nevus*
TDS >= 5,45	*Melanoma malignant*

Recently, synthesis of discussed images is based on latest results of the research executed at Kansas University [7, 8], differentiating the role of a particular color and structure within a lesion, allowing to determine the value of a new total dermatoscopy score parameter, called **New_TDS**:

$$\begin{aligned}\mathbf{New\_TDS} = {} & (\mathbf{0{,}8} * Asymmetry) + (0{,}11 * Border) + (\mathbf{0{,}5} * C\_White) \\ & + (\mathbf{0{,}8} * C\_Blue) + (\mathbf{0{,}5} * C\_DarkBrown) + (\mathbf{0{,}6} * C\_LightBrown) \\ & + (\mathbf{0{,}5} * C\_Black) + (\mathbf{0{,}5} * C\_Red) + (\mathbf{0{,}5} * D\_Pigment\_Network) \\ & + (\mathbf{0{,}5} * D\_Pigment\_Dots) + (\mathbf{0{,}6} * D\_Pigment\_Globules) \\ & + (\mathbf{0{,}6} * D\_Branched\_Streaks) + (\mathbf{0{,}6} * D\_Structureless\_Areas)\end{aligned} \quad (3)$$

3 Algorithms of Mapping Lesions' Symptoms

Initial results of our preliminary research [2] showed that the transformation of a single case from our informational database allowed to obtain only one synthetic image. Then, the application of random mapping of two selected symptoms of lesions (i.e. <***Asymmetry***> and <***Border***>) [4] enabled to generate the exhaustive number of synthesized images [9], corresponding to symptoms displayed by a given lesion. At present, developed algorithms are improved by using hybrid type (**vector-raster**) approach to synthesis of lesions images. The general technique applied for synthesis of lesion's asymmetry through the use of NURBS surfaces (i.e. **n**on-**u**niform **r**ational **B**-spline) [10], together with raster operations for mapping lesion's border has been described in [11]. Here, the attention is focused only on raster type algorithms for mapping two remaining symptoms of lesion's, namely <***Color***> and <***Diversity** of structure*>.

4 Algorithms of Synthesis Colors and Structures of the Lesion's

Synthesis of colors and structures of lesion's should consider multi-argument character of <***Color***> and <***Diveristy** of structure*> attributes, capable to create considerable number of combinations of these parameters, appearing simultaneously in a given lesion. <***Color***> can have **6** allowed values: *black, blue, dark-brown, light-brown, red* and *white*, when at the same time the <***Diversity** of structure*> attribute can have **5** logical values: *branched streaks, pigment dots, pigment globules, pigment network* and *structureless area*. The number of all possible combinations is a Cartesian product of **both parameters**. Structurally:

$$\mathbf{COLORS\ x\ STRUCTURES} = \{(\mathbf{color, structure}) \in \mathbf{P}\ (\mathbf{P}(\mathbf{COLORS} \cup \mathbf{STRUCTURES})) : \mathbf{color} \in \mathbf{COLORS} \wedge \mathbf{structure} \in \mathbf{STRUCTURES}\} \tag{4}$$

where **P(COLORS)** means power set of **COLORS** set.

These calculations lead to the conclusion that it would be required to define $\mathbf{2^{30} - 1}$ static fragments (so called textures) of an image. Generating over **one milliard** textures is virtually almost impossible; additional disadvantage of such mapping would be very frequent repetition of occurrence of selected structures in particular colors, because of its shape, size and place in the generated image. Taking these facts into consideration, the synthesis required a special approach: initially (before generating textures), there is an attempt to find which colors and structures occur simultaneously in a real lesions [2]. The results of these investigations are shown in Fig. 1.

Basing on these findings, the developed algorithms can be simplified through application of so called basic textures, having two combinations of colors only: images with color blue, appearing separately, and images with colors dark-brown and light-brown.

In the next step, for the prepared *a priori* texture, containing basic color (Fig. 2b) and binary image with previously defined NURBS surface (Fig. 2a) [11], the logical product is computed, applying following rules: every pixel of ultimate image (Fig. 2c) with coordinates (x_i,y_i) is designed by means of pixels with coordinate (x_i,y_i) of bitmap, if pixel of image with NURBS surface is white. However, if pixel of vector type graphic is black, then pixel of ultimate image is also black.

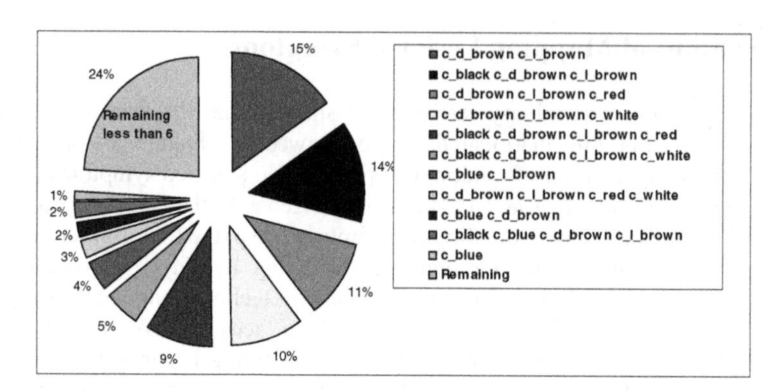

Fig. 1. Simultaneous occurrence of colors and structures in real lesions

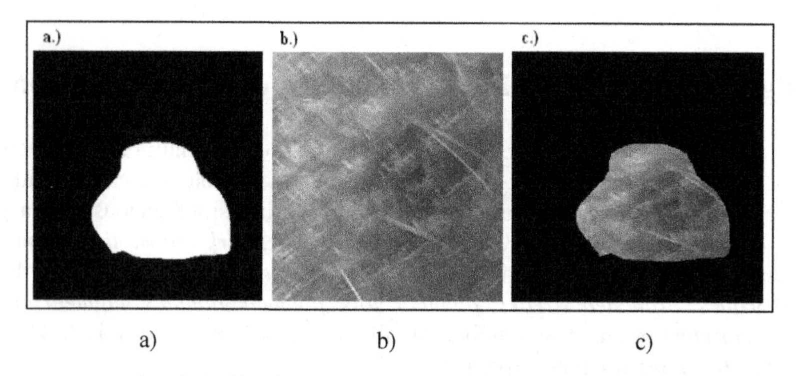

a) b) c)

Fig. 2. Adding basic color to pre-defined NURBS surface

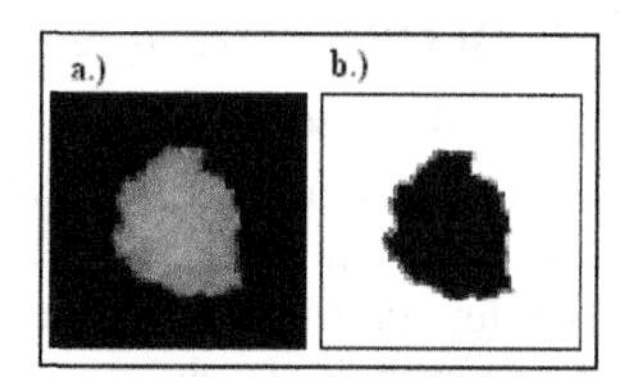

Fig. 3. Additional layer with red structureless area (a) and its mask image (b)

The remaining (i.e. additional) colors in combination with required structures are defined in additional layers (each of **5** *diversity of structures* is defined in each of **6** permitted *colors*). For each additional layer (Fig. 3a) binary images, which are a copy of these texture (but in black and white colors) are then defined; we call them image mask (Fig. 3b).

The algorithm of adding the additional layers is executed as a two-step process. First, a mask image (Fig. 4a) is placed on top of the primary (basic) texture (Fig. 4c). The white parts of image mask represents the transparent part of the mask, whereas black parts represent the solid part. It should be emphasized, that the type of blending used, causes the black parts of mask will appear on the scene only (Fig. 4d). Then blending modes is switch, and logical sum operation of image with required structure

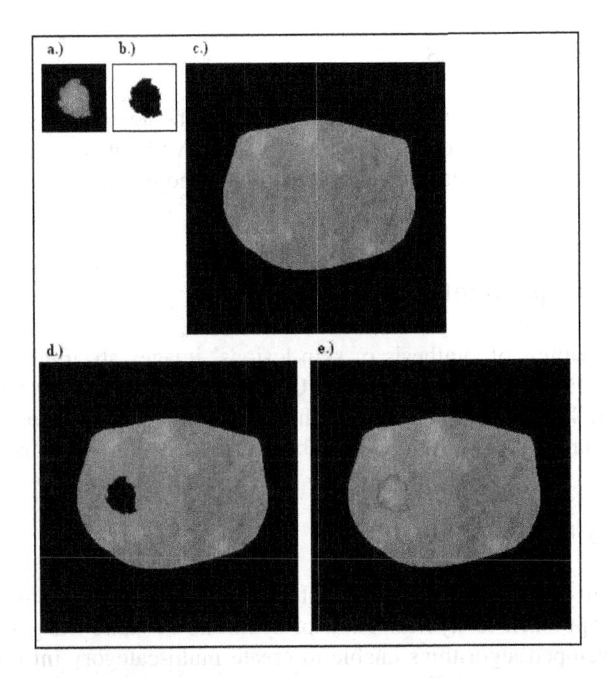

Fig. 4. An example of adding additional layer, containing required diversity of structure

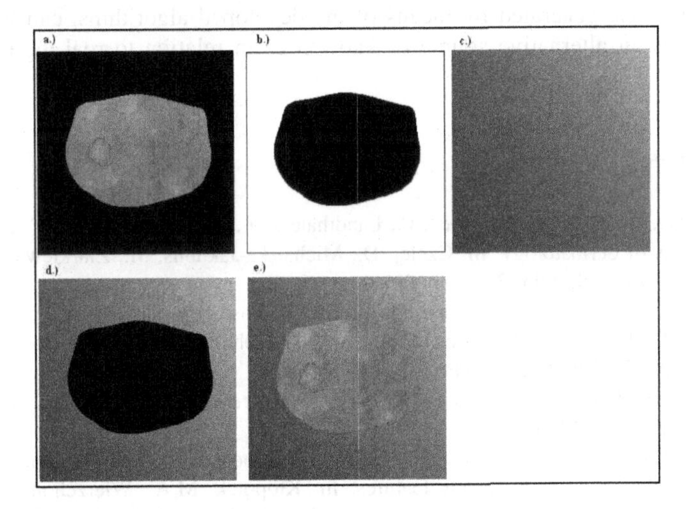

Fig. 5. Adding to lesions' image (a) new layer with healthy skin (c), using image mask (b)

(Fig. 4b) and image from Fig. 4d is applied. The final image is shown on Fig. 4e. At the end of the discussed process, a special operation is defined for adding an image of healthy skin to encircle the lesion (see Fig. 5).

5 Experimental Results

In an exhaustive set of experiments it was found that the developed algorithms enable random mapping of required colors and structures, without necessity to define all previously mentioned simultaneous combinations of both symptoms (over 1 milliard possibilities).

6 Program Implementation

Developed algorithms of synthesis of skin lesions' images are implemented in **C++** language, combined with the use of **MFC** (**M**icrosoft **F**oundation **C**lasses) library [12], and **OpenGL** graphic library [13]. The developed computer program system for synthesis of melanocytic skin lesion images is available at www.melanoma.pl.

7 Summary and Conclusion

Combination of algorithms described tentatively here (and also discussed in [11]) follow a new approach to hybridization of synthesis of static images (vector-raster type). The developed algorithms enable to create multi-category informational database, which can be successfully used not only in teaching of medicine students, but also in job practice of dermatologists and preferred medical doctors. It seems that synthetic images, generated by means of the developed algorithms, can be successfully used as an alternative source of knowledge in relation to real digital medical images.

References

1. Stolz, W., Braun-Falco, O., Bilek, P., Landthaler, M., Burgdorf, W.H.C., Cognetta, A.B.: The Atlas of dermatology. In: Czelej, D., Michalska-Jakubus, M., Ziarkiewicz, M. (eds.) Czelej Sp. z o.o., Lublin (2006) (in Polish)
2. Hippe, Z.S., Piatek, Ł.: From research on the database of simulated medical images. In: Proc. of the Conferene Databases for Science and Technology, Gdańsk, Poland, September 25-27, pp. 225–230 (2005) (in Polish)
3. Hippe, Z.S.: Computer Database 'NEVI' on Endangerment by Melanoma. TASK Quarterly 3, 483–488 (1999)
4. Hippe, Z.S., Grzymała-Busse, J.W., Piątek, Ł.: Randomized dynamic generation of selected melanocytic skin lesions features. In: Kłopotek, M.A., Wierzchoń, S.T., Trojanowski, K. (eds.) Advances in Soft Computing (Intelligent Information Processing and Web Mining), pp. 21–29. Springer, Heidelberg (2006)
5. Braun-Falco, O., Stolz, W., Bilek, P., Merkle, T., Landthaler, M.: Das dermatoskop. Eine Vereinfachung der Auflichtmikroskopie von pigmentierten Hautveranderungen. Hautarzt 40, 131 (1990)
6. Atlas of Dermatoscopy of Pigmented Skin Tumors of La Roche-Posay, `http://www.pless.fr/dermatoscopie/`

7. Alvarez, A., Bajcar, S., Brown, F.M., Grzymała-Busse, J.W., Hippe, Z.S.: Optimization of the ABCD Formula Used for Melanoma Diagnosis. In: Kłopotek, M.A., Wierzchoń, S.T., Trojanowski, K. (eds.) Advances in Soft Computing (Intelligent Information Processing and Web Mining), pp. 233–240. Springer, Heidelberg (2003)
8. Grzymała-Busse, J.W., Hoppe, Z.S.: Data Mining Methods Supporting Diagnosis of Melanoma. In: Proc. of the 18th IEEE Symposium on Computer-Based Medical Systems, pp. 371–373. IEEE Comp. Soc., Los Alamitos (2005)
9. Kulikowski, J.L.: The foundations of the structural description of distracted databes of expert knowledge. In: Proc. The Conference Databases for Science and Technology, Gdańsk, September 25-27, pp. 29–38 (2005) (in Polish)
10. Angel, E.: Interactive Computer Graphics - A Top Down Approach with OpenGL, pp. 445–446. Addison Wesley Longman Inc., Amsterdam (2000)
11. Hippe, Z.S., Piątek, Ł.: Synthesis of Static Medical Images – an Example of Melanocytic Skin Lesions. In: Kurzyński, M., Puchała, E., Woźniak, M., Żołnierek, A. (eds.) Advances in Soft Computing (Computer Recognition Systems 2), pp. 503–509. Springer, Heidelberg (2007)
12. http://www.mfc.org.pl/
13. http://www.opengl.org/

Modelling of Alveolar Recruitment Phenomena in Human Lungs

Bozenna Kuraszkiewicz

Institute of Biocybernetics and Biomedical Engineering PAS, 02-109 Warsaw, Trojdena 4, Poland
bozena@ibib.waw.pl

Abstract. This paper presents the study on a possible solution to the questions concerning the classical theory of pressure-volume (PV) hysteresis and determines the role of alveolar recruitment phenomena in it. The primary purpose of the present study is to see, whether this physical process, which can be solved by model analysis, might explain a number of experimental observations on lung and airway dynamics in term of pressure-volume and flow relationships.

1 Background

Gil and Weibel have demonstrated the importance of alveolar recruitment at relatively low inflating pressure, which has also been noted by Klingele and Staub [1-2]. These findings are incorporated into a model of alveolar mechanics, which presents a possible solution to the questions concerning the classical theory of pressure-volume (PV) hysteresis. Recruitment and de-recruitment are the important modes of volume change at low air-filled lung volumes (less than 40% TLC). Pulmonary physiologists have shown that, in the de-gassed lung, alveolar recruitment is important during the entire initial inflation as reflected by the changes in shunting. All of them have long been fascinated by the hysteresis demonstrated during inflation/deflation cycling of lungs (Fig.1).

The width of the hysteresis has some frequency dependence (i.e. it varies with the PV cycling rate), but the hysteresis remains in static curve that is in PV cycling in which the system is allowed to come to equilibrium before recording pressure and volume. It is the static hysteresis phenomenon that is of interest here. When lungs are emptied during exhalation, peripheral airways close up. For people with lung diseases they may not reopen even for significant portion of inhalation, impairing gas exchange. Knowledge of the mechanisms, that govern reinflation of collapsed regions of the lungs, is therefore central to development of ventilation strategies for combating respiratory problems.

There are two contributions to the wall tension in an alveolus: the tissue tension, which is elastic in character, and the surface tension. It is held that changes in the surface area of an alveolus during expansion and contraction of the lung lead to hysteresis in wall tension, which in turn results in PV curves similar to Fig.1.

There are several theories concerning the elasticity of the structure, which is composed mainly of reticular and collagen fibres with the bulk of elastic fibres in the

E. Kącki, M. Rudnicki, J. Stempczyńska (Eds.): Computers in Medical Activity, AISC 65, pp. 231–239.
springerlink.com

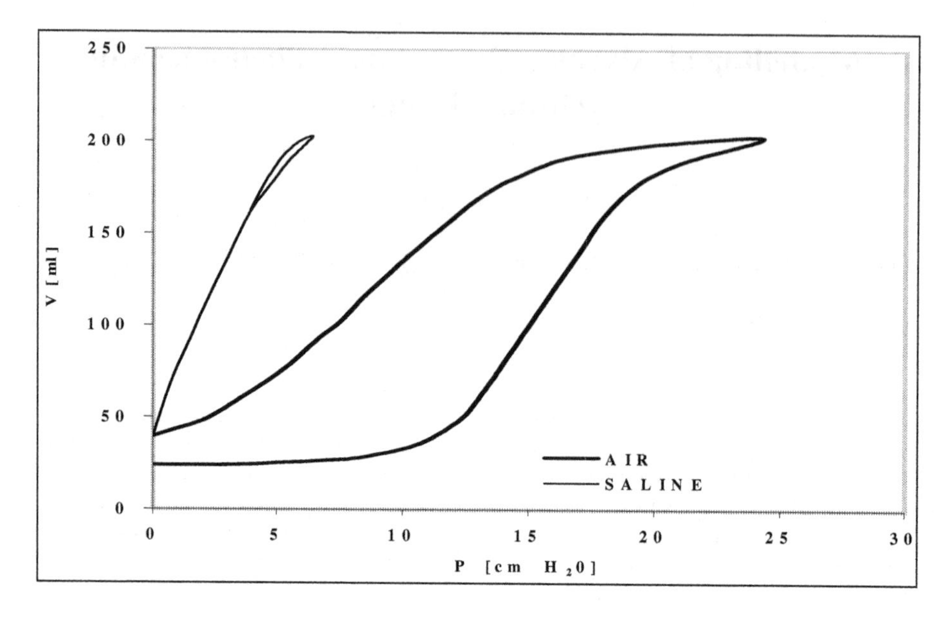

Fig. 1. PV curves for saline and air-filled lung from experimental data [14]

alveoli being found encircling the alveolar entrances. Von Neergaard was the first to postulate that a surface-active material in the lung might be responsible for pressure-volume behaviour [3]. Pulmonary surfactant has since been the subject of numerous studies attempting to define its chemical composition and physical properties, as well as its role in PV hysteresis in lungs (Scarpelli [4], Gladston [5], Blank [6], Brown [7]).

One of the most interesting properties of pulmonary surfactant is its ability to display a static hysteresis relationship of its own. Pulmonary surfactant is harvested. It is then layered on the surface of a saline solution in a Langmuir trough, a shallow container with a movable bar, which confines the surfactant at the air/fluid interface such that its surface area, can be varied. Lempert and Macklem measured surface tension as the surface area, which was varied and a hysteresis loop resulted [8](see Fig.2).

The occurrence of "hysteretic" behaviour of surfactant on a Langmuir trough and in the pressure-volume relationship in lungs has led to the conclusion that the former is directly responsible for the latter. Krahl describes the alveolar framework as being composed mainly of reticular and collagen fibres with the bulk of elastic fibres in the alveoli being found encircling the alveolar entrances [9].

There are several theories concerning the elasticity of the structure, which is composed in large part of nonelastic fibres. Bull has drawn an analogy with a nylon stocking whose elasticity results from the weave used in its construction, not from the nylon fibre, a relatively inelastic material [10]. Pierce has suggested that one function of the elastic fibres might be to act as shock absorbers in over expansion and has pointed out that the architecture of the alveolus is ideally suited to folding and unfolding, and he proposed this unfolding process as the means by which lung volume might increase during expansion [11]. Klingele and Straub found that at

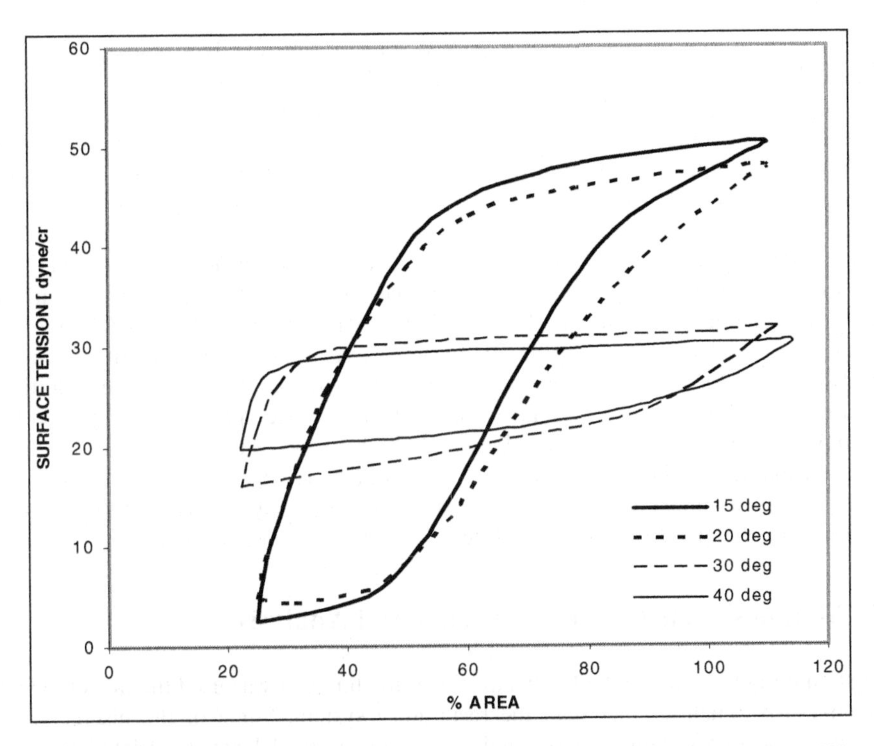

Fig. 2. Surface tension versus percent area as recorded on a surface tension balance [8]

volumes below 40% TLC alveoli tend to fold like so many small accordions and "disappear" [2]. Recently Gil and Weibel fixed rat lungs at various points during the measurement of pressure-volume relationships [1].

The lungs were analysed morphometrically for various parameters with some interesting results. Collapsed alveoli were found at all pressures used in the inflation/deflation cycles. The number of collapsed alveoli decreased with increasing pressure and *vice versa.* If alveoli expand elasticity, then the total alveolar volume of the lung should be proportional to the total alveolar surface area by the relation: $A = CV^{2/3}$, where C is a proportionality constant.

But Gil and Weibel found that alveolar surface area was directly proportional to alveolar volume at four of the five points measured. These findings indicate that total alveolar volume at relatively low pressures (max.P = 16 mmHg) is determined by the number of open alveoli, which in turn is a function of pressure. Thus, according to their work, changes in lung volume seem to occur in large part by recruitment and de-recruitment of alveoli [1].

Dunnil found that, using unspecified pressures, alveolar surface area is proportional to volume by the relation $A = CV^{2/3}$ [12]. Thus, one is drawn to the conclusion that at air-filled lung volumes greater than 50% TLC, after an initial expansion to 100% TLC, alveoli behave `elasticity`, while below approximately 40% TLC volume alveolar recruitment and de-recruitment are more important. One exception to this is the initial inflation of a de-gassed lung.

Anthonisen has shown that a de-gassed lung *in situ* exhibits marked shunting, which decreases to 3% with inflation to 100% TLC, and which point shunting begins to increase sharply [13]. This correlates with microscopic data in which alveoli are recruited, largest first, on initial inflation of a de-gassed lung with air, but then no de-recruitment is noted on deflation from TLC until relatively low volumes are reached (Radford [14]).

In an experiment performed by Pierce, it was found that a lung filled with mercury displayed PV hysteresis, which was greater than that of an air-filled lung [11]. A subsequent experiment by Hills has shown that there is no hysteresis in the surface tension measurements at the interface of mercury with surfactant saturated solution of normal saline [15]. Therefore, the PV hysteresis seen in the mercury-filled lung is probably not due to surfactant caused hysteresis in surface tension. In addition, Radford rinsed a rat lung with a non-ionic surfactant, which presumably replaced the pulmonary surfactant lining the alveoli [14]. Pressure-volume data for this lung showed significant, although diminished, hysteretic behaviour.

If it was assumed that the natural alveolar lining layer was replaced in this experiment, then PV hysteresis would be expected to disappear entirely.

2 Methods – Theory and Experimental Analysis

In attempting to simulate the PV behaviour of the lungs, it was used the model, which is obviously much simpler than the respiratory system. Some of the discrepancies between the experimental curves and the computer model can be related to these simplifications. There is a significant change in lung volume prior to the appearance of the knee in many of the experimental inflation curves; while in this model there is no volume change until the onset of alveolar recruitment. This difference is accounted for by the elastic expansion of the airways in experimental data, which is not taken in the model presented here. The interdependence of alveoli, which will account for some differences of unknown extent, was ignored.

There are some serious difficulties in re-creating the pressure-volume behaviour of air-filled lungs. In mathematical equations it has not taken into account any variation in some parameters with changes in total volume and alveolar surface area. For the case of the inflation of a de-gassed lung it may not be too serious limitation. When inflating such a lung, the collapsed alveolus is recruited at a pressure that is much higher than that minimal pressure necessary for stability and at pressures that are, in general, well advanced towards the maximal expansion portion of the lung tissue elasticity curve. Therefore, when such an alveolus is recruited, it is often almost maximally expanded, which will cause the surface tension in the alveolus to be at its highest. If such is the case, then surface tension in the open alveoli over the inflation portion of air-filled lungs, which start from zero volume, may be nearly constant.

Because of the complexity of describing the elastic behaviour of alveolar tissue, starting from basic principles a more empirical approach is used. When the lung is filled with saline, as in von Neergaard experiment, surface energy at the liquid/tissue interface is very nearly zero [3]. The pressure-volume relationship of Fig.1 for the saline-filled lung is due almost entirely to the elastic properties of the alveoli. The pressure – volume (PV) saline curve of Fig.1 can be fit empirically by the equation:

$$V = V_{max}\left[1 - \exp(-P/K)\right] \tag{1}$$

K is an adjustable parameter. It was assumed that this same equation could be used to describe elastic volume changing behaviour of a single alveolus. The value of K will increase with increasing surface tension.

The mechanical properties of a given alveolus are assumed as that is, it will open at a given pressure and close at a specific pressure, all other factors remaining the same. It is also assumed that all alveoli of a given size at a specific pressure will have the same mechanical properties. Since recruiting an alveolus exposes a surface with non-zero surface energy, the total surface energy is increased by γA_a, where γ = surface energy (erg/cm^2) and A_a is the surface area of the alveolus. Surface energy is equivalent to surface tension (dyne/cm).

The lining layer of the closed alveolus remains trapped within the lumen, according to the work of Gil and Weibel [1]. Work must be done to overcome the attractive forces between the walls in the unfolding alveolus and the amount of work necessary to do this will be proportional to alveolar surface area. Other work necessary to open the alveolus might be related to the reticular architecture. If it is assumed certain homogeneity of structure among various sizes of alveoli, then this work will also be dependent on alveolar surface area. Thus, it may be assumed that a given alveolus will open when the work done by expansion of the alveolus is approximately equal to the work necessary to open it:

$$P_o\, \Delta V = P_o V_a = \alpha\, A_a \tag{2}$$

where: $\Delta V = V_a$, V_a is the alveolar volume [ml], P_o - opening pressure [cmH$_2$O], A_a- alveolar surface [cm^2], α - the work per unit area required to open an alveolus [dyne/cm] or [cmH$_2$O·cm].

Generally, the shape of alveoli is ascribed as polyhedral. But the ratio of alveolar volume / surface area can be very well approximated by a sphere [16]. A combination of eqs. (1) and (2) finally leads to:

$$P_o = \frac{\alpha A_a}{V_a} = \frac{4\pi r^2 \alpha \left(1 - e^{-P_o/K}\right)^{2/3}}{\frac{4}{3}\pi r^3 \left(1 - e^{-P_o/K}\right)} = \frac{3\,\alpha}{r\left(1 - e^{-P_o/K}\right)^{\frac{1}{3}}} \tag{3}$$

The pressure, at which the alveolus will close or be de-recruited, can be similarly derived. Factors, which one might expect to determine the stability of the open alveolus, are also functions of alveolar surface area. Surface energy (tension) is one obvious factor. The ability of pulmonary surfactant to lower the surface energy to small values, as compared to bare surface or other surface-active materials, adds to the stability of the open alveolus [16]. Structural and other factors may play a role. At this time it is the purpose to treat those cases in which surface tension does not change.

A cursory treatment of the de-gassed lung inflated with air is attempted to illustrate the genesis of the knee in the inflation curve, which is seen in lungs deflated below 50% TLC.

The calculation of PV curves is accomplished as follows: for each species the volume of the lung ($V(r)$) corresponding to each size of alveoli is calculated and normalised, so that the total volume (V_{TOTAL}) of the sum of all alveoli is equal 100 and alveolar volume ($V(P)$) can be read directly as percent total volume. The radii are varied in 1 micrometer (10^{-4} cm) steps from 1 to 200 μm and:

$$V(r)=\frac{4}{3}\pi r^3\frac{dN(r)}{V_{TOTAL}}\times 100 \quad (4)$$

$$V_{TOTAL}=\sum_{r=1\mu}^{200\mu}\frac{4}{3}\pi r^3 dN(r) \quad (5)$$

$$V(P)=\sum_{r=1\mu}^{200\mu}V(r)\left(1-e^{-P_o/K}\right) \quad (6)$$

The distribution of alveolar size for various species has been known for some time [17]. A good approximation of the experimental data is obtained using the following equation [18]:

$$dN(r)=N_o\exp\left[-\ln 2\left\{\frac{\ln[1+2b(r-r_o)\Delta X]}{b}\right\}^2\right]dr \quad (7)$$

where:

r_o - Radius of the most numerous alveolus of a given size
N_o - The number of alveoli of radius r_o
ΔX - The width at half-height of the curve
b - An adjustable parameter which determines the skew of the curve
dr = 1 micrometer

The values of $dN(r)$ plotted *versus* radius yields a skewed Gaussian.

These equations correspond to expansion by alveolar recruitment combined with elastic inflation. The volumes and pressures for deflation in regions of de-recruitment are calculated in a similar manner, replacing α with β in calculating pressure P (where β is the work per unit area done by the collapsing alveolus).

In regions, where no recruitment or de-recruitment occurs, volume is allowed to expand or contract elasticity using eq. (6). An example of this type of region is that between the maximum volume and pressure attained during inflation and the pressure and volume, at which de-recruitment begins to occur with deflation.

The scheme of calculations is following:

Volume is set at zero, which corresponds to a de-gassed lung and remains at that pressure value from $P = 0.0$ mmHg to $P=3\alpha/200\,(1-e^{-P/K})^{1/3}$.

At the latter pressure, which is calculated by an iterative technique, alveoli of radius 200 micrometers are recruited and the volume over at that point is computed by eq. (6), where the sum is taken over only the one value of $r = 200$ µm.

Next, the total volume is computed for $P=3\alpha/199\,(1-e^{-P/K})^{1/3}$ and so on, until the volume is equal 99 % of total maximum volume. At that point all alveoli from 200 to 10µm in radius are assumed to be open.

Then, as the deflation calculation begins, the pressure will be dropped in 0,1 mmHg steps and calculate volume by eq. (6), summing from r = 10 to 200µm until $P=3\beta/10\,(1-e^{-P/K})^{1/3}$ is reached.

At that pressure all alveoli of r = 10 µm close and the de-recruitment phase of lung contraction begun.

Then the volume and pressure, at which alveoli of r = 11µm are de-recruited, are calculated and so on, to zero volume.

3 Results and Conclusion

Pressure-volume (PV) curves on Fig.1 are Radford's data for saline- and air-filled cat lung [14]. These curves represent the elasticity of the lung tissue without any contribution from surfactant. It results from the very low; probably close to zero, surface tension at the interface of saline with tissue saturated with isosmotic fluid.

The saline curve of Fig.3 is a result of computer simulation using $\alpha = \beta =$ 0.0005cmH_2O-cm and K = 2.0cmH_2O. The values of α and β were not set exactly equal to zero, because the computer will not divide into zero. The values are low enough that the value of K is a good approximation of the tissue elasticity. The residual volume in Fig.1 is not calculated in Fig.3, as it was interested only in the alveolar portion of the lung and not in the airway's contribution to total lung volume.

In Fig.3 the air-filled lung curve was calculated by adjusting α such that the knee, which marks the onset the alveolar recruitment, approximately matches that in the air-inflation curve of Fig.1. The value for β was arrived at by an examination of the data [19-20]. The value of K was increased from 2.0 until the calculated deflation curve approximately matched the experimental data. The following values arrived at: $\alpha =$ 0.030 cmH_2O-cm, $\beta =$ 0.0045 cmH_2O-cm, $K =$ 4.5 cmH_2O.

It should be noted that the values assigned to α and β for the various experiments are probably accurate to at least ± 0.0005 cmH_2O-cm and K to ± 0.5 cmH_2O, as any greater changes led to significant variations of the PV curves from reasonable reproduction of the experimental data. Also, both the experimental and computer data show represent static pressure-volume (PV) curves.

The discontinuities, which appear in some of the computer curves, are the result of the assumption of jumps of one micron in alveolar size.

The values for the parameters used in the calculations are physiologically interpretable and were arrived at on the basis of a reasonable model of alveolar

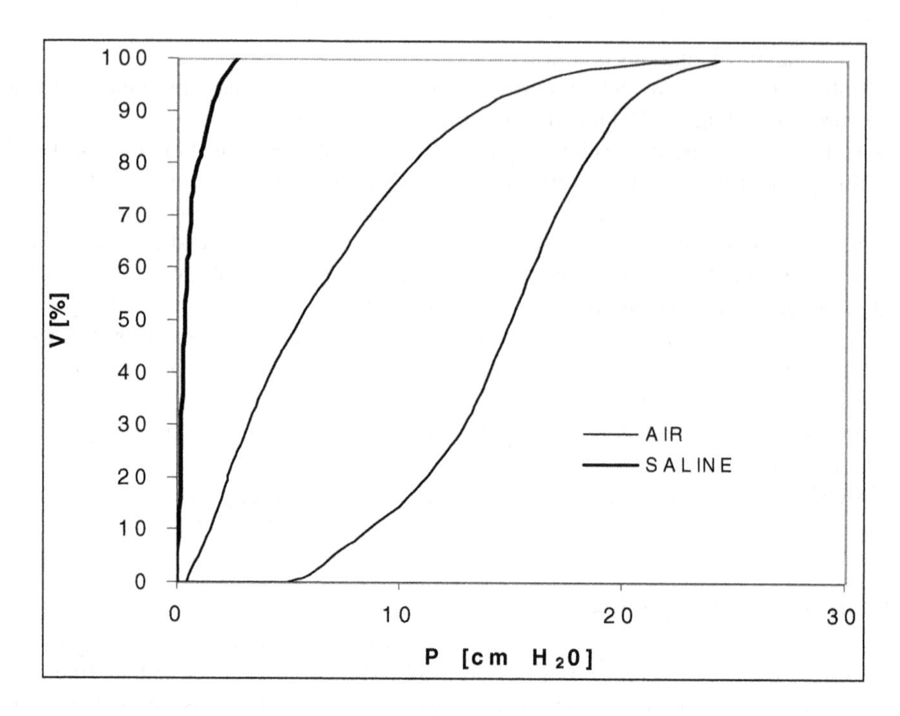

Fig. 3. PV curves of computer simulation for saline lung and air-filled lung

mechanics. The equations derived are based on experimentally observed facts. It has purposely ignored a number of factors, which, if incorporated into equations, would have enabled to better fit the experimental data. Complicating these equations with any greater number of physiologically interpretable, but experimentally unknown, parameters would not be appropriate at present.

Acknowledgments. This work is supported by a grant from the MNiSW, Grant N51801732/1217.

References

[1] Gil, J., Weibel, E.R.: Morphological study of PV hysteresis in rat lungs fixed by vascular perfusion. Respir. Physiol. 15, 190–213 (1972)

[2] Klingele, T.G., Staub, N.C.: Alveolar shape changes with volume in isolated, air-filled lobes of cat lung. J. Appl. Physiol. 28, 411–414 (1980)

[3] Neergaard, K.: Neue Auffassungen über einen Grundbegriff der Atemmechanik. Die Retraktionskraft der Lunge, abhängig von der Oberflachenspannung in den Alveolen. Z. ges. Exp. Med. 66, 373–394 (1929)

[4] Scarpelli, E.M.: The surfactant system of the lung. In: Pa, L., Febiger (eds.), Philadelphia, pp. 19-40, 45–46, 139, 241–257 (1968)

[5] Gladson, M., Shah, D.O., Shinowara, G.Y.: Isolation and characterization of a long lipoprotein surfactant. J. Coll. Interface Sci. 29, 319–333

[6] Blank, M., Goldstein, A., Lee, B.: The surface properties of lung extract. J. Coll. Interface Sci. 29, 148–154

[7] Brown, E.S.: Chemical identification of a pulmonary surface-active agent. J. Coll. Interface Sci. 21, 438–442

[8] Lempert, J., Macklam, P.T.: Effect of temperature on rabbit lung surfactant and pressure-volume hysteresis. J. Appl. Physiol. 31, 380–385 (1991)

[9] Krahl, V.E.: Anatomy of the mammalian lung. In: Fenn, W.O., Rahn, H. (eds.) Handbook of Physiology, section 3. Respiration, vol. I, pp. 267–298. Am. Physiol. Society, Washington (1995)

[10] Bull, H.B.: Protein structure and tissue elasticity. In: Remington, J.W. (ed.) Tissue elasticity, pp. 32–42. Am. Physiol. Soc., Washington (1997)

[11] Pierce, J.A.: The elastic tissue of the lung. In: Liebow, A.A., Smith, D.E. (eds.) The lung, pp. 45–46. Williams and Wilkins Co., Baltimore (1998)

[12] Dunnil, M.S.: Effect of lung inflation on alveolar surface area in the dog. Nature 214, 1031–1034 (1997)

[13] Anthonisen, N.R.: Effect of volume and volume history of the lungs on pulmonary shunt flow. Am. J. Physiol. 207, 235–238 (1999)

[14] Radford Jr., E.P.: Influence of physiochemical properties of the pulmonary surface on stability of alveolar air spaces and on static hysteresis of the lungs. In: XXII International Congress of Physiological Sciences, Symposia and Special Lectures, Leiden, vol. 1 (2002)

[15] Hills, B.A.: Effect of DPL at mercury/water interfaces and estimation of lung area. J. Appl. Physiol. 36, 41–44 (1984)

[16] Weibel, E.P.: Morphometrics. In: Fenn, W.O., Rahn, H. (eds.) Handbook of Physiology, Section 3. Respiration, vol. 2, pp. 288–290. Am. Physiol. Society, Washington (1965)

[17] Macklin, D.C., Hartroft, W.S.: Report on the sizes of pulmonary alveoli. In: Mimeograph Doc., Sub-Committee on Physiological Aspects of Chemical Warfare, pp. 156–169. Medical School Univ. Western Ontario, Canada (1983)

[18] Frazer, R.D., Suzuki, E.: Biological application. In: Blackburn, J.D. (ed.) Spectral analysis: methods and techniques, pp. 183–199. Marcel Dekker, Inc., New York (1990)

[19] Lempert, J., Macklam, P.T.: Effect of temperature on rabbit lung surfactant and pressure-volume hysteresis. J. Appl. Physiol. 31, 380–385 (1998)

[20] Bachofen, H.J., Hildebrandt, J.: Pressure-volume curves of air- and liquid filled excised lung-surface tension in situ. J. Appl. Physiol. 29, 422–430 (1998)

Comparison of Several Centreline Extraction Algorithms for Virtual Colonoscopy

Marcin Janaszewski[1,2], Michał Postolski[1], Laurent Babout[2], and Edward Kącki[1]

[1] Department of Expert Systems and Artificial Intelligence, The College of Computer Science in Lodz, Poland
[2] Department of Computer Engineering, Technical University of Lodz, Poland
janasz@kis.p.lodz.pl, postol@wsinf.edu.pl,
lbabout@kis.p.lodz.pl, e25kacki@cosmosnet.pl

Abstract. In the paper, authors report on test of three skeletonization algorithms, which could be used as centreline generators for 3D colon images. Two of them belong to the topological thinning group of skeletonization algorithms and the last one to the distance mapping group. After adaptation to centreline generation task the algorithms were tested on a real 3D colon image and obtained results are reported along with the characteristics of each algorithm performance. What is more the authors have made some improvements to the algorithms in order to obtain better results. The improved algorithms were also tested and results are reported. Moreover the paper contains comparison of the new algorithms with their original counterparts. Final discussion and presentation of future works are also included in the paper.

Keywords: Skeletonization, virtual colonoscopy, thinning algorithm, subiteration algorithm, voxel coding, centreline extraction.

1 Introduction

Visual endoscopy uses medical imaging, computer graphics and image processing technologies to examine the interior structures of human organs [3, 6]. The technique is superior to the traditional fiberoptic endoscopy because of its non-invasivity, cost-effectiveness and high accuracy. Moreover it is free of risk and side effects like perforation or infection and can be applied for some special organs which are impossible to inspect using a traditional endoscopy (e.g. blood vessels). Therefore, many prototype systems have been developed for a variety of clinical applications, including virtual colonoscopy (VC) [7], virtual bronchoscopy [13], virtual angioscopy [2].

VC procedure is quite complicated. Firstly the system takes computed tomography scan of a patient's abdomen. As a result doctors obtain several hundred high-resolution slice images, which are quickly taken during a single breath hold, forming a volumetric abdomen dataset. Then, using image segmentation algorithms, the entire colon is extracted from the abdomen dataset. After that, the colon centreline is extracted using 3D image processing algorithms. Intuitionally, centreline is a curve which goes through the centre of an organ. Then the system is ready to perform real time navigation based on volume rendering on a personal computer. The inspection

E. Kącki, M. Rudnicki, J. Stempczyńska (Eds.): Computers in Medical Activity, AISC 65, pp. 241–254.
springerlink.com

can be realized in an automatic manner, following the centreline or by interactive navigation for more accurate study of suspicious areas. A crucial component of a VC system is the extraction of the centreline. It plays several roles from providing compact colon shape description and accurate colon geometry measurement to supporting path generation for both interactive and automatic navigations. The centreline generation has been a challenging problem due to the colon complexity, presence of distortion in 3D colon images and several postulates which a centreline should meet. Therefore many centreline extraction algorithms have been developed for the last 2 decades. Most of them are derived from skeletonization algorithms because a centreline can be treated as a part of a skeleton. Unfortunately, despite of several decades of research in this field, there is not a centreline generation algorithm which is superior to all others and generates centrelines which meet all desired postulates. The literature analysis leads to the conclusion that despite of the fact that many useful algorithms have been constructed there is still the possibility to build new, faster and more accurate centreline generators e.g. algorithms which incorporate the best properties of several existing solutions. What is more, there are some skeletonization algorithms which have not been extensively tested on 3D colon images. Therefore we attempt to test three skeletonization algorithms, presented in [10, 12, 14] respectively, which application to centreline generation for VC has not been widely reported and discussed in the literature.

2 Basic Concepts of 3D Volumetric Images

Basic concepts of a volumetric image and volumetric image processing were presented in detail elsewhere e.g. [14]. In this subsection only the notions necessary to understand the following parts of the paper are introduced.

The 3D crack images are 3D binary volume data sets. A 3D binary volume set consists of voxels – the smallest unit cube in the volume. Each voxel is described by a quadruple (x, y, z, v) where (x, y, z) represents 3D location of the voxel and value v indicates its membership. $v = 0$ means that a voxel belongs to a background, $v = 1$ indicating that a voxel belongs to an object (in our case the entire of a colon). Treating a voxel as a unit cube results in three kinds of voxel neighbourhood. Following the same notations in [14], for a voxel p a voxel q is called a *F-neighbour, E-neighbour*, or *V-neighbour*, of p if it shares a face, an edge or a vertex, respectively, with voxel p. Voxels p and q are also called *F-connected, E-connected, V-connected.* Two voxels are *adjacent* or *neighbours* if they are at least V-connected. If a voxel within an object has a background voxel as a neighbour, it is considered as an *inside voxel* otherwise it is called a *boundary voxel.* A background voxel is called an *outside voxel* if all its neighbours are background voxels; otherwise it is regarded as a boundary voxel. A sequence of voxels $p_1, p_2,...,p_n$ is called a *voxel path* if it fulfils the following condition: p_i is adjacent to p_j if and only if $|i - j| = 1$, for $i, j = 1, 2...,n$ and $i \neq j$.

A set of voxels is *connected* if, for any two voxels within it, there is a path within the set connecting them. Two sets of voxels A, B are *connected* or *adjacent* if there are at least two voxels, one within set A and the other one within set B, which are neighbours.

3 Centreline Characteristics

Informally, a centreline can be defined as a curve which passes through the centre of an object interior. Some objects like colon have only one centreline but there are complicated objects with many branches like blood vessels, human lungs, cracks in materials and many others.

The notion of a centreline for any object O was introduced by Blum [1] who defined it as a result of *medial axis transformation*. According to the definition an object voxel p belongs to a centreline if and only if there is a ball $B(p) \subset O$ centred at a voxel p such that there is not any other ball $B \subset O$ which includes $B(p)$. The centreline extraction and evaluation based on Blum's definition is very difficult and time consuming therefore many authors e.g. [3, 6, 8, 14] usually define a centreline as a curve which meets the following conditions:

1. *Connectivity* – a centreline must be a voxel path according with the definition presented in the previous chapter.
2. *Centricity* – a centreline should traverse a centre of an object interior. The postulate guarantee that a centreline is not only a descriptor of an object centre but also is a safe path for colon navigation preventing a navigator from hugging a colon walls on sharp bends.
3. *Singularity* – centreline should be one wide smooth curve without any self-intersections and folds. More formal a centreline should be a voxel path.
4. *Topology preserving* – there are various definitions of topology preserving e.g. [4, 11]. Two objects have the same topology if they have the same number of connected components, holes, and cavities. The model colon dataset should consist of one object without any holes and branches. Nevertheless, in real situations narrow bowel can collapse or by twisting various colon parts can touch each other resulting in holes, branches or even separation a colon into several objects. Therefore the centreline generation algorithm should detect disconnected colon segments, branches and holes. In case of several segments the algorithm should extract centreline for each segment. In case of a hole the classical skeletonization algorithms generate a loop which consists of two connected branches, but one of the branches is false because it traverses the two walls touching area. Therefore an algorithm should detect and discard such a branch.
5. *Parameterisation* – along with a set of centreline voxels an algorithm should result with a centreline structure description. It means that the main centreline and its branches should be parameterised by their starting voxel, ending voxel and length. Such a parameterisation simplify further processing like refinement, hole detection or pruning unnecessary branches.
6. *Robustness* – the algorithm should not be sensitive to little changes in an object structure or geometric transformations such as translation or rotation. What is more extracted centreline should not fluctuate according to changes of starting and ending voxel.
7. *Automation* – The algorithm should extract a centreline fully automatically without user interaction. It concerns especially automatic determination of a colon starting and ending voxel.

8. *Cost effectiveness* – For large and complicated data computational time and memory utilisation are critical. Therefore algorithms should be fast enough to extract a centreline for complicated colon data in seconds on standard PC computer.

4 Characteristics of Virtual Colonoscopy Algorithms

In the last several decades many centreline extraction algorithms dedicated to VC have been constructed. Most of them derive from skeletonization algorithms which were refined to perform well for volumetric colon images. These algorithms can be divided into three groups:

1. *Manual extraction* – These methods require significant manual work of user who is responsible for marking a centre of a colon on each image slice of several hundreds in a dataset. Then the centreline is linearly interpolated between consecutive marked points. Unfortunately the method is time consuming, sometimes difficult to perform and does not guarantee the centricity of marked points because of possible human mistakes.
2. *Topological thinning* – these algorithms delete, on each iteration, so called simple points from the boundary of an object. A simple point is defined as an object point which deletion does not change the object topology. The process stops when no more simple points to deletion.
3. *Voxel coding based* - A voxel coding scheme is a voxel by voxel recursive propagation and assignment of integer codes to object voxels starting from a set of voxels which are called seeds. Most of these algorithms use a special voxel coding called the distance transform or an approximation of distance transform were the seed set consists of object boundary voxels. Such a distance transform results in an image called a distance field which has very useful property from centreline generation point of view. Its ridges correspond to the voxels that are local centres in the object. Based on the ridges various algorithms use various approaches to build the skeleton. Usually the set of ridges is pruned and then remaining voxels are connected in order to form one voxel wide connected centreline.

4.1 A Fully Parallel Thinning Algorithm

The first tested algorithm, developed by Ma and Sonka [5], belongs to the topological thinning group. In this section we present only general view of its way of working. The algorithm tests all border voxels on each iteration. Once a voxel is visited the algorithm checks if it meets at least one of a priori defined deleting constraints. If so the voxel is deleted. The process ends when it does not delete any voxel in the last iteration. Points which are not deleted during the process form the final skeleton. Ma and Sonka's algorithm is based on the fully parallel strategy which uses a set of predefined deleting templates to test neighbourhood of each border voxel. When a voxel and its neighbourhood match at least one template then the voxel is marked to be deleted. After examination of all border voxels the marked ones are deleted by changing their values to 0.

Deleting templates are represented as cubic grids with three types of points (see Figure 1). An object point and a background point are denoted with "•", and "o"

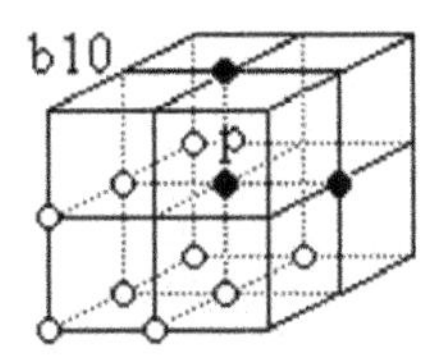

Fig. 1. One of deleting templates [12]

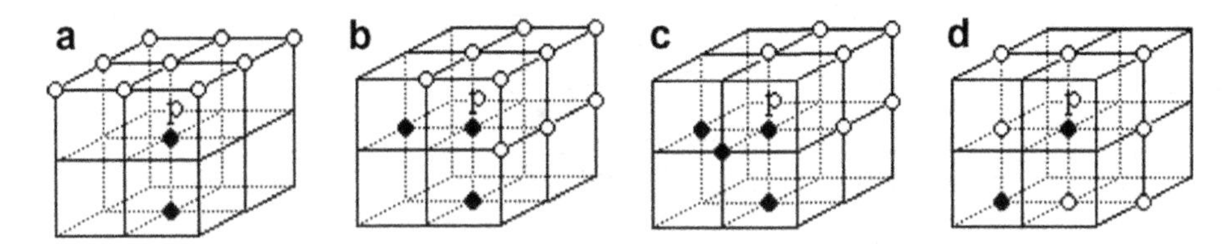

Fig. 2. Four template cores. Class A, B , C and D [12]

respectively. A "don't care point", which means that it can be either object point or background point, is unmarked. Ma and Sonka presented four classes of deleting templates (A, B, C and D). Figure 2 shows the four basic template cores. The translation of the cores results in deleting templates: six in class A, twelve in class B, eight in class C and twelve in class D [12]. We tested upgraded version of Ma and Sonka's algorithm [12]. It was proved that the original algorithm do not preserve connectivity in specific cases [12]. In new version of the algorithm 12 templates of class D were changed into new 32 ones. This change leads to the connectivity preserving algorithm. What is more in order to preserve topology the algorithm cannot delete so-called tail-points which are defined as line-end points or near-line-end points [12].

Taking into consideration all above the algorithm can be expressed as follows:

Repeat
    Mark every border point of an object
    Repeat
        Simultaneously delete every non tail-point which satisfies at least one deleting template from class A, B, C, or D;
    Until no point can be deleted;
    Release all marked but not deleted points;
Until no marked point can be deleted;

4.2 12-Subiteration Thinning Algorithm

The next algorithm which we have tested follows different thinning strategy than the first one. Detailed presentation of the strategy has been published in [9] by Palagyi. In this type of thinning strategy each iteration of a thinning process is divided into subiterations. Common subiteration algorithms use three or six subiterations, however Palagyi proposed an approach which uses twelve subiterations. In each subiteration the algorithm can use different deleting conditions. This is the main difference compared to fully parallel strategy where the thinning process uses global and predefined

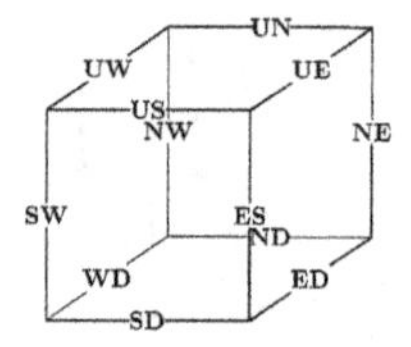

Fig. 3. 12 direction proposed by Palagyi [9]

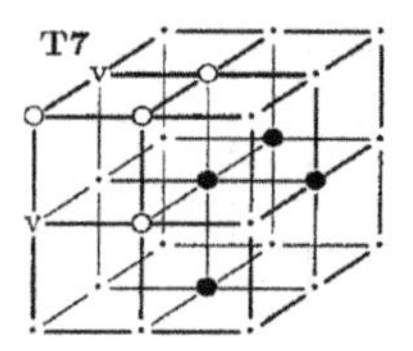

Fig. 4. One of 14 deleting templates assigned to the first subiteration in US direction [9]

delete constraints. Palagyi's algorithm uses subiterations in order to test only specific set of voxels. These sets of voxels are determined with rules called directions. Figure 3 shows twelve directions proposed by Palagyi. Each object boundary voxel in an actual direction can be tested using predefined, for this Subiteration, deleting templates. Palagyi defined 14 deleting templates which are final templates used to test voxels in US direction [9] (see figure 3). Other direction templates are formed by translation of the final US templates using rotation or reflection according to the actual direction rules. Deleting templates can be presented in similar way to Ma and Sonka ones. That is, black dots correspond to object points while white dots represent background points. Other points in template can be both object or background voxels. When all voxels which match deleting templates are marked, the algorithm deletes them and continues to the next subiteration. The algorithm stops if there is no marked voxel for deletion in each subiteration. In that case undeleted voxels form a final skeleton.

A corresponding subiteration based algorithm can be expressed as follows:

Repeat
  For $i = 1$ *to* 12 *do*
    Mark border points which match the deleting templates predefined for *i-th* direction.
  Delete all marked points
Until no point for deletion in each direction remains

4.3 Voxel Coding Algorithm

The algorithm presented here is complicated and its decryption in details exceeds the article size limitation. Therefore we are going to give only general view of the method. Interesting readers are requested to refer to [14]. The algorithm consists of two steps:

1. Initial skeleton generation
2. Refinement

The first step results in initial skeleton and utilizes a voxel coding scheme – a procedure similar to a discrete minimum distance transform. It uses the coding scheme "n_f-n_e-n_v" ("n_e-n_v" for 2D images) which is described with three integer values greater than 0: n_f, n_e, n_v, ($n_f < n_e < n_v$). First, all the object O voxels are initialized with a code (value) of infinity. Than the propagation starts from seed voxels which are given code 0. Then all the seed F-neighbours, E-neighbours, V-neighbours within an object are given a code of n_f, n_e, n_v, respectively. In the ith iteration, all neighbours of voxels which have been assigned with a code value during the ith -1 iteration are processed. Assume that voxel p is assigned with a value of n for the ith-1 iteration. Thus for the ith iteration all its F-neighbours, E-neighbours, V-neighbours within an object are assigned with value $n + n_f$, $n + n_e$, $n + n_v$, respectively, provided that the new code values are lower than the actual ones (i.e. an infinity value replaced by a code 2, or a code 4 replaced by a code 2). This method prevents voxels coded during an iteration from being coded again in the following one. This coding procedure stops when there is not any voxel to process in the next iteration or the constraint conditions are fulfilled (e.g. a particular voxel is met). The voxel coding procedure applied to 3D (2D) image results in an 3D (2D) image respectively which is called voxel field.

The skeletonization algorithm described in this section utilizes two types of voxel codings:

1. *BS-coding* which uses object boundary voxels as a set of seeds and the generated field is called *BS-field.*
2. *SS-coding* which uses a seed set which consists of only one specific object voxel called *reference point* (RP). The coding results in a field called *SS-field.*

BS-field is utilized to obtain cantered skeleton while SS-field provides useful information about object connectivity and topology. The next step consists in SS-field transformation to a collection of clusters. A *cluster* is defined as a set of connected object's voxels of the same SS-code; the SS-code is called the *cluster code.* Therefore a cluster can be considered as a connected set of object voxels which belong to the intersection between the object a sphere with center RP and radius equal to the cluster code. During initial skeleton generation one voxel of the highest BS-code is choosen from each cluster to form a centreline. Such a voxel is called *medial point.*

Unfortunately the initial skeleton comprised of medial points, lacks of connectivity therefore the second step - sophisticated refinement, which consists of three steps is utilised. The goal of the refinement first step is to restore connectivity inside branches of the skeleton. Unfortunately the side effects of the first step are folds, branch self-intersections and thick branch fragments. Therefore the second step which smoothes the skeleton has to be applied. Unfortunately the initial skeleton generation procedure gives only information which skeleton branches should be connected but does not connect them. Therefore the third step of refinement is performed which connects extracted branches.

5 Discussion of the Original Algorithm Test Results

The chapter presents test results of the above described algorithms. Moreover it contains the discussion of the algorithms properties concluded from the results. All tests have been performed, with the use of a real human colon image with size 204x132x260 voxels, on standard PC platform computer with Pentium dual core 2GHz processor.

The results are presented in figure 5. Although, FPA produces smooth and traversing a centre of a colon centreline, it also generates some unnecessary branches, loops and flat, one voxel wide surfaces (see figure 5 a). The branches are the result of the algorithm sensitivity to the object shape. The loops are the result of small holes which occur in the colon data because sometimes a colon is so twisted that walls of its two different parts touch each other. In the case a centreline extraction algorithm should not generate a path through the contact area of walls. The last problem (flat surfaces) is the results of inadequate set of deleting templates. If object is thin and flat or in

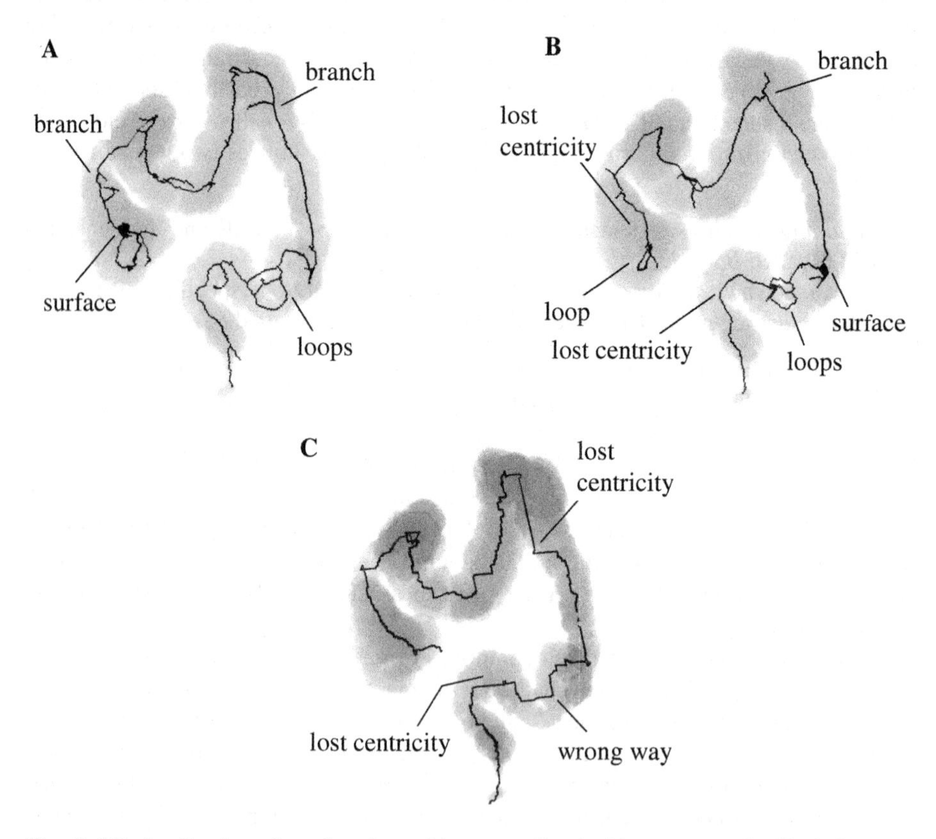

Fig. 5. 3D visualisation of a colon data with a centreline inside represented with dark curve. There are also some special areas indicated which show the interested centreline features. a) Centreline generated with FPA, b) Centreline generated with TSA c) Centreline generated with VCA.

previous iteration the algorithm generated one voxel thin surfaces than proposed deleting templates do not work properly. In such cases the remaining object voxels do not meet any deleting condition. Therefore the fully parallel algorithm needs significant refinement to produce acceptable centreline for VC.

TSA belongs to the same category of skeletonization algorithms but subiteration strategy produce more sharp and simple skeleton than FPA (see figure 5 b). Although, the algorithm is less sensitive to shape of an object and does not generate many branches and flat surfaces, it detects each hole and generates a loop around it. Therefore the algorithm also needs significant improvements in order to generate high quality centreline for VC.

The last tested algorithm generates the main skeletal path on the first separated step and then extracts its branches. Therefore it is very easy to remove unnecessary branches. It is only a matter to finish the algorithm after the main skeletal path is generated. The result of VC application is presented in the figure 5 c. Unfortunately, two significant drawback of the centreline can be noticed in figure 5 c; losing of centricity or even touching of the colon walls and passing of the colon wall contact areas. Unfortunately VCA also needs significant improvements but the type of improvements is totally different than in case of TSA and FPA.

Another important aspect of centreline generation algorithms for VC is computational cost which strongly depends not only on the size of an object but also on its shape. The fast centreline generation algorithm can lead to realisation of virtual colon examination immediately after CT scanning of a patient. Working times of tested algorithms for the image presented in figure 2 are included in the table 1. In case of thinning algorithms the time of working strongly depends on the amount of deleted voxels on each iteration. In some specific cases when an algorithm deletes only few voxels on each iteration, the computation time can be very long. FPA is usually faster than TSA. In our tests FPA has been almost 6 times faster than TSA (see table 1). Unfortunately, directional strategy applied in TSA results in the fact that TSA deletes less voxels on each iteration than FPA.

In case of VCA the time of working does not depend so strongly on the features of an object but for complicated objects, with many thin branches, generation of voxel field needs far more time than for simple objects. The most important problem which concerns VCA computational cost is extensive utilisation of connected component labelling procedure (CCL) - a bottleneck of many well known algorithms. The VCA uses CCL many times especially in refinement. This results in the fact that VCA is the slowest algorithm of all tested. Another reason for which VCA works slowly is the fact that the algorithm does not generates unordered set of discrete voxels which form a skeleton, (like PFA and TSA) but it extracts paths of voxels which represents main centreline and branches. Moreover the algorithm return information about structure of the skeleton like starting and ending voxel of each branch, pairs of branches which are connected, length of each branch and so on. The information is useful in further

Table 1. Times of working of tested algorithms represented in seconds. The algorithms were examined based on the real colon structure of size 204x132x260 presented in the figure 5.

Algorithm	FPA	TSA	VCA
Total time(sec):	3	17	600

processing of generated skeleton. The authors use it in implementation of the algorithm improvements.

6 Improvements of Tested Algorithms

The chapter presents the author original improvements of the algorithms presented and tested in the previous chapters. As it was shown in previous chapter, the tested original skeletonization algorithms do not generate acceptable centrelines when applied to a real human colon 3D image. Moreover the generated centrelines have serious drawbacks which lead to a conclusion that the algorithms need significant improvements.

In case of FPA and TSA the improvements have been implemented as post processing procedures which analyse skeletons generated by the original algorithms and refine them to obtain acceptable centrelines. Because these two algorithms generate skeletons represented in the same form with similar faults, the authors have implemented and applied one refinement procedure for both algorithms.

The implemented refinements extensively uses a procedure which extracts the *shortest path* (according with the definition of path presented in one of the previous chapters) within the object O, between two voxels p and q from O [14]. The procedure consists of two steps. First the *SSCode* with the q as a seed is extracted until the p voxel is reached. Then in the second step the path is generated starting from p. Assume that on the *i-th* iteration the v_i was added to the path, then on the next iteration the v_i's neighbour with the smallest SSCode is chosen as the next path voxel. The last point of the path must be q since the next point extraction is a code-decreasing process and q has the smallest code in the field.

The whole refinement procedure for FPA and TSA can be divided into three main steps:

1. The aim of the first step is to indicate two ending voxels of a centreline. In order to do so the algorithm generates *SSField* within the skeleton extracted by FPA or TSA, with the seed chosen randomly. The point $e_1$which has the highest SSCode is set as the one of two end points. Then the procedure is used once again starting from the e_1 voxel and the skeleton voxel of highest SSCode is meant to be the second end point e_2.
2. This step aim is to remove all unnecessary branches. To do so the procedure generates shortest path inside a skeleton from e_1 to e_2. The step results in clear unit wide centreline without any branches, surfaces and loops. Unfortunately, this path is wrong if some loops occur in the skeleton. Therefore the path has to be corrected in third step of our refinement procedure.
3. The last step of refinement analyses loops in order to discard false branches which go through the wall connection areas. Indeed, in each loop two paths can be indicated. The longer one which represents entire of a colon and the shorter one which is initially selected in the previous step and trespass the wall connection area. The procedure takes as an input initial skeleton S_{init} generated by FPA or TSA and centreline $C \subset S_{init}$ generated on the step 2 of the refinement. C is a path of voxels which can be represented with the following series: e_1, $v_0,...,v_k,...,e_2$. On the first

iteration the procedure deletes v_0 and attempts to generate the shortest path form e_1 to e_2 inside S_{init}. If the procedure cannot reach e_2, it means that v_0 cannot be deleted. Then the next voxel in C is deleted and the shortest path generation form e_1 to e_2 is performed. Assume that v_k is the first deleted voxel for which the algorithm is able to generate shortest path C_1 from e_1 to e_2 inside S_{init}. It means that there is a loop l in S_{init} which shorter branch b_s was broken by deletion of v_k. Thus C_1 contains longer branch of l which traverses interior of the colon as opposed from b_s which traverses the wall connection area. Therefore, better centreline C_1 replaces the worse C. On the next iteration voxel v_{k-1} from C_1 is deleted and the shortest path is generated form e_1 to e_2 inside S_{init}. The deletion of consecutive voxels and propagation of the shortest paths is repeated until e_2 is the next voxel to delete. The procedure results in the centreline C_{end} obtained in the last successful shortest path extraction. C_{end} does not contain any false branch which goes through a wall connection area.

The VCA improvements concern not only refinement procedure but also the core part. The one of the most serious drawback of the core part of the approach is lack of connectivity between consecutive centreline voxels which significantly complicates refinement. It is a result of the fact that two consecutive centreline voxels v_{i-1} and v_i are chosen from two neighbour clusters c_{i-1}, c_i respectively and have the highest BSCode in the clusters. Unfortunately, the procedure does not guarantee that v_{i-1} and v_i are neighbours. Conducted experiments showed that this lack of connectivity between consecutive voxels occurs very frequently. What is worse the distance between consecutive skeletal voxels very often is amounted to several tens voxels. Such initial skeletons are very difficult to refine and even refined, using original algorithm, do not meet most of the postulates presented in the centreline characteristics section.

Therefore we changed the strategy for choosing the next skeletal voxel. Assume that the voxel v_{i-1} from cluster c_{i-1} was added to the skeleton on the last iteration. Then on actual iteration from the neighbour cluster c_i of code one less than c_{i-1}*'s* the voxel v_i which has the highest BSCode is chosen. If distance between v_{i-1} and v_i is less than twenty then v_i becomes the next skeletal voxel. Otherwise the next skeletal point is the closest to v_{i-1}, local maximum of BSField which belongs to c_i. If there is not any local maximum of BSField among c_i voxels then v_i becomes the next skeletal point.

Another modification of VCA concerns refinement procedure which unfortunately is time consuming and does not give good results for complicated objects. Thus the three steps of VCA refinement procedure have been changed into one. The new refinement procedure for each two consecutive non neighbouring, skeletal voxels builds a voxel path which links these two voxels. Assume that on i-th iteration of the procedure voxel v_{i-1} was added to a linking path then on the i-th iteration the next voxel v_i is chosen based on the following formula:

$$F(v_i) = \min_{v \in N(v_{i-1})} F(v) \quad \text{and} \quad \mathrm{F(v_i) < F(v_{i-1})} \tag{1}$$

$$\text{where}: \ \forall v \in O: \quad F(v) = \frac{SSfield(v)}{BSfield(v)+1} \tag{2}$$

$$N(v_{i-1}) - \text{set of all neighbours of voxel } v_{i-1}$$

If there is no v from $N(v_{i-1})$ for which $F(v) < F(v_{i-1})$ than the voxel from $N(v_{i-1})$ with the minimum *SSCode* is added to the linking path.

Such a refinement procedure is faster than the original one and gives better results in performed tests (see the next section).

7 Test Results of Improved Algorithms

All improved algorithms have been tested on the same volumetric image as original ones. The results are presented in figure 6. Centrelines generated by improved

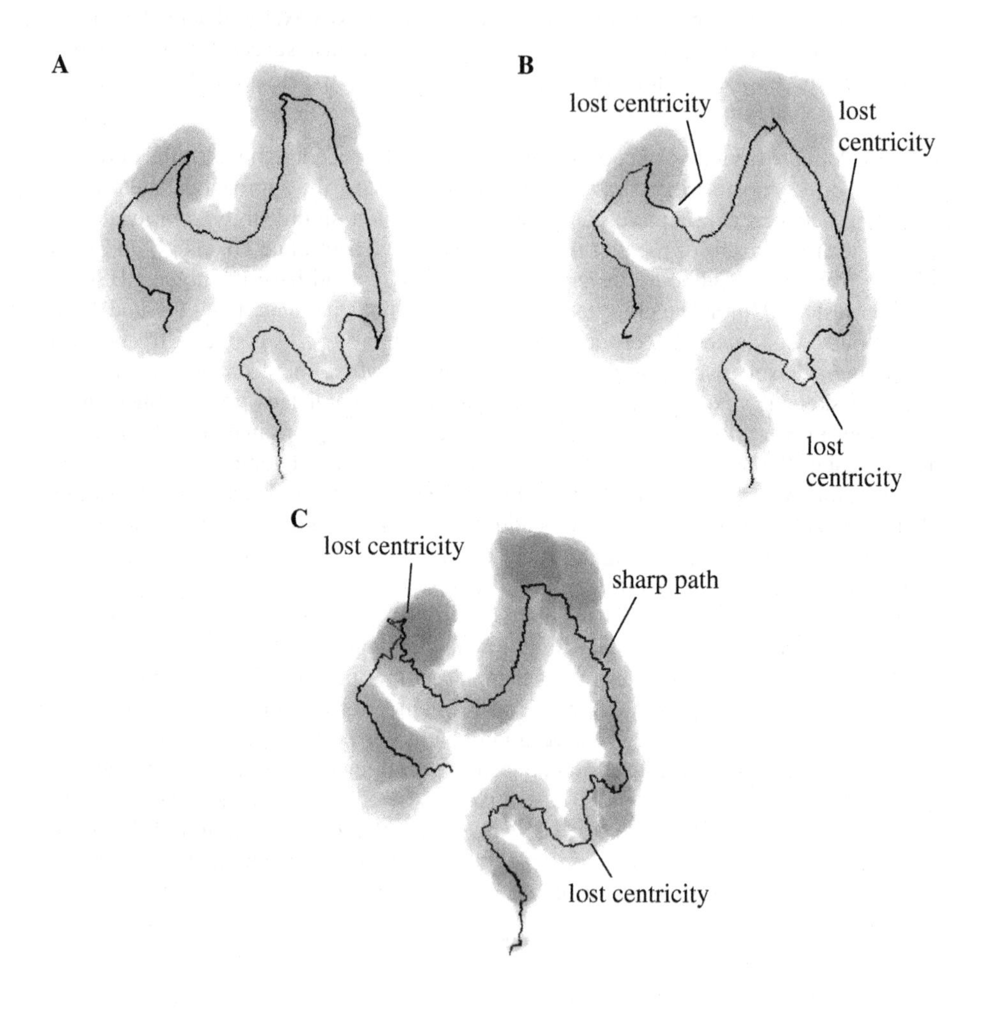

Fig. 6. 3D visualisation of a colon data with a centreline inside represented with dark curve and generated with improved versions of tested algorithms. There are also some special areas indicated which show the interested centreline features. a) Centreline generated with IFPA, b) Centreline generated with ITSA c) Centreline generated with IVCA.

Table 2. Times of working of improved versions of tested algorithms represented in seconds. The algorithms were examined based on the real colon structure of size 204x132x260 presented in the figure 6.

	IFPT	ITSA	IVCA
Total time(sec):	20	35	200

algorithms are definitely better than centrelines generated by their original equivalents. They do not have any branches and loops. What is more, in case of a hole, improved algorithms reject false branch and leave the proper one which traverses the real bulk of the colon. Unfortunately, centrelines generated by improved TSA (ITSA) and improved VCA (IVCA) still suffer from approaching the colon walls especially near holes. What is more centreline extracted with IVCA is not as smooth as others. It is the result of refinement procedure applied in the algorithm which does not guarantee centricity of restored parts of the centreline. Therefore in some areas centreline voxels oscillate around the centre of the colon.

The time of working of improved algorithms applied to the colon image presented in figure 6 are reported in table 2. Comparison of results obtained for improved algorithms and their original equivalents show that refinement procedures significantly extend working time of FPT and TSA. Interesting results were obtained for IVCA which is three times faster than VCA. It is a result of changing refinement procedure to faster one which do not use connected component labelling algorithm. The new refinement procedure is not only faster but also results in better centreline. In spite of significant acceleration, IVCA is still the slowest algorithm of all tested.

8 Conclusions

In this article three skeletonization algorithms applied to VC were compared. Unfortunately, preliminary examinations showed that original algorithms generate centrelines with many loops and branches. What is more in some areas centrelines are represented by one voxel wide surfaces and have tendency to approach walls of a colon on sharp bends. Therefore the authors have made some improvements to tested algorithms based on their own conceptions. As the result the improved algorithms generate one voxel wide centrelines without any loops and unnecessary branches. The only problem which has not been completely eliminated is local loosing of centricity, in case of centrelines generated with ITSA and IVCA. Finally the best of the tested algorithms is IFPT because it generates centrelines which meet the most postulates in comparison with centrelines generated by other tested algorithms and is fast enough to work on standard PC computer. Unfortunately very promising VCA algorithm has not met the authors' expectations, who have faced a lot of problems with its improvements. The reason for the fact is the wrong assumption that generated clusters approximately represent consecutive cross-sections of the object perpendicular to its centreline which is a basis of the method. The authors have found out that clusters generated on sharp bends of the colon are far away from such cros-sections and are the source of insufficient centreline voxels.

In the future the authors plan to compare more centreline generation methods and made some improvements if necessary to obtain centrelines which meet all postulates presented in the third chapter about centreline characteristic.

References

1. Blum, H.: Transformation for Extracting New Descriptions of Shape. In: Dunn, W. (ed.) Models for the Perception of Speech and Visual Form, pp. 362–380. MIT Press, Cambridge (1967)
2. Do Yeon, K., Jong Won, P.: Virtual Angioscopy for Diagnosis of Carotid Artery Stenosis. Journal of KISS: Software and Applications 30, 821–828 (2003)
3. Guangxiang, J., Lixu, G.: An Automatic and Fast Centreline Extraction Algorithm for Virtual Colonoscopy. In: 27th Annual International Conference of the IEEE Engineering in Medicine and Biology Society, Shanghai, China (2006)
4. Kong, T.Y., Rosenfeld, A.: Digital Topology: Introduction and Survey. Computer Vision, Graphics, and Image Processing 48, 357–393 (1989)
5. Ma, C.M., Sonka, M.: A Fully Parallel 3D Thinning Algorithm and Its Applications. Computer Vision and Image Understanding 64, 420–433 (1996)
6. Ming, W., Zhengrong, L., Qi, K., Lichan, H., Bitter, I., Kaufman, A.: Automatic Centerline Extraction for Virtual Colonoscopy. IEEE Transaction on Medical Imaging 21, 1450–1460 (2002)
7. Nain, D., Haker, S., Kikinis, R., Grimson, E.L.: An Interactive Virtual Endoscopy Tool. In: Satellite Workshop at the Fourth International Conference on Medical Image Computing and Computer-Assisted Intervention (2001)
8. Palagyi, K.: A 3-Subiteration 3D Thinning Algorithm For Extracting Medial Surfaces. Pattern Recognition Letters 23, 663–675 (2002)
9. Palagyi, K., Kuba, A.: A Parallel 3D 12-Subiteration Thinning Algorithm. Graphical Models and Image Processing 61, 199–221 (1999)
10. Palagyi, K., Kuba, A.: A Parallel 12-Subiteration 3D Thinning Algorithm to Extract Medial Lines. In: 7th Computer Analysis of Images and Patterns, pp. 400–407 (1997)
11. Saha, P.K., Chaudhuri, B.B.: 3D Digital Topology Under Binary Transformation with Applications. Computer Vision and Image Understanding 63, 418–429 (1996)
12. Wang, T., Basu, A.: A Note on a Fully Parallel 3D Thinning Algorithm and Its Applications. Pattern Recognition Letters 28, 501–506 (2007)
13. Wegenkittl, R., Vilanova, A., Hegedust, B., Wagner, D., Freund, M.C., Groller, E.M.: Mastering Interactive Virtual Bronchioscopy on a Low-End PC. In: Proceedings Visualization 2000, Salt Lake City, USA, pp. 461–464 (2000)
14. Zhou, Y., Toga, A.W.: Efficient Skeletonization of Volumetric Object. IEEE Transactions on Visualization and Computer Graphics 5, 196–209 (1999)

"Algorithm for Treelike Structures Generation"

Anna Romanowska-Pawliczek[1,2,3], Piotr Pawliczek[3], and Zbigniew Sołtys[1]

[1] Department of Neuroanatomy, Institute of Zoology, Jagiellonian University
[2] Department of Industrial Computer Science, AGH University of Science and Technology
[3] Department of Computer Science, AGH University of Science and Technology

Abstract. Treelike structures are very common in nature. They are defined as structures which bifurcate but do not form any cycles. Apart from trees examples of such structure are neurons, snow flakes, river deltas, bronchial trees, corals, cardiovascular systems and many more. One of the aims of mathematical modeling of the natural systems is establishment of effective description and generation methods of treelike structures. In the midst of such methods Diffusion Limited Aggregation, L-systems as well as heuristics dedicated to certain issues produce desired results. A great deal of treelike structures reveals self-similarity features that indicates possibility of fractal geometry utilization in order to their description.

In a number of cases treelike structure generalization method is based on a recurrent algorithm. Structures generated according to this approach usually show fractal features, therefore it leads to question if living systems are generated recurrently. Concerning living systems relatively inconsiderable amount of genetic information gives rise to highly sophisticated structures creation. It could be suspected that recurrent mechanisms are crucial in the growth process of complex organic structures.

Keywords: L-system, DLA, fractals, treelike structure.

1 Natural Examples of Treelike Structures

Numerous natural objects have a treelike structure. Such structures are clearly prevalent among plants. They are widespread also in the animal world. Quite frequently arborescent organization is characteristic for visceral systems. Corals, mosses, lichens, shrubs, branches of a tree, root systems, mammalian tracheobronchial airways, cells of the nervous system, veins and arteries forming cardiovascular system are complicated branching systems. Despite the ubiquity of such forms evolution of branching patterns and the way they are being formed remain uncertain.

The treelike figures are also encountered in inanimate objects. An example of a physical deposition pattern is the air that displaces a high-viscosity fluid between two glass plates forming a viscous-fingering pattern. Treelike branching form is observable in lightning flashes and in electrical spark.

Many marine sessile organisms can be characterized as arborescent moreover modular organisms. Modular organisms are typically built of repeated units, the modules, which might be a polyp in a coral colony or a frond in seaweeds. In many cases

E. Kącki, M. Rudnicki, J. Stempczyńska (Eds.): Computers in Medical Activity, AISC 65, pp. 255–263.
springerlink.com

the growth process in modular organisms leads to complex shapes. In literature these forms are only described in qualitative and rather vague terms, such as "thinly branching", "tree-shaped" and "irregularly branching" [Kaandorp].

Self-similarity is the property of having a substructure analogous or identical to an overall structure. For example, a part of a line segment is itself a line segment, and thus a line segment exhibits self-similarity. Fractals such as the Sierpinski triangle are self-similar to an arbitrary level of magnification. Biological structures are self-similar to some degree. This self-similarity is rather statistical. In bryozoans, the tendency toward consistency results in a kind of self-similarity different from that in trees. Rather than being a miniature, a distal piece of a bryozoan is more or less a close representation of the whole branching structure at a less-developed stage of growth [Cheetham].

Forms generated using Diffusion Limited Aggregation algorithm (DLA) are excellent examples of the self-similar structures. Growth pattern of a colony of the bacteria *Paenibacillus dendritiformis* remarkably resembles the DLA fashion [see following context].

Ubiquity of such forms in completely different natural objects implies some kind of essential principles conditioning formation of treelike structures.

Considering living organisms at first we have to analyze the mechanisms responsible for generation of particular treelike structures. Moreover, unlike inanimate matter it has to be acknowledged that organisms undergo evolution. Thus natural selection is an additional factor in charge of prevalence of such structures in nature. In this paper we focus on neurons and glial cells.

Comparative study of the morphology and growth process of arborescent animals and plants can yield insights into their structural organization, mechanical design and its adaptive and evolutionary significance. Detailed comparison of arborescent organisms requires a set of parameters which would allow describing completely the branching structure.

Treelike structures ramify without forming any cycles [Figure 1.a]. There is only one path along the structure between any two points. According to the mathematical graph theory these structures may be generalized as tree diagram in which lines branch out from a central point or stem without forming any closed loops. Ramification points and segments designate diagrams` nodes and edges respectively [Figure 1.b].

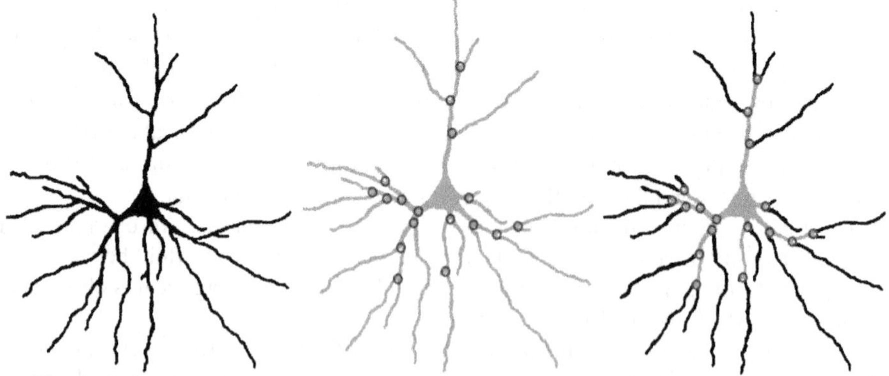

Fig. 1. a). Outline of a treelike structure b). manifesting nodes and c). terminal segments.

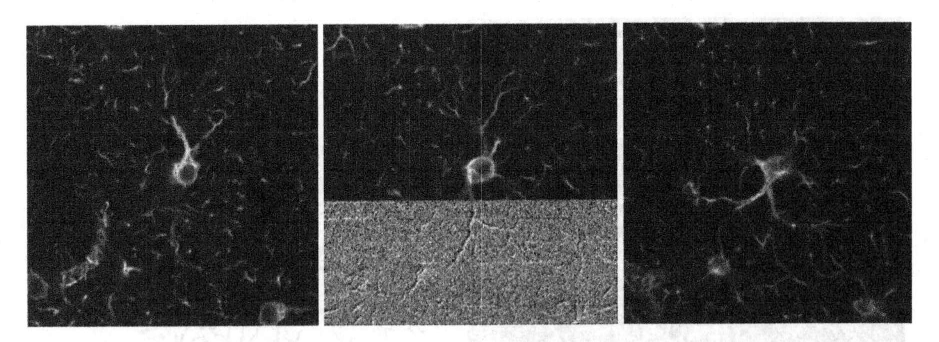

Fig. 2. Images of the same glial cell at different focus planes

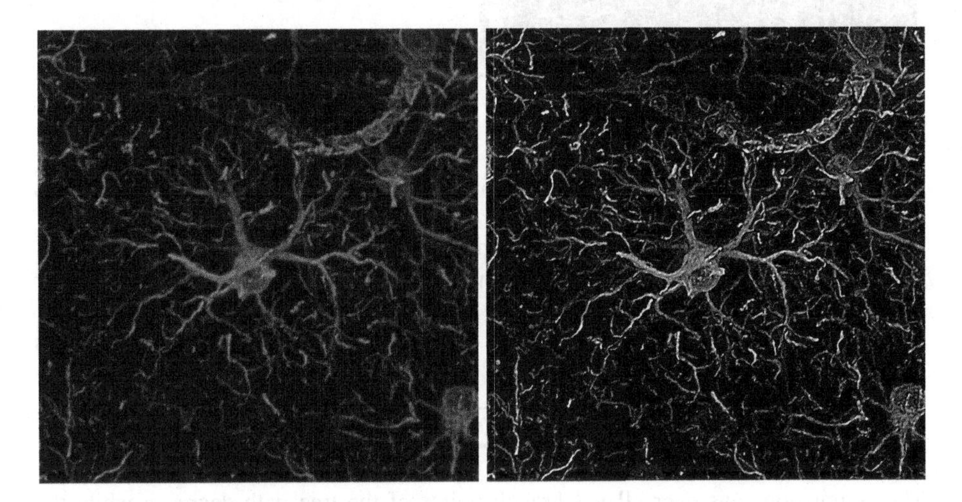

Fig. 3. Raw projection from 47 slices **Fig. 4.** After filtering

In order to verify simulation models a morphological comparison between actual and simulated forms is essential. We present briefly a number of methods suitable for the quantitative morphological comparison of branching forms. Nevertheless, there is no unequivocal way to choose the best quantitative descriptor of neural geometry or topology.

Reconstruction of 3D morphology is a complex and time-consuming task. Sophisticated microscopic equipment and multilevel image processing are required for biological object reconstruction [Figure 2, 3, 4, 5 and 6]. Confocal microscopes and technical software such as Neurolucida and ImageJ are very helpful.

Later on these reconstructed and digitalized structures can be used for verification of algorithms generating treelike structures.

Segments stretching between bifurcations are called intermediate segments. Tips of the structure, meaning branches without ramifications, are called terminal segments [Picture 1.c]. Number of segments may be reckoned as another parameter; *IntSN* – intermediate segment number and *TerSN* – terminal segment number. Number of

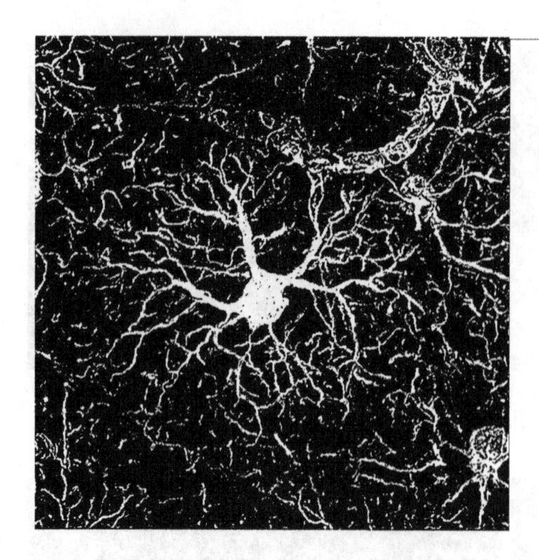

Fig. 5. Preliminary thresholding

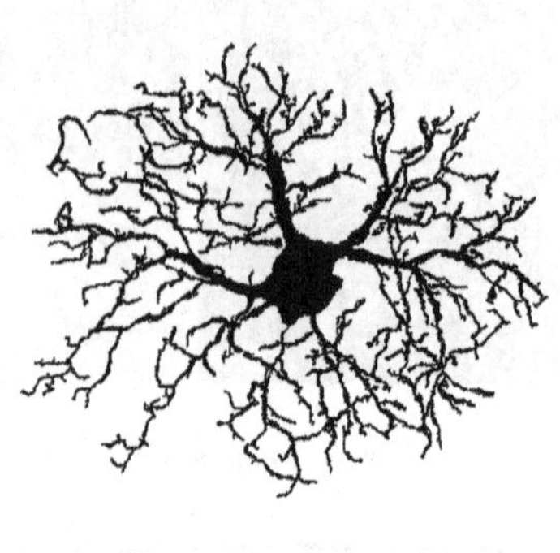

Fig. 6. Final binary image

terminal segments is always greater by one than number of intermediate segments while considering a binary tree diagram. *TotSN* is the total segments number.

In such binary trees all ramifications are formed by two daughter branches: bifurcations. *AsInx* - asymmetry index, and *AvAng* - average angle may be counted for structures forming bifurcations exclusively.

Asymmetry Index *AsInx* is defined as the mean value of the asymmetry of its partitions (subtrees).

$$AsInx = \frac{1}{n-1} \sum AsInx_p(r_i, s_i)$$

The summation runs over all *n-1* branch points of the tree with degree *n* while the partition (r_i, s_i) denotes the degrees of both subtrees at branch point *i*, and $AsInx_p$ denotes the partition asymmetry

$$AsInx_p = \frac{|r-s|}{r+s-2} \quad \text{for } r + s > 2 \text{ and } AsInx_p(1, 1) = 0$$

The values of tree asymmetry range from zero, for perfectly symmetrical structures, to approaching one, for most asymmetrical forms [van Pelt].

The distance between two nodes can be considered as Euclidian distance *EucDs*, if measured along a straight line, or as a segment length, if measured along the structure: *IntSL* – intermediate segment length and *TerSL* – terminal segment length. Segment lengths added all together inform us about total lengths of the structure; *TotSL*. In order to reckon following nodes and state the height of a tree, the reference point has to be placed in the center of analyzed form. Parameter *MaxH* denotes supreme value calculated this way. Analogical value, with a reference point abandoned, refers to the longest path in the graph; *MaxP* – maximal path.

Ramification factor *RF* is the relation between the number of all the segments and value coding the highest branch in the structure

$$RF = \frac{TotSN}{MaxH}$$

Another mathematical description of purely branching networks is the Horton-Strahler branch ordering method. Branching networks are hierarchical structures because they do not form any closed cycles. The discussed method was first developed in the study of river networks by Horton. A later improvement by Strahler led to the methodology known as Horton-Strahler steam ordering. According to this method branches, branch cross-sections, numbers of branches, etc. have indices of significance assigned. The first step is to identify all terminal branches called "first order branch". After pruning new terminal branches appear; "second order". This new set of outer branches is being removed. The ordering process is iterated until all branch segments are labeled and a steam appears.

Since treelike structures are often characterized as self-similar therefore we use estimation of fractal dimension to describe their complexity [Romanowska-Pawliczek]. Generally, to calculate the fractal dimension (D) of any self-similar fractal the Box Counting Method could be used. By covering a structure with boxes [Figure 7] of length l_b the fractal dimension D_b is given by

$$D_b = -\lim_{l_b \to 0} \frac{\log N_b(l_b)}{\log(l_b)}$$

where $N_b(l_b)$ is number of boxes needed to completely cover the structure. D_b corresponds to the slope of the plot $logN_b(l_b)$ versus $logl_b$.

According to Sholl analysis the reference point is placed in the soma of neuron cell. Concentric circles are drawn through the dendritic field [Figure 8.a.]. The number of intersections within each circle is counted. The graph showing the relationship between the mean number of intersections per unit area falls off exponentially with

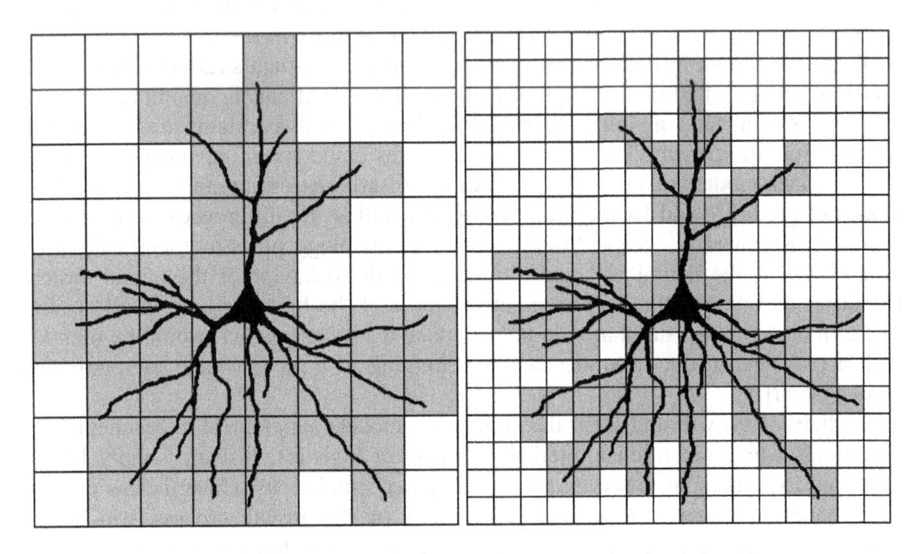

Fig. 7. Structure covered by boxes with decreasing box's length

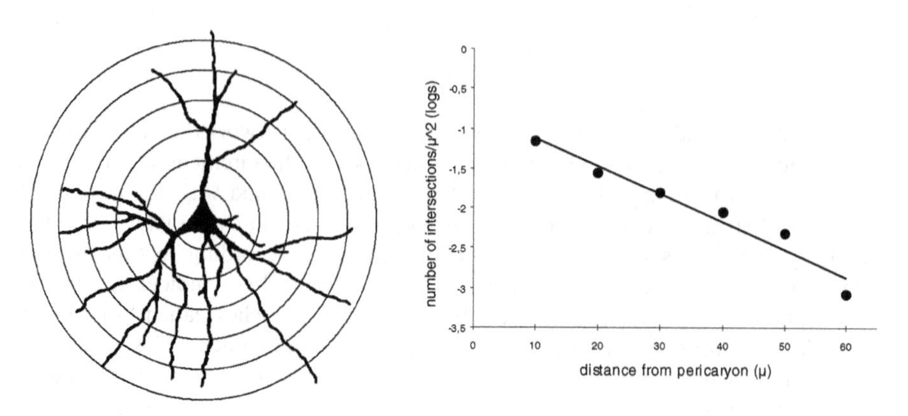

Fig. 8. a. Diagram of a cell with series of circles [Piechota]; b. Graph showing the relationship between the number of intersections/unit area and the distance from the pericaryon.

the distance. Plotting the logarithms of these numbers against the distance results in a linear relationship [Figure 567.b.].

The plotting line is fitted to the logarithmic form of $y = ae^{-kx}$, where a is a parameter of position and k of slope [Sholl].

When concerning a 3D structure concentric circles are replaced by spheres.

2 Simulation Purpose

One of the fundamental questions in biology is how the interplay between the genome and the physical environment controls morphogenesis. Recently there is a great interest in many branches of science to study in a quantitative way the geometrical description of structures, both static and in development, and from that knowledge to probe further into the functioning and justification of those forms.

There are certain inflictions for scientists dealing with such structures. It is necessary to elaborate effective description methods that would enable quantitative growth characterization, carrying out comparative analysis, as well as establishing methods of virtual structure growth. The simulated structures could be an advantageous device for computer models of growth and evolution of arborescent organisms. Underlying modes of growth could be important in understanding the differences in mechanical design. It is generally accepted that dendritic morphology plays a crucial role in the functioning of the neural cell and ultimately in the behavior of the neural system. Dendrites and axon collaterals account for most of the brain volume in all species. The aim of computer simulation is not to create a structure which would be identical with a real neuron but structure clearly belonging to a recognizable morphological class [Ascoli].

In study of growth and form the simulation models supplement experimental observations, which are often limited by expense or logistics. It could simply lead to replacing experimental observations by computer simulations. Nevertheless creating such models requires very specific information on the growth process, which is in general not available in the biological literature. Simulations not referring to the reality go nowhere.

3 How to Generate Virtual Treelike Structures

There are certain kinds of virtual neurons generation mechanisms derived throughout the years. L-systems seem to be an exceptionally effective solution. An L-system or Lindenmayer system is a formal grammar. It is based on a set of rules and symbols. The recursive nature of the L-system rules leads to self-similarity and thereby fractal-like forms which are easy to describe with an L-system [Prusinkiewicz]. Recurrence is an immanent feature of L-system's algorithms therefore it could be conjectured that substantial mechanisms designating embodied structures are similar.

L-Neuron, created by group of G. A. Ascoli, is a software package for the generation and study of anatomically accurate neuronal analogs. It is based on sets of recursive rules (L-systems). It also brings into play such laws like Rall's "power rule", Hillman's algorithm that calculates diameters and measures angles, Tamori's concept of "effective volume" and Burke's method of encoding the length of a branch in the probabilities to elongate or to bifurcate. L-Neuron is likewise equipped with an external directional "bias" on the angles, called tropism [Prusinkiewicz]. In L-systems tropism is used in aim to simulate the effect of gravity or wind in growing botanical trees. In L-Neuron, tropism responds to the effect of neurotrophic factors. It can be directional or centrifugal [Ascoli].

Another interesting method of treelike structure generation is a Diffusion Limited Aggregation (DLA). The growth form, the branching structure, is represented in this simulation by lattice sites in a square lattice. Growth of this object proceeds by releasing particles from a circle surrounding the cluster. The particles make a random walk

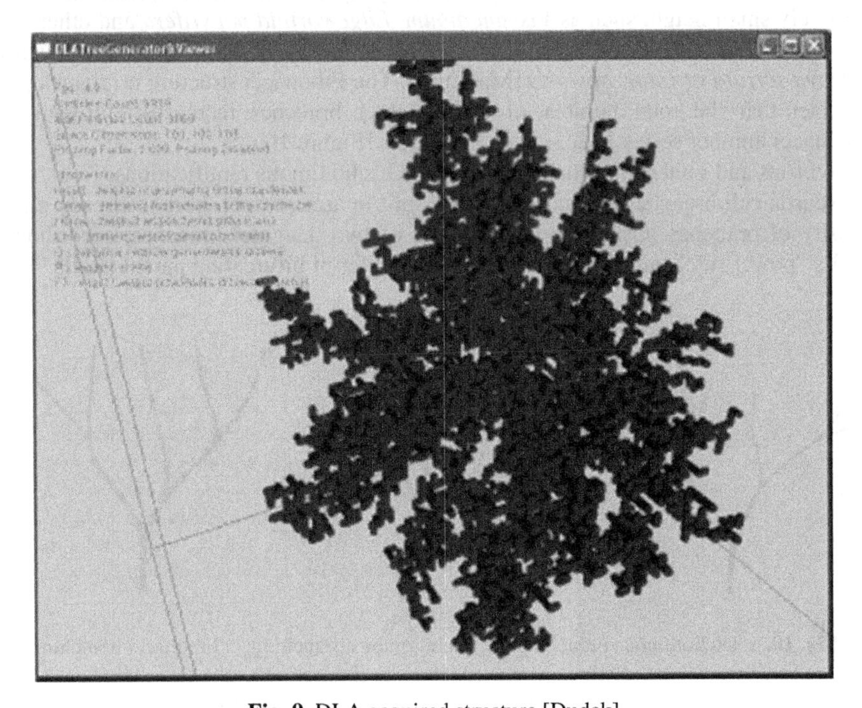

Fig. 9. DLA acquired structure [Dudek]

through the square lattice. The random walk stops as soon as a particle sticks to the growing structure [Peitgen]. The simulation of the growth process results in an irregular branching object [Figure 9]. It has been proved theoretically [Smailer] that in this not complicated growth process predicting the growth at a certain point in time is intractable. Therefore the only way to find growth at a certain point in time is by explicit simulation of every growth step. As far as L-systems are generally deterministic, Diffusion Limited Aggregation is stochastic from its assumption. In effect the growth form cannot be predicted analytically.

Models in general can be assigned to either diameter-dependent or branch order group [Ascoli, 2002]. Particular shape of the probability functions, the assignment of daughter diameters at bifurcations, and the determinations of the internal and terminal lengths are parameters that vary in different approaches.

Models are based on the empirical observations. In most growth processes the only way to predict growth forms in models is to simulate every growth step in the mathematical model. In many cases large-scale computing techniques will be needed in these simulations.

4 Growth Rules

In biological systems the branching is usually dichotomy [Figure 10.a] with rare occurrences of trichotomy [Figure 10.b] or polychotomy. Daughter segments can be equal or can vary in size [Yeh].

The dichotomous or trichotomous branching structure is found in plant trees with relatively small height such as *Viscum album*, *Edgeworthia papyrifera* and others. On the other hand, Fibonacci branching is found in relatively large erect trees such as *Zelcova serrata* or *Celtis sinensis* [Masahiro]. The Fibonacci structure originates from the fact that the total number of the daughter branches increases following the Fibonacci number series 1, 2, 3, 5, 8, 13, 21, etc [Figure 10.c].

Neurons and glial cells usually do not form trichotomous ramifications.

Neuron cell branches are more likely to split in areas where there is already a high density of branches [Carriquiry]. Diameters of two daughter branches, according to Rall's "power rule", are determined by the diameter of bifurcating parent [Rall].

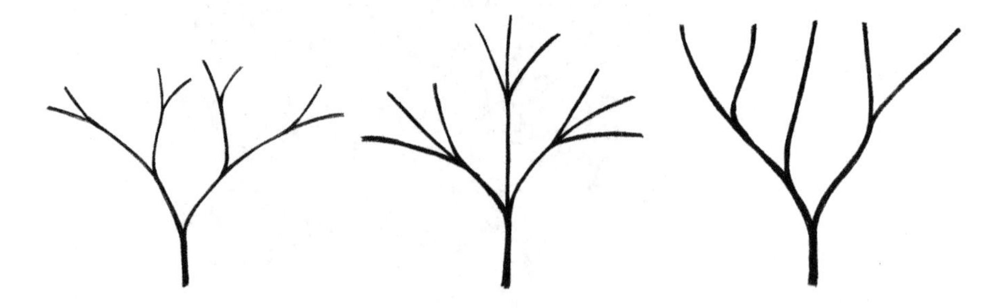

Fig. 10. a. Dichotomous branching, b. Trichotomous branching, c. Fibonacci branching.

5 Neuronal Shape Coherence

Neural geometry is the major factor that determines connectivity and, possibly, functional output from a nervous system [Acebes]. There are certain developmental constraints. Ultimate shape is an effect of joint action of two factors: genetic factors responsible for shape generation and factors of interaction with other cells that form a nervous system during its creation.

Neurons have ability to form expanded networks of synaptic junctions. It is a consequence of their treelike fashion which increases radically possibility of creation a connection.

Specifically, among other indicators, a decreased complexity in the dendritic trees of cortical pyramidal neurons has been associated with mental retardation [Barbosa].

AGH founds 11.11.110.728.

References

Acebes, A.: Cellular and molecular features of axon collaterals and dendrites. Trends Neurosci. 23, 557–565 (2000)

Ascoli, G.A.: Neuroanatomical algorithms for dendritic modelling (2002)

Ascoli, G.A., Krichmar, J.L.: L-neuron: A modeling tool for the efficient generation and parsimonious description of dendritic morphology (2000)

Barbosa, M.S., da Costa, L.F., Bernardes, E.S., Ramakers, G., van Pelt, J.: Characterizing neuromorphologic alterations with additive shape functionals (2007)

Cayal, S.R.: Textura del sistema nervioso del hombre y los vertebrados, pp. 1894–1904. Oxford University Press, Oxford, English translation by N. and L. W. Swanson

Carriquiry, A.L., Ireland, W.P., Kliemann, W., Uemura, E.: Statistical evaluation of dendritic growth models, pp. 579–589. Springer, New York (1991)

Cheetham, A.H., Hayek, L.C., Thomsen, E.: Branching Structure in Arborescent Animals: Models of Relative Growth (1980)

Dudek, Ł., Jaje, K., Basista, A., Romanowska-Pawliczek, A.: Zdecentralizowane Systemy Informacyjne. AGH University of Science and Technology (in progress)

Kaandorp, J.A., Kubler, J.E.: The Algorithmic Beauty of Seaweeds, Sponges, and Corals. Springer, Heidelberg (2001)

Agu, M., Yokoi, Y.: A stochastic description of branching structures of trees (1984)

Peitgen, H.-O., Jurgens, H., Saupe, D.: Granice Chaosu Fraktale (2002)

Piechota, M., Romanowska-Pawliczek, A., Sołtys, Z.: Analiza fraktalna w badaniu morfologii komórek tkanki nerwowej: metody i problemy, Episteme (2007)

Prusinkiewicz, P., Lindenmayer, A.: The Algorithmic Beauty of Plants. Springer, New York (1990)

Rall, W.: Branching dendritic trees and motoneurons membrane resistivity. Exp. Neurol. 1, 491–527 (1959)

Romanowska-Pawliczek, A., Piechota, M., Sołtys, Z.: Analiza fraktalna w badaniu morfologii komórek tkanki nerwowej: zastosowania, Episteme (2007)

Sholl, D.A.: Dendritic organization in the neurons of the visual and motor cortices of the cat (1953)

Smailer, I., Machta, J.: Exact enumeration of self-avoiding walks on lattices with random site energies. The American Physical Society (1993)

van Pelt, J., Schierwagen, A.: Morphological analysis and modeling of neuronal dendrites. Mathematical Biosciences, 147–155 (2004)

Yeh, H.C.: Modeling of biological tree structures (1979)

Computer System for Robust Evaluation of Medical Tests

Mariusz Klencki

Department of Morphometry of Endocrine Glands,
Chair of Endocrinology and Metabolic Diseases, Medical University of Lodz,
Sterling Str 5, 91-495 Lodz, Poland
marklen@tyreo.am.lodz.pl

The paper describes the computer system for the evaluation of test examinations organized by Centre for Examinations in Medicine. The system consists of the optical mark reader (OMR) and originally developed Windows-based application. The application supports up to 600 multiple choice questions with 4 or 5 answers to choose from. There can be two versions of test with the same questions in different orders. After reading the cards, necessary checks are performed (e.g. for multiple or missing answers). The application allows to efficiently input necessary corrections and then to calculate the individual scores. The statistical features of the whole test are also calculated (including KR20, mean difficulty index, mean discrimination index) as well as characteristics of every question, including its difficulty and point biserial correlation coefficients.

1 Introduction

The efficient evaluation of test results in case of hundreds of examinees is not possible without an automated reading of the answers and a suitable computer application which allow to handle properly the data read from answer forms. Computerization of the evaluation process allows not only to obtain the individual scores in a reliable and efficient way. It can also provide a quick access to some important statistics describing the difficulty and reliability of a whole test (a set of test items or questions) as well as statistics regarding individual test items. The latter statistics can be very useful in the assessment of questions quality and correctness.

The uncompromised reliability and efficiency are especially important in state examinations, like those organized be Center for Examinations in Medicine (CEM). CEM is a Polish governmental institution responsible for the organization of state examinations related to post-graduate medical education of physicians, dentists, pharmacists, laboratory diagnosticians and other related health care professionals. The scale of test examinations organized by CEM is well characterized the two most important ones. The state examination for specialization is organized twice a year and includes test examination consisting of 120 multiple choice questions (MCQ). Test are carried out separately for each of about 40 specializations. The total number of examinees is about 2500 per session. The largest exam is organized for internal medicine and it is attended by as much as 800 physicians. Even larger examination is LEP – state examination of doctor. This examination is also organized twice a year and its

E. Kącki, M. Rudnicki, J. Stempczyńska (Eds.): Computers in Medical Activity, AISC 65, pp. 265–270.
springerlink.com

passing is necessary to obtain the license to practice medicine. In autumn sessions the number of examinees exceeds 2000 young medical doctors.

Generally, multiple choice questions used commonly for test examinations can be divided into true or false items and so-called one-best answer items [1]. In examinations organized by CEM we always use the latter type of MCQs. A simple form of such MCQ can be exemplified as:

"Arteries are blood vessels which carry:	<– stem
A. blood to the heart.	<– distracter
B. blood from the heart.	<– correct answer
C. oxygenated blood.	<– distracter
D. deoxygenated blood."	<– distracter

In this form MCQ consists of the question (usually called stem), which is followed by the correct answer surrounded by 3 or 4 distracters. Writing MCQs is often regarded an easy task but it is not. A good MCQ should a clear and unambiguous stem, a single answer which is correct and several distracters which should appear plausible to examinees without the ability to recognize a correct answer. Distracters which are incredible make the question easy even for examinees without any significant knowledge.

2 Hardware

As it was mentioned above, quick and reliable evaluation of the results of large test examinations requires to employ a suitable computer system. A very important part of such system is scanner which allows to input the contents of answer forms into the computer. There are two main types of such scanners: optical mark recognition (OMR) scanners and image scanners (e.g. based on video camera). OMR is claimed to be the fastest and most accurate of the data collection technologies [2]. The most important feature of OMR technology (in comparison to image scanners) is a detection of the absence or presence of a mark, but not the shape of the mark. Thus, OMR scanner cannot recognize hand-printed or machine-printed characters. Forms which are scanned through an OMR scanner contain small ovals or rectangles, referred to as 'boxes' that are filled in by the examinee and there are strict requirements regarding the position of these boxes. The use of OMR scanner imply the necessity of separation between the question form and answer form. When image scanner is used, it is possible to put questions and boxes for marking answers into a single form. On the other hand, important advantages of OMR scanners are their higher portability and lower cost in comparison with image scanners.

OMR scanner hardware interprets the output from the optical scanner and translates it into the desired ASCII output. An OMR scanner can maintain a throughput of 1,800 to 10,000 forms per hour. This activity can be controlled and processed by a single workstation, which can handle any volume the scanner can generate. More sophisticated OMR scanners allow a precise measurement of the darkness of a mark, and then mark discrimination algorithms can be used for determining whether a mark is an erasure or a mark.

The system used in CEM employs OMR scanner and is compatible with 2 types of scanners produced by Chatsworth Data Corporation (USA; http://www.omrsys.com):

OMR-2000 and ACP-100. These scanners can be connected to computer by serial or USB ports and have similar programmatic interface. The OMR-2000 scanner is a desktop model with auto-feeding of answer forms and ACP-100 is very light-weighted and portable model with manual feed of forms.

3 Software

For the whole evaluation system to be working it is necessary to provide a suitable computer software. The main tasks of such software are: controlling the scanner and handling data read from it, verification of that data, calculation of the test results as well as the statistics related to the test and to each of the questions. Such software can be now purchased from most scanner vendors but it was more convenient for CEM to prepare custom software which could fit perfectly specific needs of state examinations.

This application has been named 'Egzaminator' and it was written in c++ using Microsoft Visual Studio package. Its design was optimized for the sake of efficiency. For example the number of keystrokes needed for the input of correct answers or other similar data has been lowered to absolute minimum. Another important point for CEM is the possibility of printing documentation of answer data at each step of test evaluation. The 'Egzaminator' provides also the secure storage of the list of correct answers. It also supports two versions of test which differ in the sequence of questions. The application is capable of exporting results data in various formats including direct connection to SQL server. The 'Egzaminator' is also capable of performing tasks which are not directly related to the test evaluation itself. It can print the code numbers in headers of answer forms and it allows to check the packs of forms preprinted for the examination.

Main steps of test evaluation with the use of 'Egzaminator' application include: 1. definition of the test, 2. reading answer forms, 3. checking for correctness of the data from each form, 4. checking for completeness of the data, 5. manual correction for apparently missing or multiple answers, and 6. calculation of the results. The 'Egzaminator' application has got a very user-friendly help system which guides user through the necessary steps during the evaluation of test results. If for any reason user tries to perform action which should be preceded by yet undone operation a suitable alert is displayed. User can also ask for a suggestion by pressing single button on the toolbar.

The evaluation of the test must be started by definition of number of test versions, number and type of answer forms, the total number of questions, the number of examinees together with the ranges of their code numbers. It is possible to define how these data are coded in the form headers. The application supports 4 and 5 choice questions. It is also possible to assign marks to the test scores according to several different algorithms. The next step (step 2) is reading the contents of answer forms. The connection with a scanner is very easy to configure: the only thing to be done by the user is to select the appropriate serial port (USB connected scanners emulate serial ports). A separate process is created for reading data from a scanner what assure application stability if communication problems occur. Data read from the scanner can be corrupted - nearly always because of dirtiness of answer forms. The area which is the most susceptible is the margin area with strobe marks. Any additional marks made by examinee in this area result in false rows read by scanner. Checking whether examinee code number, test version and length of data is correct (step 3) successfully discovers such errors. Step 2 and 3 can be repeated iteratively. Step 4 should be performed after scanning all answer forms and is useful especially when more than 1 answer form per examinee is used. In this step the data from answer forms are assigned to examinees. This operation allows to create the list of absent examinees, to find examinees with code numbers outside the range defined in step 1, as well as to check for the correct number and type of answer forms scanned for each examinee. In that way missing forms can be indicated and erroneous double scanning of the form can be excluded. Answers to the questions are marked with a pencil and it is allowed to erase the marking and to select another answer. In cases when erasing is not complete the scanner reads apparently multiple answer. If marking is not complete or too weak it can be missed by the scanner. Such situations are revealed by application and must be verified by manual inspection of answer forms. That is why step 5 can be very time-consuming. But it is necessary for reliable evaluation of the examination. The corrections can be entered and are considered when calculating the results. To minimize the risk of input errors voice confirmation of selected answer is possible.

Somewhere between the first and the last step the list of correct answers must be input or imported by application. If there are two versions of test also the relation between versions must be input and it is checked for consistency. The last step of test evaluation is calculation of the results. Not only individual scores are calculated but also some statistics regarding each of test questions as well as the whole test are given. More detailed description of these statistics is presented in the following section. The questions may be grouped into custom categories which allow to calculate separate statistics for each category. Each question can be canceled (for example when unrecoverable errors are found in the text of questions). The answers to cancelled questions are disregarded and points may be rewarded or not (depending on the selected option).

4 Statistics Used in Test Evaluation

There are some statistics which are commonly used in evaluation of the test examination and were introduced to 'Egzaminator' application. They can be divided into those regarding individual test questions (item statistics) and those referring to the test as a whole (test statistics). The latter group includes mean values of some statistics from the former group but there is also a specific statistic meaningful and calculable only at the level of the set of questions.

4.1 Item Statistics

For each test item the correct answer is given which is followed by frequency of response to each choice. The next statistic given is difficulty index. This index is based on the results two extreme groups of examinees, namely, 27% of examinees with the best test score and 27% of examinees with the worst score. It is defined as a ratio of the total number of correct answers in both groups to the number of examinees in these groups:

$$IDI = \frac{Ns + Ni}{2n} \tag{1}$$

where: n is the number of examinees within each of extreme groups, Ns is the number of correct answers in superior group and Ni is the number of correct answers in inferior group. This index ranges from 0 to 1, and unlike its name suggests, it closes to 1 in case of easy questions [3].

Another important item statistics calculated by 'Egzaminator' application is discrimination index. It provides the information on the power of a given question to make a distinction between good and poor examinees and is defined as:

$$DI = \frac{Ns - Ni}{n} \tag{2}$$

with the same variables which were used for calculation of the difficulty index. Discrimination index ranges from -1 to1 and its negative values indicate that group of examinees with the worst test scores passed that particular question better than those who achieved top test scores. The power to discriminate depends on the difficulty of the question and it is the highest if IDI equals to 0.5. In case of extremely easy or extremely difficult questions, DI approaches 0 [3].

The last item statistic is the point biserial correlation coefficient which is abbreviated as RPBI [4]. This statistic is calculated for each item choice, according to the following formula:

$$RPBI = \frac{Mp - Mq}{S_t}\sqrt{pq} \tag{3}$$

where: Mp is the whole test mean score for examinees who selected the considered choice, Mq is the whole test mean score for examinees who selected another choice, St is standard deviation of the test scores, p is percentage of examinees who selected the considered choice and q is percentage of examinees who selected another choice. This statistic also ranges from -1.00 to +1.00. An item which discriminates well has an RPBI for the correct response which is at least 0.30. RPBI coefficients for the incorrect choices should be negative. One should not be too concerned about RPBIs computed from groups of less than about 200 examinees. The RPBI is not very stable for groups smaller than this.

4.2 Test Statistics

The majority of test statistics calculated by the application describe the distribution of the test scores. These include mean score, standard deviation of scores, minimal and maximal score. The mean value of item difficulty index (equation 1) for all questions in the test is also provided. Another important statistic is calculated according to the following formula:

$$KR20 = \frac{k}{k-1}\left(1 - \frac{\sum_{i=1}^{i=k} p_i q_i}{\delta^2}\right) \tag{4}$$

where p is percentage of examinees who passed the item i, q is percentage of examinees who didn't pass the item i, δ^2 is variance of the total score of this test, k is the number of test items. This formula was devised by Kuder and Richardson in 1937 [5] and now it is a standard for estimating test reliability for single administration of a single form. Kuder-Richardson measures inter-item consistency and can be interpreted like a correlation coefficient, i.e. the closer to 1 is KR20 value the better test consistency and thus its reliability.

5 Conclusion

'Egzaminator' application has been successfully used in Center for Examinations in Medicine for 5 years. It is also used in 2 medical universities in Poland, in Katowice and in Kraków. It has been used to evaluate the test results of nearly 100.000 examinees and has proved to be an efficient and reliable tool.

References

[1] Case, S.H., Swanson, D.B.: Constructing written test questions from basic and clinical sciences, pp. 13–18. NBME, Philadelphia (2003)

[2] NCS Pearson. OpScan® optical mark read (OMR) scanners. NCS Pearson Inc. (2003), `http://www.pearsonncs.com/scanners/`

[3] Zurawski, R.M.: Making the most of exams: procedures for item analysis. National Teaching and Learning Forum 7, 1–4 (1998)

[4] Magnusson, D.: Wprowadzenie do teorii testów, pp. 299–305. PWN, Warszawa (1981) (in Polish)

[5] Kuder, G.F., Richardson, M.W.: The theory of the estimation of test reliability. Psychometrika 2, 151–160 (1937)

Author Index

Author Index